Biopsychosocial Perspectives and Practices for Addressing Communicable and Non-Communicable Diseases

Simon George Taukeni
University of Namibia, Namibia

A volume in the Advances in Medical Diagnosis, Treatment, and Care (AMDTC) Book Series

IGI Global
DISSEMINATOR OF KNOWLEDGE

Published in the United States of America by
IGI Global
Medical Information Science Reference (an imprint of IGI Global)
701 E. Chocolate Avenue
Hershey PA, USA 17033
Tel: 717-533-8845
Fax: 717-533-8661
E-mail: cust@igi-global.com
Web site: http://www.igi-global.com

Library of Congress Cataloging-in-Publication Data

Names: Taukeni, Simon George, 1973- editor.
Title: Biopsychosocial perspectives and practices for addressing communicable and non-communicable diseases / Simon George Taukeni, editor.
Description: Hershey PA : Medical Information Science Reference, [2020] | Includes bibliographical references and index. | Summary: "This book addresses the psychological/mental, emotional, social, and spiritual factors that influence communicable and non-communicable diseases"-- Provided by publisher.
Identifiers: LCCN 2019036398 (print) | LCCN 2019036399 (ebook) | ISBN 9781799821397 (hardcover) | ISBN 9781799821403 (ebook)
Subjects: MESH: Behavioral Medicine--methods | Mental Health | Culturally Competent Care | Attitude to Health | Health Behavior
Classification: LCC RA418 (print) | LCC RA418 (ebook) | NLM WB 103 | DDC 362.1--dc23
LC record available at https://lccn.loc.gov/2019036398
LC ebook record available at https://lccn.loc.gov/2019036399

This book is published in the IGI Global book series Advances in Medical Diagnosis, Treatment, and Care (AMDTC) (ISSN: 2475-6628; eISSN: 2475-6636)

British Cataloguing in Publication Data
A Cataloguing in Publication record for this book is available from the British Library.

For electronic access to this publication, please contact: eresources@igi-global.com.

Advances in Medical Diagnosis, Treatment, and Care (AMDTC) Book Series

ISSN:2475-6628
EISSN:2475-6636

MISSION

Advancements in medicine have prolonged the life expectancy of individuals all over the world. Once life-threatening conditions have become significantly easier to treat and even cure in many cases. Continued research in the medical field will further improve the quality of life, longevity, and wellbeing of individuals.

The **Advances in Medical Diagnosis, Treatment, and Care (AMDTC)** book series seeks to highlight publications on innovative treatment methodologies, diagnosis tools and techniques, and best practices for patient care. Comprised of comprehensive resources aimed to assist professionals in the medical field apply the latest innovations in the identification and management of medical conditions as well as patient care and interaction, the books within the AMDTC series are relevant to the research and practical needs of medical practitioners, researchers, students, and hospital administrators.

COVERAGE

- Alternative Medicine
- Emergency Medicine
- Medical Procedures
- Patient Interaction
- Disease Management
- Experimental Medicine
- Critical Care
- Disease Prevention
- Cancer Treatment
- Internal Medicine

IGI Global is currently accepting manuscripts for publication within this series. To submit a proposal for a volume in this series, please contact our Acquisition Editors at Acquisitions@igi-global.com or visit: http://www.igi-global.com/publish/.

The Advances in Medical Diagnosis, Treatment, and Care (AMDTC) Book Series (ISSN 2475-6628) is published by IGI Global, 701 E. Chocolate Avenue, Hershey, PA 17033-1240, USA, www.igi-global.com. This series is composed of titles available for purchase individually; each title is edited to be contextually exclusive from any other title within the series. For pricing and ordering information please visit http://www.igi-global.com/book-series/advances-medical-diagnosis-treatment-care/129618. Postmaster: Send all address changes to above address.

Titles in this Series

For a list of additional titles in this series, please visit:
http://www.igi-global.com/book-series/advances-medical-diagnosis-treatment-care/129618

Ethnopharmacological Investigation of Indan Spices
Neha Mishra (Sam Higginbottom University of Agriculture, Technology, and Sciences, India)
Medical Information Science Reference • © 2020 • 300pp • H/C (ISBN: 9781799825241) • US $295.00

Advanced Pharmacological Uses of Medicinal Plants and Natural Products
Ajeet Singh (National Dairy Research Institute, India) Padam Singh (Vaccine and Infectious Disease Research Centre, Translational Health Science and Technology Institute, India) and Navneet Bithel (Gurukul Kangri Universit, India)
Medical Information Science Reference • © 2020 • 540pp • H/C (ISBN: 9781799820949) • US $425.00

Quality Control of Cellular Protein in Neurodegenerative Disorders
Md. Sahab Uddin (Southeast University, Bangladesh) and Ghulam Md. Ashraf (King Abdulaziz University, Saudi Arabia)
Medical Information Science Reference • © 2020 • 515pp • H/C (ISBN: 9781799813170) • US $295.00

Multidimensional Perspectives and Global Analysis of Universal Health Coverage
Yeter Demir Uslu (Istanbul Medipol University, Turkey) Hasan Dinçer (Istanbul Medipol University, Turkey) and Serhat Yüksel (İstanbul Medipol University, Turkey)
Medical Information Science Reference • © 2020 • 499pp • H/C (ISBN: 9781799823292) • US $265.00

Examining Biological Foundations of Human Behavior
Barre Vijaya Prasad (Dharwad Institute of Mental Health and Neurosciences, India)
Medical Information Science Reference • © 2020 • 266pp • H/C (ISBN: 9781799828600) • US $285.00

IGI Global
DISSEMINATOR OF KNOWLEDGE

701 East Chocolate Avenue, Hershey, PA 17033, USA
Tel: 717-533-8845 x100 • Fax: 717-533-8661
E-Mail: cust@igi-global.com • www.igi-global.com

Table of Contents

Detailed Table of Contents

Primary health care is an approach adopted for the delivery of health services to the Namibian population. In terms of this approach, these services are made universally available, accessible, affordable, acceptable, and appropriate to meet the needs of communities. The health care delivery system in Namibia comprises services provided by both the Ministry of Health and Social Services (MoHSS) and the private sector. In addition to these services, some people consult traditional health care providers. All in all, health care comprises a combination of promotive, preventive, curative, and rehabilitative services. In addition to government funding, donations and technical support are also provided by non-governmental organisations. The MoHSS health care delivery system is coordinated at national, regional and district levels. This chapter elaborates on the Namibian health care delivery system, the structure and functions of each coordinating level, primary health care services in Namibia, as well as successes and challenges experienced.

Global health issues are a global burden and are relatively common in industrialized societies. The World Health Organization and researchers have developed and rebuilt tools to report the burden of disease affecting mortality and health of the people. Apart from America and Europe, which are at an average of global burden for mental health disease, in some regions it is a major priority to be addressed globally. In South East Asia, one of the affected regions is Kashmir, Northern Indian. Disasters have manifested in various forms encompassing the natural calamities of earthquake, flood, landslides and manmade calamities of violence. Trauma due to manmade calamities has taken over as a leading cause of morbidity and mortality among the most productive working age group of 12-35 years. The chapter aims to understand the patterns of resilience in people surviving war and conflict in Kashmir over last 60 years. The focus is on the young population of society. Generations in Kashmir have faced the psychosocial impact of ongoing political conflict since the 1980's.

Malaria is transmitted by the female Anopheles mosquito and is a parasitic disease which is caused by the Plasmodium species. It is a serious communicable disease in sub-Saharan Africa (SSA). The most vulnerable group is children aged 0-5 years. Malaria is responsible for most outpatient visits, hospital admissions and the main cause of school and work absenteeism. Knowledge, attitudes, and practices (KAP) are essential for control programmes being the educational diagnosis and perception of a community about a disease which affects their attitudes and practices. This chapter reviews that the KAP of most communities in SSA have existing gaps which impacts on the control of malaria. A sound and adequate understanding of malaria and its proper recognition are crucial to its control. The inclusion of malaria education in

Smoking

Section 5
Diabetes

Preface

AN OVERVIEW OF THE SUBJECT MATTER

The bio-psychosocial model seeks to address the psychological, mental, emotional, social, and spiritual factors that influence health. While there are best medical and clinical practices for treating communicable and non-communicable diseases, there is an urgent need to integrate bio-psychosocial perspectives and practices in order to promote comprehensive healthcare. Current research reports that diseases such as HIV/AIDS, malaria, tuberculosis, cancer, diabetes, cardiovascular diseases, and chronic lung and heart diseases are a growing threat to the heath and quality of life of individuals across the globe. Considering that nearly all these diseases are directly related to lifestyle of an individual, prevention and intervention should be devised to address psychological, emotional, social and spiritual factors.

A DESCRIPTION OF WHERE YOUR TOPIC FITS IN THE WORLD TODAY

The main objective of this book is to provide relevant theoretical frameworks and the latest bio-psychosocial practical intervention results as informed by the current global trends of communicable and non-communicable diseases. It will be written for professionals and by professionals who want to promote good health and quality of life through psychosocial interventions to address psychosocial problems facing the individuals such as discrimination and stigma, stress, depression, alcohol and drug abuse, smoking, lack of physical activity, poverty and many other socio-economic factors. Overall, the benefit of the book will include interventions that have potential to empower the caregivers and their families towards increased ability to cope better with a health condition faced.

A DESCRIPTION OF THE TARGET AUDIENCE

The target audience of this book are professionals and researchers working in the field of Health Sciences and other related disciplines such as public health, mental health, nursing, community-based healthcare, health psychology, psychiatry, HIV/AIDS education, human movement education, and sport psychology.

A DESCRIPTION OF THE IMPORTANCE OF EACH OF THE CHAPTER

This book consists of eleven important chapters and they are placed in seven sections.

The first chapter presents the overview of health care in Namibia. Authors elaborated on the Namibian health care delivery system, the structure and functions of each coordinating level, primary health care services in Namibia, as well as successes and challenges.

The second chapter talks about mental health. The chapter aims to create awareness regarding the patterns of resilience in people surviving war and conflict in Kashmir over last 60 years. The focus is on young population of society, generations in Kashmir have faced the psychosocial impact of on-going political conflict since 1980's.

Chapter three focuses on malaria in sub-Saharan Africa. This chapter advocates that a sound and adequate understanding of malaria and its proper recognition are crucial to its control. The inclusion of malaria education in pupil's curriculum and effective information on the electronic and social media can change the misconceptions about malaria and correct attitudes and practices to intensify control efforts.

In the fourth chapter, the authors discussed the importance of HIV care continuum in fighting HIV and AIDS. Specific efforts are directed into the need to implement comprehensive HIV care continuum. The chapter also includes specific solutions and recommendations and future research directions.

The fifth chapter covers elderly grandparents as caregivers of children affected or infected by HIV and AIDS in Namibia. This foundational chapter attempts to provide readers with content to assist in their understanding of the characteristics, role, and experiences of kinship elderly caregivers of children affected and/or infected by HIV and AIDS. In addition, the chapter highlights what is known about children living with HIV in Namibia. Finally, the chapter offers suggestions for policy and practice

Smoking is addressed in chapter six of the book. This chapter provides readers with vital knowledge on smoking including its effects in the human body which in return could lead to positive smoking behavioural change for a reader's own health as well as to caution non-smokers on the danger of exposure to second-hand smoke.

The chapter further highlights factors related to smoking from national, continental and global perspectives.

The seventh chapter deals with diabetes. There is increasing evidence that diabetes mellitus is associated with a number of psychological and psychiatric conditions. This chapter addresses the distinctive biological, psychological and sociocultural factors such as social support, socioeconomic status and family interaction encountered by diabetic patients. Recommendations are provided that can enhance diabetic care and include improving current screening of psychological conditions as well as treatment practices.

Stress is another important subject which is discussed in chapter eight. The chapter focuses on stress, defining the concept, outlining the causes, as well as identifying the warning signs and symptoms and its effects on health. The impact of stress in the workplace and strategies for managing stress are also discussed.

Chapter nine further expands on stress and trauma. In particular, the chapter singles out different types of stress, the neurological changes that can occur as a result of adversity, common and paradoxical reactions to trauma, and the ability of coping skills and resilience to change the trajectory from negative outcomes to opportunities for positive growth.

In the tenth chapter, the authors focused primarily on the tension type headache (TTH). Stress, especially tension type headaches, are a serious problem in today's world. Now, every person in this world is facing headaches and stress-related problems in daily life. To measure the stress level, the authors have introduced the concept of EEG, EMG, and GSR biofeedback.

The last chapter eleventh is about depression. This chapter provides a broad overview of depression in adults. The purpose of this chapter is to outline the link between various contributory factors and depression among the adult population. Optimal management processes, including self-care, reduce the risk of relapse and improve the quality of life.

CONCLUSION

Written especially for health sciences students and academics, this book serves as an essential resource for bio-psychosocial model of health. Each chapter was critically well detailed, argued and researched. This book is indeed a must have for everyone concerning health and quality of life.

Acknowledgment

First of all, I would like to extend my heartfelt appreciation for the support provided by the IGI Global team.

Secondly, I would also like to acknowledge the support provided by both Dr. Joyce Mathwasa and Dr. Zoleka Ntshuntshe from the University of Fort Hare for spending their limited time to review some of the chapters of this book.

Finally, if it were not for the contributors, this book would not be what it is. I therefore thank all the contributors to this book. Thank you once more. May God bless you.

Section 1
Healthcare and Mental Health

Chapter 1
Healthcare System in Namibia:
An Overview

Vistolina Nuuyoma
https://orcid.org/0000-0002-5744-1355
School of Nursing, University of Namibia, Namibia

Daniel Opotamutale Ashipala
University of Namibia, Namibia

ABSTRACT

Primary health care is an approach adopted for the delivery of health services to the Namibian population. In terms of this approach, these services are made universally available, accessible, affordable, acceptable, and appropriate to meet the needs of communities. The health care delivery system in Namibia comprises services provided by both the Ministry of Health and Social Services (MoHSS) and the private sector. In addition to these services, some people consult traditional health care providers. All in all, health care comprises a combination of promotive, preventive, curative, and rehabilitative services. In addition to government funding, donations and technical support are also provided by non-governmental organisations. The MoHSS health care delivery system is coordinated at national, regional and district levels. This chapter elaborates on the Namibian health care delivery system, the structure and functions of each coordinating level, primary health care services in Namibia, as well as successes and challenges experienced.

DOI: 10.4018/978-1-7998-2139-7.ch001

INTRODUCTION

On gaining independence in 1990, Namibia inherited a health care delivery system that was segregated along racial lines, was fragmented and based entirely on curative health services while simultaneously being inefficient and inadequate. Since then, the government of Namibia (GRN), through the Ministry of Health and Social Services (MoHSS), has adopted a primary health care (PHC) approach for the delivery of health services to the Namibian population. These services are made universally available, accessible, affordable, acceptable and appropriate to meet the needs of communities. Communities are the focal point for action and all planning and allocation of resources must take into account community needs such as safe water supplies, sanitation, adequate housing, immunisation, the prevention of epidemics, health education, maternal and childcare services and curative services.

Chapter Objectives

After reading this chapter, you should be able to:

§ Describe the health care system in Namibia
§ Identify how Primary Health Care approach is integrated into the Namibian health care system
§ Illustrate the structure, composition and functions of the health care system

MAIN FOCUS OF THE CHAPTER

This chapter describes the health care delivery system used in Namibia. In this section, the public health care system, health care services in the private sectors and the traditional health care in Namibia are described in detail. Moreover, the role of non-governmental organizations in the health care system are briefly introduced. Lastly, the structure, composition and functions of different levels in the health care delivery system are described.

The Health Care Delivery System in Namibia

Health care services in Namibia are provided by the government through the MoHSS, the private sector and traditional health care service providers. Such health care provides a combination of promotive, preventive, curative and rehabilitative services. In order to render these services, the MoHSS has divided the country into 14 operational health regions which correspond with the 14 delimited political and administrative regions. These regions are further divided into 34 districts. In the public sector, health care services are provided by 29 district hospitals, four intermediate and referral hospitals, 309 health centres, as well as 1150 clinics and outreach points. In addition, there are private health care facilities in some regions. The districts are managed by district coordinating committees which are responsible for providing basic health care services. These basic services are managed on three levels: nationally through the MoHSS from its head office in Windhoek, regionally through regional management teams and at district level by district management committees.

Namibia's health care system aims to improve and maintain the wellbeing of all its citizens to attain the MoHSS goal of "forward with health for all Namibian by the year (2005) and beyond". The aim of the health care services is to prevent and cure disease, rehabilitate those who have suffered illness and promote good health for all citizens. Since independence, the area of coverage within a 10-kilometre radius of a health facility has more than tripled as a result of an increase in the number of health facilities in the country. Consequently, 80% of the population now lives within 10 kilometres of a clinic. However, this still leaves 20% or over 300 000 people in remote areas, particularly Omaheke and Kunene, without ready access to health services.

Health Care Services in the Private Sector

The private health care sector in Namibia is found mainly in the urban areas and provides such services as medium-sized hospitals, pharmacies, medical practices, ambulances, radiology units, nursing homes, as well as physiotherapy and biokinetic services among others (Ashipala, Wilkinson, & Van Dyk, 2016). Private sector healthcare facilities comprise private nursing homes, hospitals and clinics, frail-care facilities and doctors in private practice. In addition, some registered nurses and supplementary health personnel, for example physiotherapists and occupational therapists, run independent private practices. A private sector service functions as a business with a profit motive, and in addition is subject to the Health Act and must be registered. The private sector in Namibia includes about 850 facilities registered with the MoHSS, which include 13 hospitals, 75 clinics and eight health centres. These services are accessible to people with medical aid and insurance, as well as people who can afford to pay the fee required before a service is provided. In addition, faith-based health care services exist that are provided by the Roman Catholic Mission and the Anglican churches; however, these are subsidised by the government. Although the public health sector is the main provider of health care services to the public, there has been strong intersectoral collaboration between the private and the public sectors. Accordingly, the private health care sector is a major partner in the Namibian health care sector and has made a significant contribution to the benefit of people who cannot afford private care services.

Traditional Health Care in Namibia

Although public and private health care facilities are available in most areas in Namibia, there are individuals who prefer to seek health care services from traditional healers. Such decisions are generally influenced by cultural and religious beliefs and practices in relation to health and illness, as well as clients' experiences or perceptions of the health care services provided by the public and private sectors. To date there is no information regarding the numbers of traditional healers practising in Namibia, as most consultations and practices are conducted in secrecy. Furthermore, not all healers are registered with the traditional healers' associations such as the Namibia Eagle Traditional Healers Association (NETHA) and no compulsory accreditation is required to practise as a traditional healer in Namibia. On a positive note, the public health sector has collaborated with traditional health service providers in areas of training, health care kits and safety equipment such as gloves (MoHSS, 2013). Traditional health care providers in Namibia include traditional birth attendants, herbalists, faith healers, homeopaths and masseuse/masseurs.

Non-Governmental Organisations (NGOs)

Non-governmental organisations (NGOs) are privately funded by donor agencies. At times, the MoHSS contracts an NGO to perform activities or run a project on its behalf. In such cases, the ministry signs a memorandum with thc donor concerned and takes responsibility for expenditure accounting. NGOs employ health personnel of all categories and contribute to their training to ensure that they are equipped with the knowledge and skills needed to run the project. In addition, training is provided to orientate the new personnel to the projects.

Structure, Composition and Functions of the Health Care System

The post-apartheid government that came to power in 1990 in Namibia was faced with many challenges. One of these was to transform the highly segregated health system, which was curative in nature and run along racial lines. Subsequently, the health care system was changed to a comprehensive, equitable and non-racial system intended to address social and economic injustices, eradicate poverty, reduce waste and the duplication/fragmentation of services, increase efficiency and promote greater control by communities and individuals over all aspects of their lives. The national level comprises a single ministerial structure that coordinates all aspects of health care delivery, both in the public and the private sector, at national, regional, district and local levels. Table 1 indicates the structure and composition of the national health system.

ORGANISATIONAL STRUCTURE OF THE HEALTH CARE SYSTEM IN NAMIBIA

The government aim is to decentralise the management of health care delivery services to regional, district and local PHC in order to increase the efficiency and effectiveness of health care provision. Through the primary health care approach, the system puts emphasis on health prevention and not on cure, with health promotion, prevention, curative care and rehabilitation inherent in its operation. Thus, the responsibilities of the various authorities are as follows:

National Level

Composition of the national health management teams (NHMTs)

- Permanent secretary
- Deputy permanent secretaries
- **Director:** Primary Health Care
- **Director:** Specialised Services
- **Director:** Planning and Human Resources
- **Director:** Administration
- **Director:** Social Services

The functions of the national level are as follows:

- Identification of service priorities and priority groups and the articulation of policies to meet those needs.
- Budget and financial management of revenue and expenditure levels for PHC services.
- Personnel administration which includes guidelines on appointment, posting, promotion, career development and evaluation of all categories of staff.
- Information and reporting of routine statistical systems covering service utilisation, morbidity, revenue and expenditure, and providing summaries of these data to lower levels of the health system. Conducting national health

Table 1. Organisation of the health care system in Namibia

MINISTER

DEPUTY MINISTER

PERMANENT SECRETARY

DEPUTY PERMANENT SECRETARY: Planning and Administrative Support Services	DEPUTY PERMANENT SECRETARY: Health Care Services	DEPUTY PERMANENT SECRETARY: Social Services

DIRECTOR:	DIRECTOR:	DIRECTOR:	DIRECTOR:	DIRECTOR:	REGIONAL DIRECTORS:
Primary Healthcare Services	Specialised Health Services	Social Services	Administrative Support Services	Planning & Human Resource Development	Oshana Omusati Ohangwena Oshikoto Kunene Otjozondjupa Omaheke Khomas Erongo //Kharas Kavango East Kavango West Zambezi

DIVISION: PRIMARY HEALTH CARE	DIVISION: SPECIALISED SERVICES	DIVISION: PLANNING & HUMAN RESOURCES	DIVISION: ADMINISTR ATION	DIVISION: SOCIAL SERVICES
-Family & community health -Epidemiology & public health -Nursing services	-Windhoek State Hospital -Pharma services -Laboratory services -Radiographic services -Orthopaedic workshop	-Planning -Human resource department	-Finance -Auxiliary services -Personnel	-Professional social services -Social service administration

Source: Adopted from MoHSS (1995)

surveys to fill gaps in information about health needs in Namibia such as the National Health Demographic Survey (NHDS).

- Human resources development through pre- and in-service training strategies and balancing the human resources requirements with supply.
- Supervisory support visits to the regional level through review and strengthening of activities to personnel, thus bringing improvements to lower levels
- Logistics and supply of goods achieved through the selection, procuring, storing and distribution of supplies such as pharmaceuticals, vehicles, medical equipment and stores.
- Setting standards and monitoring the quality of services provided in the health sector.

Regional Level

Composition of the regional management teams (RHMTs)

- Regional Director
- Chief Health Programme Administrator – Family Health
- Chief Health Programme Administrator – Special Programmes
- Control Administrative Officer
- Chief Human Resource Practitioner
- Chief Regional Pharmacist
- Chief Social Worker
- Other persons may be co-opted to the teams whenever necessary. These may include experts from other divisions such as laboratory technicians, NGO representatives, community members and representatives of other sectors.

The RMHTs are responsible for the following:

- Identification of needs and planning to meet the needs of the region
- Planning and implementation of health services and programmes in the region
- Supporting the district health management teams (DMHTs) in planning health programmes, as well as implementation, budgeting, training, logistics and medical supply
- Monitoring and evaluating of health services as well as responsibility for all regional plans
- Conducting supervisory support visits in the district
- Creating a link between the directorate and district operations by planning and controlling the functions of the referral system

- Collecting and analysing data, and giving feedback to the directorate and to the districts
- Overall decision-making in regard to health issues at the regional level
- Planning and managing a regional health information system by capturing and storing health data from the district level
- Supporting the national level with its health programmes
- Human resource provision and development for both in-service and pre-service training
- Ensuring quality control of health services and facilities by conducting supervisory support visits to the regional and district level
- Formulating guidelines for combating disease outbreaks
- Promoting intersectoral collaboration with stakeholders within the region
- Undertaking research and making recommendations to the national level
- Monitoring and evaluation of health care services throughout the region.

District Level

Composition of the district health coordinating committees (DHCCs)

- Senior Medical Officer (SMO)
- Hospital Matron
- District Primary Health Care Supervisor
- Senior Hospital Clerk
- Principal Social Worker
- Pharmacist
- Health Inspector/Environmental Health Officer

The overall functions of the DHCCs are listed below:

- Identification of the health needs of the community
- Planning to meet the health needs of the community
- Implementation of health activities in the district
- Monitoring and evaluation of health plans made at national, regional and district levels
- Problem-solving in relation to the challenges in the implementation of health activities
- Promotion and support of community committees
- Community mobilisation of resources and involvement in the implementation of health activities
- Allocation and utilisation of health personnel

- Link between region and community
- Provision for community mobilisation and engagement
- Keeping records of health data from the district
- Planning, implementation, monitoring and evaluation of PHC services at the district hospital, health centres and clinics
- Referral of health matters to regional level when advice is required

The key functions of the MoHSS in the Namibian national health care system are summarised in the figure below:

National level
- Policy making
- Guideline development
- Programme management

Directorate level
- Programme management
- Coordination of regional and district activities
- Policy implementation

Regional level
- Coordination of activities in the districts of the region
- Supervisory support for the districts

District level

IMPLEMENTATION OF DISTRICT OPERATIONAL ACTIVITIES

Proposed Restructuring of the National Health System in Namibia

The presidential commission of inquiry conducted in the MoHSS in 2013 observed that the structure currently used in the ministry is not responsive to the current health demands. The low staffing norms and inadequate skill mix in health facilities are regarded as being a result of this inappropriate structure. Consequently, a new structure has been proposed for all the three levels in the Ministry's organisational hierarchy (national, regional, and district levels). This new structure is yet to be finalised and forwarded to the Office of the Prime Minister for approval and for the implementation plan to be put in place. What is currently included in the proposed structure seems to have addressed the above deficiencies as it is a product of extensive consultation.

Primary Health Care Services in Namibia

The health care services in Namibia have slowly transited from a hospital-based and curative-based system to a promotive, preventive, community and home-based system (MoHSS, 2010a). PHC was adopted as it offers the most efficient and cost-effective means of improving the health of all the people in the country. To ensure that the adoption of a PHC approach was successful, the government restructured the health care system, as indicated in Flow Chart 2, and also ensured that the functions of all coordinating committees were clearly stipulated. In addition, provision was made for home-based health services and community health care services such as immunisation, health education and nutritional assessments of pregnant and breastfeeding women, as well as children under the age of five. In Namibia, PHC approach entails promotive, preventive, curative and rehabilitative strategies addressing communicable and non-communicable diseases. Concurrently, these strategies encompass biological, psychological and social aspects in addressing communicable and non-communicable dieseases.

As a measure to facilitate the transformation of the health services to a PHC approach, more emphasis was placed on the district level by revising the service packages provided through the district health system so that most services are decentralised. Moreover, the districts have been given a mandate to gather health data, analyse them and then re-plan their activities in order to provide solutions to the most pressing issues.

The services provided at the district levels consist of the categories of health professions indicated in Table 2; however, the nurse remains the major role player or the core of health service provision. Services listed in Table 2 are provided at clinics, health centres and district hospitals. However, certain categories of health professions such as dieticians and psychologists are not available at the district level; clients requiring their services are referred to the national and regional levels where they are available. In some instances, clients covered by medical insurance/ medical aid or those who can afford the cost are referred to private practitioners in the district to avoid travelling long distances (Blockmeyer, 2012).

Home-Based Care Services

The MoHSS recognises the key role that community home-based care (CHBC) plays in providing care for people with HIV (human immunodeficiency virus) and AIDS (acquired immunodeficiency syndrome) and other chronic and life-threatening illnesses and their affected family members, particularly children. CHBC for chronically or terminally ill clients and their families is primarily available from both trained and untrained care providers supported by various faith-based organisations and their health facilities, community-based organisations, NGOs and the MoHSS. CHBC facilitates the continuity of client care between the health facility, the home and the community (MoHSS, 2010b).

In 2006, community-based volunteers reached a total of 39,330 people living with HIV/AIDS, equivalent to 69% of those eligible, providing mostly HIV/AIDS-related care. However, coverage was not uniform and 29 of the 107 constituencies in Namibia were not covered at all by CHBC programmes (MoHSS, 2006).

These standards have been developed in response to the implementation of the CBHC Policy. The frameworks for these standards are the National HIV/AIDS Policy, 2007, the National Policy on Disability, the National Community-Based Care and Rehabilitation Programme, 2006, the National Orphan and Vulnerable Children Policy, 2005, the National Plan of Action for Children, 2007, National Community Based Health Care Policy, 2008 and MoHSS, 2010c) respectively.

Community Health Care Services

Outreach to deep rural communities is conducted by a team of health workers from the district hospital in each region through the local clinic. These workers visit various villages to deliver medical health services to the inhabitants and those of neighbouring villages. The team conducts outreach tasks at the outreach points once a month. The district office has the responsibility for the smooth administration and flow of all the medical care needs of these health facilities. Outreach teams are able to refer patients to a doctor if necessary. The teams provide the comprehensive health care services required by the community, including services like family planning, immunisation, screening, dressing of wounds, antiretroviral treatment (ART) and the like.

Staffing of the Health Care Delivery System

Health services in the public facilities are provided by about 10,000 employees. Nurses, medical doctors, pharmacists and all other allied health practitioners are trained in Namibia at the University of Namibia (UNAM), the International University of Management (IUM), the National University of Science and Technology (NUST), Welwitchia University (WU), and the National Health Training Centre (NHTC) of the MoHSS. The same categories of staff are also available in the private health care facilities. Over half of all the doctors employed are expatriates (about 125), highlighting the shortage of skilled personnel in the public health system. All health

Table 2. Primary health care services in Namibia and categories of health professions at district level

Services provided	Categories of health professions available
Promotive, preventative and curative services: Screening for common diseases Health education Personal curative services for acute minor ailments, trauma, as well as endemic and other communicable and some chronic diseases Nutrition assessment and dietetic services Provision of family planning Immunisation	PHC/community nurses Community health care workers Nutritionists and dieticians (available from private practices) Medical doctors
Maternal and child health services: Antenatal care Health education Intrapartum care Postnatal and neonatal care Provision of essential drugs	Midwives PHC/community nurses Community health care workers Pharmacists and assistant pharmacists Traditional birth attendants (preferred in some communities)
Basic rehabilitative therapy services:	Physiotherapist and assistants Occupational therapists and assistants Rehabilitation care workers
Basic oral health services:	Dental therapists Dentists
Health education Health-related nutritional support Communicable, non-communicable and endemic disease prevention and control	PHC nurses General doctors
School and institutional health services for children: Oral health Hearing tests Eyc tcsts	PHC nurses Dental therapists Ophthalmology nurses Private audiology technicians Private optometrists
Health-related water and sanitation services and other environmental health services:	Environmental health officers
Community mental services:	PHC nurses Social workers Medical doctors
Occupational health and safety services:	Health inspectors Medical doctors Environmental health officers Occupational health officers Nurses
Community nursing and home-care services, including care for the terminally ill:	PHC nurses Community health care workers Social workers
Accident and emergency services:	Nurses Ambulance drivers Paramedics and basic life supporters

continued on following page

Table 2 continued

Services provided	Categories of health professions available
Outbreak responses and care: Epidemiology and health information system Investigation and health monitoring Planning and administration Basic and medico-legal services	Nurses Data clerks Health programme administrators Pathologists from district laboratory Medical doctors Environmental health officers Medical rehabilitation worker Community health care workers

professions are required to be registered or enrolled with the Health Professions Council of Namibia, as a requirement to practice in both private and public health care facilities.

Achievements and Challenges

Since independence, access to health services in Namibia has greatly increased and the health of children has improved, not least because of expanded immunisation programmes. Some diseases such as measles, neonatal tetanus and polio have virtually been eradicated. Instances of malnutrition and diarrhoea have declined, reflecting better education, nutrition and water supply. On an international World Health Organisation ranking, the efficiency of Namibia's health service (the level of health of people compared to what 'should' be achieved for the money) came in at 189 out of 191 countries (Bell, & Louw, 2002). Since Namibia ranked 66th in terms of per capita expenditure, obviously the level of health should be much higher for the money spent. While the health system is now more equitable and accessible, it is still lagging behind in its quality and efficiency (MoHSS, 1995). People are the most important resource within the health system and Namibia's progress continues to be hampered by a shortage of skilled health workers, managers and other technical professionals. Providing appropriate training is therefore a big priority. Other challenges are the high teenage pregnancy rate, inadequate essential equipment, poor access to health facilities due to long distances and poor road infrastructure (Victor, 2002). The biggest challenge, however, is caused by the effects of the HIV/AIDS pandemic on the health care system and the population in general.

SOLUTION AND RECOMMENDATIONS

Challenges in the Namibian health care delivery system presented above requires an adequate number of health care workers in order to tackle pressing issues at all levels of care. Most financial resources should be directed to training and equipping health professionals with basic skills needed to plan, implement and evaluate the preventive and health promotion projects in the communities. Moreover, since high teenage pregnancy rate was pointed out as one of the challenging issues, there is a need for the Ministry of Health and Social Services to partner with the Ministry of Education in designing programme aiming to educate teenagers on sexual and reproductive issues.

FUTURE RESEARCH DIRECTIONS

Health research in Namibia is developing, and in recent years a number of studies in the areas of HIV/AIDS, adolescence health, child and maternal health were conducted. However, there seems to be limited scientific information on access to health care facilities and access to health care services. The authors encourage future research exploring the community needs in terms of provision of services and availability of health services that are responsive to the public health needs. In addition, there's a need to study the role of traditional health care system in provision of preventive and promotion health services to population groups without access to health care facilities and services.

CONCLUSION

On attaining its independence in 1990, Namibia adopted a PHC approach which made provision for services that are accessible, affordable, acceptable and appropriate to meet community needs. The national system is coordinated at national, regional and district levels, each of which has clearly specified functions. There are various categories of health professions that are available in the public and private sectors. Private health care providers tend to provide services to those with medical aid and insurance. The health care system in Namibia has recorded some success stories, nevertheless, major challenges are still experienced such as the effects of the HIV/AIDS epidemic on various sectors in the society.

ACKNOWLEDGMENT

The authors wish to thank colleagues from the MoHSS who provided us with incredible insight into the structure of health care services in Namibia, which has culminated in this chapter; as well as our colleagues at the School of Nursing, Rundu Campus for the encouragement and moral support they gave us during the drafting of the chapter. Behind every successful person lies a good mentor; we wish to thank Prof. Louise Pretorius, Associate Dean for the School of Nursing, who inspired us to engage in research, merit publication and extension services.

REFERENCES

Victor, A. A., Jim, A. W., Uusiku, P., Abdisalan, M. N., Robert, W. S., & Peter, M. A. (2012). Spatial modelling of healthcare utilisation for treatment of fever in Namibia. *International Journal of Health Geography, 11 (6), 1 -13*. https://doi.org/10.1186/1476-072X-11-6.

Ashipala, D. O., Wilkinson, W. & Van Dyk, A. (2016). Mental health policy implementation as an integral part of primary health care services in Oshana region, Namibia. *Journal of Nursing Education and Practice*, *11*(6), 53–59. doi:10.5430/jnep.v6n11p53

Bell, R., & Louw, A. (2002). Improving equity in the provision of primary health care: Lessons from decentralized planning and management in Namibia. *Bulletin of the World Health Organization*. doi:10.1590/S0042-96862002000800013 PMID:12219160

Blockmeyer, B. (2012). The health system in Namibia: Deliberation about an affordable national health insurance for the low workforce in Namibia. Retrieved from http://cms.my.na/assets/documents/p19p2lof2lsi2moqo2tsjfbp5a.pdf

Ministry of Health and Social Services. (2008). *National Policy on Community Based Health Care*. Windhoek: Directorate of Primary Care Services.

Ministry of Health and Social Services (MoHSS). (1995). *Integrated health care delivery: The challenge of implementation. A situational analysis and practical implementation guide*. Windhoek, Namibia: Government of the Republic of Namibia.

Ministry of Health and Social Services (MoHSS). (2006). *Progress Report on the Third Medium Term Plan on HIV/AIDS 2004–2006*. Windhoek: Directorate of Special Programmes, MOHSS.

Ministry of Health and Social Services (MoHSS). (2010a). *PHC Guidelines for Namibia*. Windhoek: Government of Republic of Namibia.

Ministry of Health and Social Services (MoHSS). (2010b). *National Community Based Care*. Windhoek: Government of Republic of Namibia.

Ministry of Health and Social Services (MoHSS). (2010c). *National Health Policy Framework 2010–2020*. Windhoek: Government of Republic of Namibia.

Ministry of Health and Social Services (MoHSS). (2013). *Namibia demographic and health services*. Windhoek: Government of Republic of Namibia.

WHO. (2018). Primary health care in Western Pacific. Retrieved from https://www.who.int/westernpacific/health-topics/primary-health-care

ADDITIONAL READING

Grigorov, V. (2009). Healthcare in Africa. *Cardiovascular Journal of Africa*, *20*(5), 275–277. PMID:19907798

Kasilo, O., & Trapsida, J. (2010). An overview of the traditional medicine situation in the African Region. *African Health Monitor*, *13*(5), 7–15.

Katuu, S. (2018). Healthcare systems: Typologies, framework models, and South Africa's health sector. *International Journal of Health Governance*, *23*(2), 134–148. doi:10.1108/IJHG-10-2017-0054

Olujide, A. (2016). Quality in Primary Health Care Services in Sub-Sahara Africa: Right or Privilege? Keywords. *Journal of Community Health and Primary Health Care*, *28*(1), 25–30.

Rajfur, P. (2019). Selected models and the classification of health care systems. *Medical Science Pulse*, *13*(1), 48–54. doi:10.5604/01.3001.0013.0513

Tumusiime, P., Gonani, A., Walker, O., Asbu, E. Z., Awases, M., & Kariyo, P. C. (2012). Health systems in sub-Saharan Africa: What is their status and role in meeting the health Millennium Development Goals? *African Health Monitor*, (14), 14–24.

WHO. (2008). Review of primary health care in the African region. Retrieved from https://www.eldis.org/document/A36616

Willcox, M. L., Peersman, W., Daou, P., Diakité, C., Bajunirwe, F., Mubangizi, V., ... Mant, D. (2015). Human resources for primary health care in sub-Saharan Africa: Progress or stagnation? *Human Resources for Health*, *13*(1), 1–11. doi:10.118612960-015-0073-8 PMID:26358250

Yoong, J., Burger, N., Spreng, C., & Sood, N. (2010). Private sector participation and health system performance in sub-Saharan Africa. *PLoS One*, *5*(10), 1–9. doi:10.1371/journal.pone.0013243 PMID:20949054

Chapter 2
Mental Health:
A Global Issue Affecting the Pattern of Life in Kashmir

Shazia Ali
https://orcid.org/0000-0003-3116-9194
Sheri-Kashmir Institute of Medical Sciences, India

Amat Us Samie
Superspeciality Hospital Shireen Bagh, Government Medical College,Srinagar j&k India

ABSTRACT

Global health issues are a global burden and are relatively common in industrialized societies. The World Health Organization and researchers have developed and rebuilt tools to report the burden of disease affecting mortality and health of the people. Apart from America and Europe, which are at an average of global burden for mental health disease, in some regions it is a major priority to be addressed globally. In South East Asia, one of the affected regions is Kashmir, Northern Indian. Disasters have manifested in various forms encompassing the natural calamities of earthquake, flood, landslides and manmade calamities of violence. Trauma due to manmade calamities has taken over as a leading cause of morbidity and mortality among the most productive working age group of 12-35 years. The chapter aims to understand the patterns of resilience in people surviving war and conflict in Kashmir over last 60 years. The focus is on the young population of society. Generations in Kashmir have faced the psychosocial impact of ongoing political conflict since the 1980's.

DOI: 10.4018/978-1-7998-2139-7.ch002

INTRODUCTION

A healthy mental condition is described as a normal standard of life in which a person realises his/her own abilities coping with the hardships of life, working productively and, fruitfully, and is able to contribute to his/or community ("world Health Organization," 2001d). Mental illness is an abnormal affair or health condition that is defined by any change in thinking, mood or behaviour associated with distress and/or impaired functioning ("US Dept. of Health and Human Services," 1999; Kessler et al., 2005). Mental disorders affect people from all countries and societies involving people from all age groups, men and women; poor and rich; urban and the rural populations. People living in conflict zones experience more mental disorders. Recently, the world has received an increased change in terms of warfare and violence to civil society resulting in unstable situations. Introduction of advanced weapons have resulted in grave human concerns. People are disappeared, tortured, forced to migrate, and starved to death. Globally, mental health disorders are among the leading causes of illness and disability. Mental illness leads to decreased productivity and has a negative impact on the quality of life of affected individuals and their families ("World Federation for Mental Health," 2015). Annually, over 450 million people have been reported to be affected by mental disorders, and only a few have access to cure. There are barriers to accessing the treatment created by social stigma and negligence. Mental health is determined by several factors of psychological illness and is influenced by society governed by political instability leading to number of events (Miller et al., 2010; Silove et al., 2014; Steel et al., 2009; Summerfield et al., 2000).

The chapter presents the support that strengthens the patterns of resilience in people who have survived war and conflict in Kashmir (India) over the last 60 years. Peace in Kashmir has been repeatedly interrupted due to conflicts between India and Pakistan. Generations in Kashmir have faced the psychosocial impact of ongoing political conflict from last 60 years. There are reports of human rights violations and their impacts. There has been research, though limited, on losses faced by the community, psychosocial impacts of exposure to violence and impact on mental health, socio-economic functioning and health service usage. In Kashmir, many women have lost their husbands to the conflict. Currently, it is believed that there is no reliable, comprehensive and factual survey about the number of widows and orphans in Kashmir. There are different estimates by different sources. Over the years, people living in Kashmir have been accustomed to the circumstances and have adapted themselves to survive in such situations. Gradually, the role of civil society becomes imperative to increase support systems, especially related to health services, children's needs care and persons with disabilities and women should be protected.

OVERALL POPULATION SCENARIO AND CONFLICTS IN KASHMIR VALLEY

The Kashmir Valley is situated in north region of the Indian state of Jammu and Kashmir between Jammu (to the south) and Ladakh (to the east) with the line of control (border with Pakistan) along its northern and western borders. It covers a geographical area of 15,948 km^2, with a population density of 430/km^2. The total population is 6.9 million, with 73% living in rural areas and 27% living in urban centers (2011 census). The majority (97%) of the population is Muslim, with Hindus, Sikhs, Buddhists and Christians making up the other 3% ("Human Rights Watch," 2006). Since partition of India in 1947, the Kashmir has faced political instability. Following three Indo-Pakistani wars (1947, 1965 and 1971) and one Indo-Chinese war (1962), the wars were consequences of an internal movement for determining freedom. In 1989, an insurgency began, resulting in 27 years of movement of gun-men group (fighting for self-determination) and military activity. By 2012, approximately 70,000 Kashmiris had lost their lives in the conflict and 10,000 people had been reported missing ("History of Kashmir," n.d.).

MENTAL HEALTH: INFLUENCE OF CONFLICT

Conflict influences lives of people and the society by having a negative impact. Irrespective of age, sex, career, residence the emotional and psychological effects of violence are deeply felt by many individuals. The conflict has brought about insecurity and breakdown of social relations, it has destroyed families in Kashmir and forced the youth of Kashmir to switch to drugs and to undertake anti-social activities. Kashmir has been regarded as "heaven on earth" for the nature and beautiful scenery. Over the past three decades, Kashmir has been affected with conflict and violence which has led to mental malfunctioning. Mental well-being is related to physical, social livelihood and economic disability. People who are affected by a conflict environment are burdened under mental and physical stress and suffer from post-traumatic stress problems (Amin et al., 2005; Amin et al 2004). Political instability creates an atmosphere of negativity, with long lasting effects on social, economic and livelihood of common people (Sack et al., 199; Amin et al., 2004; Margoob et al., 2006). A nationwide survey undertaken by the Ministry of Labour and Employment in 2012-2013 reported that Kashmir has the highest rate of unemployed people in India. At state level, the number of job seeking people increased by 190% between 2008 and 2013. Employment-generating sections like private sector, industry, agriculture, horticulture have been reduced due to present instability in region. Tourism was one of the main paths for employment among young people which has reduced in past 27 years. In 2011, a Kashmir-based report by Mercy Corps reported that unemployment leads to stress, social pressure, delay in marriages. The expression and behavior of people in such zones lead to stress, mental illness and tendency to suicide among youth ("Mercy Cops," 2011; Hassan et al., 2013).

For the past decade, a tremendous increase in mental illness has been reported in the Kashmir Valley. IMHANS, Institute of Mental Health and Neuroscience in the valley's capital, Srinagar, has a large number of patients being treated from an average of 100 per week in 1980 to 850 per week in 2016 (Dar et al., 2016). In 2005, in cross sectional study of 548 individuals in the districts of Kupwara and Badgam, researchers reported a prevalence rate of 33% for distress in patients having psychological effect (De Jong et al., 2008) In another study involving 3000 individuals from all districts in 2006, there was a prevalence of 7.3% for PTSD and a lifetime prevalence of 15.2% (Margoob et al., 2006). The year 2009, have shown a prevalence rate of 55.7% for depression in a study of 2728 individuals across all districts of the valley. A retrospective study on suicide demonstrated an increase of over 250% in suicide attempt cases between 1994 and 2012 (Shoib et al., 2012). Another study was reported on behavior of PTSD patients treated in Government Psychiatric Diseases Hospital in Srinagar reportedly having a lag time from symptoms occurred and treatment of such patients of 32 months in women and 48 months in men. The authors also stated that such patients seeking care was highly incongruent with the prevalence of PTSD in the community (Margoob et al., 2006).

As per the Kashmir Mental Health Survey Report 2015, a report prepared by MSF, Medecins Sans Frontieres, 1.8 million (45%) adults in the Valley had mental ill health symptoms. Approximately 1.6 million adults (41%) in the valley are facing depression with 415,000 (10%) susceptible to severe depression. An estimated 1 million adults (26%) in the valley are living with anxiety problems. Nearly 1 in 5 adults (19%) or 771,000 individuals are having PTSD symptoms, with 248,000 (6%) meeting the diagnostic criteria for PTSD. There are increased rates of co -morbidity depression, anxiety and PTSD symptoms found in adults in the valley. The districts of Baramulla and Budgam reported increased prevalence rates of mental ill health ("Kashmir Mental Health," 2015).

ARMED CONFLICT AND MENTAL HEALTH STATUS IN KASHMIR

Armed conflict is present in most of the Asian parts (Gates et al., 2012). War has catastrophic effects on health and well-being of human beings. Studies have reported that wars have long lasting effects on mankind, livelihood, households, and hunger.

It affects the psychology of people involved, decreasing their working and social ability of a normal life. WHO reflects that 10% of the population are subjected to trauma or war having psychological effect and 10% of those exposed to war have behavioural problems (Laxaminarayna et al., 2006). Studies have shown that the common people including young and adults suffer from trauma and psychological disorders. The common symptoms found were mental disorder, anxiety and PTSD. The children in Gaza have been affected by psychological disturbance and sleeping disorders (Hein et al., 1993). Social supports for such affected people have played an important role but people are affected and destroyed in war zone areas. The social support would have acted as a buffering zone for conflict and psychological disorder if present ("Sustainable Development UNICEF," 2013).

Kashmir has been in conflict for decades now. Deaths, Disappearances, killings, and harassment have been an outcome of conflict in Kashmir. About 8000 persons are reported to be disappeared and more than 70000 persons have been killed, and more than 6000 have been buried in graves ("Alleged Perpetrators JKCCS," 2012). The most affected group is that of the young and children. About 97000 to 100000 children turned orphans. The widows are increasing in number from 16000 in 2000 to 32400 in 2008 (Double) (Rather et al., 2013). This has reportedly increased the number of deaths and mental disorders in Kashmir affecting the young population. As a result, psychiatric admissions to one of the hospital increased from 6 per day in 1990 to 250-300 per day in 2000. The total number of patients rose from 1760 in 1990 to 18000 in 1994, to over 50000 in 2003. In 2006, the number of patients had increased to 82000 (Wani et al., 2006). According to the report documented by MSF, it was shown that about 45% of the adults in Kashmiri have a mental disorder. About 41% in the valley are affected by depression, with 10% having more serious depression. Almost 26% population in the valley have anxiety disorders. About 19% of population is having PTSD (Gates et al., 2012). Exposure to trauma leads to behavioural problems, having psychological and emotional distress to population. However, a different prevalence rate is reported with respect to gender and location. The women are suffering from depression more (60%) as compared to men (51%). Women suffered from increased prevalence of depression in all the age groups, particularly among 26 to 35 years, the reproductive years of their lives. Besides depression, PTSD is common in Kashmir population with symptoms of depression associated with it (Amin Syed et al., 2009). The conflict is one of the main reasons for mental ill heath population (Margoob et al., 1993). In addition to this, suicide rates and drug abuses are on high rate (Yaswi et al., 2008). About 25% of people in Kashmir are having depression (Hassan et al., 2013). Measuring the levels of depression, anxiety among the groups exposed to such conflict is more than non-exposed groups. About 90% of the population who are affected by such psychological disturbance do not intend to return home because of fear of being accepted in society.

There are major health issues like gastritis, headache, and weakness (Dilnaz et al., 2014). As a result, the children and youth develop a self-made mind governed by their rules and regulations and react on every small problem (Zahid et al., 2017). It results in children's who do not find their interest in education and normal livelihood, they wander after some self-made life and social set up.

USE OF WEAPONS IN KASHMIR AND IMPACT ON MENTAL HEALTH

The conflict has led to mental disturbance among children and youth. They do not look for jobs or education is not completed. They have psychological disturbances and mental disorders. They react inappropriately to any outbreak or cannot handle critical circumstances and have sleeping disorders. Their social life is affected. They are not able to cope up with normal social life, economically weak. They have lost hope of life, and have difficulty in concentrating on anything (Bilkis et al., 1996). Some of this may be linked to weapons use by law enforcement in Kashmir.

TERRORISM AND THE IMPACT ON MENTAL HEALTH

For the past three decades, 'terrorism' has spread and engulfed the entire world. In the face of escalating tensions created by terrorism and the after-shocks and trauma of violent crime, the psychological aspects of communities who confront terroristic incidents constantly and a terrorizing environment have mental imbalance. While cultures differ, it is amazing how many people are alike. Citizens of all cultures perceive threats to their security and safety in a negative manner. They long for stability and peace in their homelands. Most people want to be able to provide themselves with necessities, rather than fight. There is no dearth of evidences related to the worldwide terrorism. 4220 terroristic incidents were reported by the International Association of Chiefs of Police (IACP) worldwide for 1987. The data plainly indicate that terrorism is increasing and that multiple deaths and destruction are increasing enormously. Terrorism in India still occupies the center-stage in many parts of the country specially Jammu and Kashmir where it has dominated almost every aspect of the life of its citizen for years. Terrorism creates a state of mind where anxiety and fear dominate the people's thinking and behavior. Terrorist succeeded in creating such an effect in Kashmir for the last three decades. Most of the studies have emphasized the post-traumatic stress disorder (PTSD) of the people who have survived the terrorist attacks. Poor Mental health and Depression are highlighted in many related studies along with other related psychological abnormalities. A study was carried to report number of mental health of 58 refugees (18-64 years old) of war who were victimized by trauma. Study reported that 70.7 percent of the people had trauma. While a prevalence of psychiatric disturbance was found in 64.1 percent. Results inferred that age had a major factor related to mental disorder (Hassan et al., 2013). A study on terrorism, trauma and mental health suggests that the effects of violence lead to lack of hope, social ability and support. Another study was on psychology of terror and how this affects the livelihood of common people with lasting effects. One more study was on mental and behavioral problems associated with such outbreak of mental ill-health [39-40-53].

CONCLUSION

Operational Possibilities in Case of Mental Health

It is widely recognized that women and young people are main population who are affected. In most conflict situations, gender plays an important role, women are more vulnerable than other groups including children, they are the primary care, education and home builders and once they are targeted, a family gets affected and which leaves a mark in society. It is evident that very few studies have focused substantially on the life of women in the cultural context of Kashmir, with conflict, and psychosocial interventions, as the primary background. Studies based on Social Work principles and mental health perspectives, hopes to address this gap.

Questions Need to be Addressed

1. What do young women and men from Kashmir have in mind about the current situation there?
2. What are the lifestyle patterns young women and men, from Kashmir, which help them, cope and survive in the conflict zone?
3. What are the similarities and differences in these patterns among young women and men in different age groups say for example 16-21years, and 21-26 years?

Mental Health and Psychosocial Support: Any type of local or outside support that aims to protect or promote psychosocial well-being and/or prevent or treat mental disorder can be incorporated (Ashraf et al., 2008; Haji et al., 2018).

Interviews and Observation: Interviews should be held for these age group populations, observational studies on their behaviour, way of thinking, and pattern of living should be focussed. The data should be kept confidential. Further process of consulting experts, who have relevant experience related to gender and conflict, should be included. The data sheets should be prepared and analysed in the focussed age group. On the basis of these methodologies and data collection, mental health can be studied and evaluated in a conflict zone region. One can take necessary measures in order to prevent such disease affecting mental ill health and how they can be diagnosed by mood, behaviour, and distress. Mental, physical and social health, are vital strands of life that are closely interwoven and deeply interdependent and are important for normal functioning of body and livelihood. This needs to be protected as an important component of life for survival of a population in a region. There has been research, though limited, on losses faced by the community, psychosocial impact of exposure to violence, including impact on mental health, socio-economic functioning and health service usage. Further, the political and economic instability fuelled by unemployment has added to the mental disturbances in the valley. Gradually, the role of civil society groups has also grown in order to increase support systems, especially related to health services, children in need of care and protection, persons with disabilities, and women. Mental health disease is one of the fatal types to be measured and detected at an early stage. Educational set up and working settings need to be reformed to check behavioural parameters collaborated to lifestyle, its affect in community named as a mental illness (Price et al., 2018; Mohan et al., 2018; Soomro et al., 2019).

ACKNOWLEDGMENT

We acknowledge the authors for contributing in the chapter and Dr. Mushtaq Margoob for sharing his view on the topic and his experience on the area of interest.

REFERENCES

Amin, S. & Khan, A,W. (2009). Life in conflict: characteristics of Depression in Kashmir. Retrieved from www.ncbi.nlm.nih.gov/pmc/articles/PMC3068807/

Ashraf, M. (2008). *Kashmir First- Kashmir Story, A collection of commentaries, Politics & History* (Vol. I). India: Gulshan Books.

Boga, D. (2014). No Juvenile Court in J&K. Retrieved from http://infochangeindia.org/children/features/no-juvenile-courts-in –j&k/

Dar, M. M. (Ed.). (2016). Presentation on mental health work at the Institute of Mental Health and Neurosciences, Srinagar. In *Symposium on the results of the Kashmir Mental Health Survey*. Academic Press.

De Jong, K., Van de Kam, S., Ford, N., Lokuge, K., Fromm, S., Van de Galen, R., & ... (2008). Conflict in the Indian Kashmir Valley II: Psychosocial impact. *Conflict and Health*, *2*(11), 11. doi:10.1186/1752-1505-2-11 PMID:18854027

Gates, S., Hegre, H., Nygård, H. M., & Strand, H. (2012). Development consequences of armed conflict. *World Development*, *40*(9), 1713-1722. Retrieved from https://www.sciencedirect.com/science/article/pii/s0305750x12001015

Government of India. (2012). 2011 Indian National Census Online: Census Organization of India. Retrieved from www.census2011.co.in

Haji M. (2018). Killing One Colonial Law at a Time – After Section 377, It's Time to Repeal AFSPA. The Wire.

Hassan, A., & Shafi, A. (2013). Impact of conflict situation on mental health in Srinagar, Kashmir. *Bangladesh e-Journal of Sociology*, *10*(1), 101–126.

Hassan, A., & Shafi, A. (2013). Impact of Conflict Situation on Mental Health in Srinagar, Kashmir. *Bangladesh e-Journal of Sociology*, *10*(1).

Hein, F. A., Qouta, S., Thabet, A., & El Sarraj, E. (1993). Trauma and mental health of children in Gaza. *BMJ: British Medical Journal*, *306*(6885), 1130.

Human Rights Watch. (2006). *Everyone Lives in Fear: Patterns of Impunity in Jammu and Kashmir*. New York: Human Rights Watch.

Inter-Agency Standing Committee. (2006). *IASC guidelines on mental health and psychosocial support in emergency settings*. Geneva, Switzerland: IASC.

Kessler, R. C., Chiu, W. T., & Demler Walters, E. E. (2005). prevalence, severity, and comorbidity of 12- month DSM-IV disorders in the National comorbidity survey Replication. *Archives of General Psychiatry*, *62*(6), 617–627. doi:10.1001/archpsyc.62.6.617 PMID:15939839

Laxaminarayna, R., & Murthy, S. (2006). Mental Health Consequences of war: A Brief Review of Research Findings. *World Psychiatry; Official Journal of the World Psychiatric Association (WPA)*. PMID:16757987

Margoob, A. M., & Ahmad, S. A. (2006). Community prevalence of adult post traumatic stress disorder in south Asia: Experience from Kashmir. *Jammu Kashmir Practitioner*, *13*(1), S18–S25.

Margoob, A. M., Firdosi, M. M., Ali, Z., Hussain, A., Mushtaq, H., Khan, A. Y., & ... Muzamil, M. (2006). Treatment seeking post-traumatic stress disorder patient population - Experience from Kashmir. *Jammu and Kashmir Practitioner*, *13*(1), S57–S60.

Margoob, M. A., Beg, A. A., & Dutta, K. S. (1993). Depressive disorders in kashmir; A changing Socio Demographic and Clinical Profile of patients over the past two decades. *JK Practitioner*, 22–24.

Mercy Corps. (2011). *Youth Entrepreneurship in Kashmir: challenges and opportunities. Kashmir*. Mercy Corp.

Miller, K. E., & Rasmussen, A. (2010). War exposure, daily stressors, and mental health in conflict and post-conflict settings: Bridging the divide between trauma-focused and psychosocial frameworks. *Social Science & Medicine*, *70*(1), 7–16. doi:10.1016/j.socscimed.2009.09.029 PMID:19854552

Mohan, D., Mander, H., Singh, N., Philipose, P., & Bose, T. (2018). Unending trauma: The heavy toll of ongoing violence on mental health in Kashmir. In Blood, censored: When Kashmiris Become the 'Enemy.' Yoda Press.

MSF. (n.d.). Kashmir Mental Health Survey-2015.

Price, G. (2017). *Is India Getting Serious About Dialogue in Kashmir?* Chatham House.

Quraishi, H. (2004). *Kashmir- The Untold Story*. India: Penguin Books.

Rather, F. (2013). Armed conflict in j&k and its impact on society: A case study of Kashmir valley. *International journal of Scientific and Research Publications*, *3*(2).

Sack, W., Him, C., & Dickason, D. (1999). Twelve year follow up study of khmer youths who suffered massive war trauma as children. *Journal of the American Academy of Child and Adolescent Psychiatry*, *38*(9), 1173–1179. doi:10.1097/00004583-199909000-00023 PMID:10504817

Shah, A. V. (1982). Integration of mental health. *Indian Journal of Psychiatry*, *24*, 3–7. PMID:21965877

Shoib, S., Maqbool, D., Bashir, H., Qayoom, G., & Arif, T. (2012). Psychiatric morbidity and the socio-demographic determinants of patients attempting suicide in Kashmir Valley: A cross-sectional study. *International Journal of Health Sciences and Research*, *2*(7), 45–53.

Silove, D., Liddell, B., Rees, S., Chey, T., Nickerson, A., Tam, N., ... Steel, Z. (2014). Effects of recurrent violence on post-traumatic stress disorder and severe distress in conflict-affected Timor-Leste: A 6-year longitudinal study. *The Lancet. Global Health*, *2*(5), 293–300. doi:10.1016/S2214-109X(14)70196-2 PMID:25103168

Soomro, A. (2019, August 17). Fear and uncertainty around Kashmir's future. *Lancet*, *394*(10198), 542. doi:10.1016/S0140-6736(19)31939-7 PMID:31423985

Steel, Z., Chey, T., Silove, D., Marnane, C., Bryant, R.A., & van Ommeren, M. (2009). Association of torture and other potentially traumatic events with mental health outcomes among populations exposed to mass conflict and displacements: A systematic review and meta-analysis. *American Medical Association*, *302*(5), 537-549.

Summerfield, D. (2000). War and mental health: A brief overview. *British Medical Journal*, *321*(7255), 232–235. doi:10.1136/bmj.321.7255.232 PMID:10903662

Sustainable Development starts with safe, healthy and well educated children. (2013). UNICEF.

Syed, H. R., Zachrisson, H. D., Dalgard, O. S., Dalen, I., & Ahlberg, N. (2008). Concordance between Hopkins Symptom Checklist (HSCL-10) and Pakistan Anxiety and Depression Questionnaire. *BMC Psychiatry*, *8*(59). PMID:18647394

Tabish, A. (2004). Mental Health: Science and sensibility. In *The Future of Health* (1st ed., pp. 179–207). New Delhi: Paras Medical publishers.

Tabish, A. (2005). Mental Health: Neglected for far too long. *JK Practitioner*, *12*(1), 38–42.

The World Health Organization. (2003). Department of mental health and substance Dependence.

U.S Department of Health and Human Services. (1999) Mental health: A Report of the surgeon general. Rockville, MD: U.S. Department of Health and Human Services; Substance Abuse and Mental health services Administration, enter for mental Health Services, National institute of Health, National institute of mental health.

Wani, Z. A., & Margoob, M. A. (2006). Family study of Adult PTSD patients in south Asia: Experiences from Kashmir. *JK Practitioner*, 61–64.

Wikipedia. (n.d.). History of Kashmir online. from https://en.wikipedia.org/wiki/History_of_Kashmir

World Federation for Mental Health. (2015).

World Health Organization. (2001d). strengthening mental health promotion. Geneva, World Health Organization (fact sheet no. 220).

Yaswi, A., & Haque, A. (2008). Prevalence of PTSD symptoms and Depression and level of coping among the victims of the Kashmir conflict. *Journal of Loss and Trauma, 13*(5), 471–480. doi:10.1080/15325020802171441

Zahid M. (2017). Judicial Independence and Accountability of Judiciary in Pakistan. *International Journal of Research in Social Sciences, 7*(12).

KEY TERMS AND DEFINITIONS

Disorder: A disorder is a practical irregularity or trouble. Medical disorders can be characterized into mental illnesses, physical disorders, genetic disorders, emotional and behavioural disorders, and functional disorders.

Mental Health: Mental health comprises our expressive, psychosomatic, and communal well-being. It affects how we reflect, sense, and act. It also helps regulate how we handle anxiety, relate to others, and make selections. Mental health is significant at every phase of life, from childhood and adolescence through maturity.

Psychology: Psychology is the discipline of behaviour and awareness. Psychology comprises the study of conscious and unconscious occurrences, as well as sensation and thought. It is a theoretical discipline of immense scope. Psychologists seek an understanding of the developing belongings of brains, and all the variability of phenomena related to those emergent belongings, joining this way the wider neuroscientific group of researchers.

Section 2
Malaria

Chapter 3
Malaria:
Knowledge, Attitude, and Practices in Some Sub-Saharan African Communities

Omolade Olayinka Okwa
Lagos State University, Nigeria

ABSTRACT

Malaria is transmitted by the female Anopheles mosquito and is a parasitic disease which is caused by the Plasmodium species. It is a serious communicable disease in sub-Saharan Africa (SSA). The most vulnerable group is children aged 0-5 years. Malaria is responsible for most outpatient visits, hospital admissions and the main cause of school and work absenteeism. Knowledge, attitudes, and practices (KAP) are essential for control programmes being the educational diagnosis and perception of a community about a disease which affects their attitudes and practices. This chapter reviews that the KAP of most communities in SSA have existing gaps which impacts on the control of malaria. A sound and adequate understanding of malaria and its proper recognition are crucial to its control. The inclusion of malaria education in a pupil's curriculum and effective information on the electronic and social media can change the misconceptions about malaria and correct attitudes and practices to intensify control efforts.

DOI: 10.4018/978-1-7998-2139-7.ch003

INTRODUCTION: MALARIA AS A VECTOR TRANSMITTED DISEASE

Malaria meaning "bad air' is one of the oldest and re-emerging disease in the world today (Awolola, 2017). Human malaria is a leading infectious disease which is caused by apicomplexan coccidian which are haemosporinas of the family Plasmodidae and genus *Plasmodium*. Apicomplexa are characterized by being exclusively parasitic and without locomotory organelles. Five species of *Plasmodium* parasitizes humans such as *P. falciparium*, *P.ovale*, *P. malariae*, *P. vivax* and the zoonotic *P. knowlesi* of Southeast Asia (Okwa, 2019). However, *P. falciparium* is the most virulent and prevalent of the malaria parasites in sub-Saharan Africa (SSA) accounting for 99.7% of estimated malaria cases in 2017 alone (World Health Organization; WHO, 2018). Malaria is a complex disease due to its complicated transmission process being transmitted by the infectious bites of the female *Anopheles* mosquitoes which are considered as the deadliest creatures on planet Earth (WHO, 2016; Okwa & Savage, 2018).

The spread of malaria needs conditions which are favorable to the survival of the *Anopheles* mosquito and the *Plasmodium* parasite (Okwa & Savage, 2018). Female *Anopheles* mosquitoes carry infective sporozoite stages of the *Plasmodium* parasite in their salivary glands, which they transfer to the blood stream of their host during a blood meal. The source of the malaria problem is the diverse breeding sites of the *Anopheles* mosquito which indiscriminately oviposits and breeds in any available stagnant or still waters in the presence of favourable environmental conditions such as temperature, rainfall and humidity typical of that found in SSA (Okwa, 2019). Malaria is no respecter of persons as all classes and groups of people are exposed to the infectious bites of the female *Anopheles* mosquito (Awolola, 2017; WHO, 2018). Apart from vector control, human behavior in terms of their knowledge, attitudes and practices (KAP) of prevention and control of malaria are crucial for control programmes.

BACKGROUND: THE GLOBAL PICTURE OF MALARIA

Globally, malaria remains the most important parasitic disease and a social public health problem being a major threat in the world today (Centre for Disease Control; CDC, 2019). In 2016, it was reported that the disease was present in about 97 countries covering half the world's population causing up to a million deaths a year (WHO, 2016). In 2017, malaria was estimated to infect over 300-500 million people yearly, so an estimated half of the world's population were at risk (WHO, 2017). The World malaria report, estimated that there were 219 million cases of malaria in 2017, in 87 countries and 10 highest burden African countries had an estimated 3.5 million more malaria cases in 2017 than in 2016 (WHO, 2018). According to Tambo (2019), the estimated number of malaria deaths stood at 435 000 in 2017 alone and 11 countries accounted for approximately 70% of estimated malaria cases and deaths globally in 10 SSA countries and in India (WHO, 2018)

According to Salomon (2014), the disability-adjusted life year (DALY) is a measure of overall disease burden, expressed as the number of years lost due to ill-health, disability or early death. It is a way of comparing the overall health and life expectancy of different countries. Almost 3% of DALYS are due to malaria mortality globally, with 10% burden in Africa (WHO, 2019). The global malaria burden indicates that endemicity of malaria in SSA alone is more than an estimated 80% of cases. Over 90% of deaths of the global burden are restricted to 30 countries in SSA (WHO, 2017). The global malaria picture is very disturbing because it is a huge economic and intolerable burden that calls for global action to eliminate it. By and large, conquering malaria, a deadly scourge and human formidable foe is still a great challenge to the whole world, today (CDC, 2019).

THE STATUS OF MALARIA IN SUB-SAHARAN AFRICA

According to Kampala (2019), SSA is the region of Africa that lies south of the Sahara, and consists of 46 of the 54 African countries excluding Algeria, Djibouti, Morocco, Libya, Egypt, Somalia, Sudan and Tunisia. Politically, these countries are part of the Arab world, so they are not considered as nations of SSA. Geographically, all the regions of the African continent excluding North Africa are regarded as SSA. Africa is the hottest continent on earth, and the climate of SSA is hot and semi-arid in the Sahel, and tropical in Central and West Africa. In SSA, temperature could be as high as 40°C -57.8°C in the Northern parts and -20.1°C- 2.8°C in the Southern parts of the region.

WHO (2019) reported that the risk of malaria as an efficient and unrepentant killer exists throughout the region of SSA, where it is a disease of public health concern. Nigeria in West Africa and the Democratic Republic of Congo (DRC) in Central Africa, are the two mostly affected countries in SSA, accounting for over 40% of the estimated total of malaria deaths, globally in 2017 (Umwangange et al., 2018; WHO, 2018). Ethiopia, in North Eastern Africa and Ugandan, in East Africa, are next in line, accounting for high prevalence of malaria deaths (Onah et al., 2017). In 2018, these four countries account for 50% of global mortality: Nigeria (19%), DRC (11%) and 20% for both Ethiopia and Uganda (WHO, 2019).

P. falciparium is the most virulent species of malaria parasite in SSA. For instance, in Nigeria with the highest malaria burden in SSA, *P. falciparium* causes 95% of infections while *P. malariae* causes 5% of infections. *P. ovale* is rarely seen in Nigeria while *P. vivax* is absent in most parts of West Africa (WHO, 2017). Several species of *Anopheles,* especially *An. gambiae s.s* and *An. funestus s.s* can transmit malaria in Nigeria as well as other countries in SSA (Awolola, 2017; Nigerian Centre for Disease Control; NCDC, 2016; WHO, 2018).

SOCIAL COST OF MALARIA IN SUB- SAHARAN AFRICA

Malaria is the second leading cause of death from infectious diseases in Africa, after Human Immunodeficiency Virus (HIV) /Acquired Immune deficiency syndrome (AIDS) and is also a leading cause of mortality in under-five aged children accounting for 20% of deaths (Onah et al., 2017). It has been estimated that every two minutes a child dies, so malaria kills over a million children every year in SSA (WHO, 2018). According to the report of the United Nations International Children Emergency Fund (UNICEF, 2018) about 61 per cent deaths in 2017 (266,000) were children under five years of age which is a daily toll of nearly 730 children under age five. Umwangange et al. (2018) also reported that malaria is the fourth cause of child death in SSA, remaining one of the main killers of children in every 2 minutes. Immunosuppressed people such as pregnant women and HIV/AIDS patients are also very susceptible to malaria infection (Atulomah et al., 2014; Owusu et al., 2018; Yalewayler et al., 2019).

Undoubtedly, malaria has remained a deadly scourge SSA where it has the reputation of causing fever, teeth chattering chills, head and body aches, loss of appetite, cough, catarrh, vomiting and nausea (Umwangange et al., 2018). Health care is a key challenge in SSA and morbidity and mortality due to malaria have been increasing due to deterioration in the health system, growing drug and insecticide resistances, periodic changes in weather pattern, human migration and population displacement (Deaton and Tortora, 2014). Much more, malaria imposes immense morbidity and mortality as well as grave socio- economic burdens on both individuals and the nations at large in SSA. Hence, the degree and extent of malaria impacts on the clinical, social and economic conditions of people living in the endemic area and cuts across all age groups and social classes (WHO, 2019).

In 2010, in Nigeria deaths from malaria were the highest recorded worldwide. This was a bizarre phenomenon since so much effort has been geared towards eradicating this dreaded disease in the country (Onah et al., 2017). According to the Federal ministry of health (FMoHN, 2015), in Nigeria, malaria is responsible for 100 million cases and about 300,000 deaths every year and about 30% of this occurs in children mostly under the age of five. This is in line with the report of UNICEF (2018).

Okwa et al. (2009) reported that Malaria is holoendemic in Nigeria where it is a public health problem accounting for 25% infant mortality and 30% childhood mortality. The disease is well known in Nigeria, a household name which is often underestimated and taken with levity, but a big contributor to economic burden. Malaria also exerts a heavy toll on lives and wasted days of labour loss in Nigeria (FMoHN, 2015). The disease is the commonest cause of work and school absenteeism and a serious impediment to economic, political, social, and educational development in Nigeria (FMoHN, 2014; NCDC, 2016).

In a report by Okwa et al. (2011) school absenteeism due to malaria was as high as 70% and students missed an estimated 3-12 school-day per year which is 2-6% of academic year. Okwa & Ibidapo (2010) reported that the disease causes about 50% of outpatient visits, 40% of hospital admission and 11% of maternal mortality in Nigeria. In 2012, hospitalized malaria patients were 40% of admitted patients while malaria outpatients were 93% (Okwa et al., 2012a). Okafor & Oko-Ose (2012) also conducted a study in Benin City, Nigeria and observed that malaria has adverse impact on school performances and learning among school children.

The situation in Nigeria gives a picture of thc situation in other countries in SSA. For example, the West African region published prevalent figures ranging from 83% in Mali and far above in some nations within the region (Umwangange et al., 2018). In Mauritania, North West Africa within the year 2016, among an estimated population of 3,537,368, malaria incidence was 78/1,000 persons at risk and malaria-associated mortality was 30 deaths/100,000 persons (Deida et al., 2019)

The prevalence of malaria in the East African region among school children ranged from 9% to 23% in Tanzania, 15% in Ethiopia to about 49% in Kenya, where the age group of 7-10 years was significantly associated with malaria infections (Umwangange et al., 2018). Malaria patients in Kenya accounted for 19% of hospital admissions, 3–5% of in-patient deaths and between 30–50% of out-patient cases and an estimated 74% of the population were at risk of infection with the disease (Ernst et al., 2016). Kenyan primary school students missed 11% of school days per year and secondary school students missed 4.3% of school days due to malaria thereby 13-50% of school absenteeism was due to malaria (Diiro et al., 2016). In Central Africa, the prevalence of malaria among school children was between 16% in DRC and 42% in Equatorial Guinea. Similarly, a higher prevalence rate of malaria among school children in Southern Africa was in the range of 43% in Zambia, South Central Africa and 60% in Malawi, South Eastern Africa (Umwangange et al., 2018). According to WHO (2018), Rwanda has noted estimated reductions in its malaria burden, with 430 000 fewer cases in 2017 than in 2016.

ECONOMIC COSTS OF MALARIA IN SUB-SAHARAN AFRICA

Malaria imposes substantial costs to both individuals and governments in SSA. The costs to individuals and their families is in terms of cost of drugs for treatment, expenses for travel to, and treatment at, dispensaries and clinics, lost days of work, expenses for preventive measures and school absenteeism which could affect general performances and lead to poor grades (WHO, 2018).

The effect on investment in education should not be undermined: Loss in school days represents a huge loss on academic standard and loss on the families, communities and nations investments in education. Apart from the incapacitating effect of malaria attack, the direct economic costs of malaria that result from absence from school and treatment are enormous and the overall economic impact is likely to be more substantial (Okwa et al., 2012b) . The cost of the illness is represented by the cost of the treatment and time loss by the patient and the caregiver and the expenses for burial in case of deaths while psychosocial costs are difficult to quantify and even compensate (WHO, 2019). Direct costs (for example, illness, treatment, premature death) have been estimated to cost at least US$ 12 billion per year (CDC, 2019)

According to WHO (2018), costs to governments include maintenance, supply and staffing of health facilities, purchase of drugs and other supplies, public health interventions against malaria, such as insecticide spraying or distribution of insecticide-treated bed nets (ITNS), lost days of work with resulting loss of income, and lost opportunities for joint economic ventures and tourism.

In 2017, an estimated US$ 3.1 billion was invested globally in malaria control efforts by governments of malaria endemic countries and international partners – an amount slighter higher than the figure reported for 2016. Nearly three quarters (US$ 2.2 billion) of investments in 2017 were spent in the WHO African Region and in 2017, US$ 1.4 billion was invested in low-income countries at 87%. The governments of endemic countries contributed 28% of total funding (US$ 900 million) in 2017, a figure unchanged from 2016 (WHO, 2018).

Two thirds of domestically sourced funds were invested in malaria control activities carried out by National malaria programmes. As in previous years, the United States of America was the largest international source of malaria financing, providing US$ 1.2 billion (39%) in 2017. To reach the Global Technical Strategy (GTS) 2030 targets, it is estimated that annual malaria funding will need to increase to at least US$ 6.6 billion per year by 2020. Stepping up investments in malaria research and development is key to achieving the GTS targets. Information on the economic burden of malaria in Africa is needed to target interventions efficiently and equitably, and to justify investment in research and control (WHO, 2019).

KNOWLEDGE, ATTITUDE AND PRACTICES OF MALARIA IN SSA

Working Definitions: For the purpose of this chapter, knowledge is information, understanding, enlightenment and awareness of something. Attitude is a predisposition or a tendency to respond positively or negatively towards an acquired knowledge, belief, idea or situation. It influences an individual's choice of action and responses to the knowledge, belief, idea or situation. Attitude is therefore the way and manner people demonstrate this knowledge, belief or idea by their actions. Practices are what people do regularly or constantly as a normal part of their life.

The KAP of malaria prevention and control has unfortunately remained a pervasive problem in different countries of SSA (Amir & Beyene 2018; Umwangange et al., 2018) Malaria is unique among diseases because its roots lie so deep within human communities (Awolola, 2017). Studies on KAP have demonstrated that, direct interaction with community plays an important role in circumventing malaria spread (Adedotun et al., 2010). Community knowledge about malaria and mosquito behavior is critical for successful malaria intervention, appropriate treatment, and prevention and control methods (Oyedeji et al., 2009). Malaria beliefs and practices are often related to culture, and can influence the effectiveness of control strategies thus, local knowledge and practices related to malaria is important for the implementation of culturally appropriate, sustainable, and effective interventions(s). The failure to consider a community KAP about malaria has contributed to the inability of programmes to achieve sustainable control (Oyedeji et al., 2009; WHO, 2017). People's behavior may increase malaria risk, but it is not easy to change such behavior. Indeed, there are many reasons why particular behaviors exist, and they are often tied to considerable benefits in areas which are quite distinct from health. It is pertinent to note that most health beliefs and behaviors are developed and maintained within the families in SSA (Deaton and Tortora, 2015).

Community perceptions, beliefs, and attitudes about malaria causation, symptom identification, treatment of malaria and prevention influence efforts to address malaria and are often overlooked in control efforts which vary from community to community and among individual households (WHO, 2010). Local etiology is important and has been shown in several cases to influence treatment seeking, but it is by no means the only influence. Wrong knowledge and perception, cultural and social factors have also been identified and reported as factors that can cause delay in seeking treatment for malaria (Jombo et al., 2010). Understanding these issues is an important step to develop control strategies.

CASE STUDY OF SOME COMMUNITIES IN SUB-SAHARAN AFRICA

Previous studies have identified a need for improving malaria control measures by taking into account local beliefs and practices of the common man. These studies had found a relationship between socio-demographic factors, exposure and the knowledge of malaria. Many past studies have shown the relevance of people's illnesses, recognition of symptoms, explanation of causes, and treatment seeking behavior, even at household level (Adedotun et al., 2010; Oyedeji et al., 2009). In a comparative study in SSA, the knowledge of the cause and transmission of malaria ranged from 19.2% in Zimbabwe to 85% in Nigeria. The researchers concluded that misconceptions of malaria causes and malaria transmission still exist in many countries of SSA (Umwangange et al., 2018). Except for Southern Africa countries, many other countries in SSA do not have successful malaria control programmes, due mainly to the magnitude of the problem and the lack of adequate health infrastructure, as well as financial and human resources (Khumbulani et al., 2009)

KAP of Some Communities in Nigeria

A cross sectional survey on KAP of malaria among 50 artisans (all males) and 50 traders (78% female) was carried out in five selected areas of Lagos, Nigeria. The use of local herbs was especially common among traders, who were more educated and predominantly female. The artisans and traders surprisingly had some erroneous believes about malaria (Okwa et al., 2012b). A community-based study on KAP among expectant women in a teaching hospital in Ogun State, South western Nigeria, revealed that majority of women with non-formal education did not know the cause of malaria and that the level of education influenced how malaria was defined. In their study, they found that home remedies were the most popular method of controlling malaria among these women. The women also believed that headache was the major recognized symptom, and malaria etiology was attributed to erroneous causes (Atulomah et al., 2014).

In another study, there was a correlation between level of education, marital status and knowledge of malaria among women in Ibadan, south-western, Nigeria. In this study, uneducated women constituted the majority of those who visited traditional healers or used herbal concoctions or other local remedies (Oladimeji et al., 2019). However, Okwa et al. (2011 & 2012a) reported that there existed wrong misconceptions about malaria and gaps in seeking treatment even among students and highly educated people in two different studies they carried out in Lagos State, Nigeria.

Jombo et al. (2010) reported that educational level and marriage had a positive impact on knowledge of malaria and the burden in north -central Nigeria. In another study in Kebbi State, north -western Nigeria, Singh et al. (2014) found that the knowledge of the cause of malaria was low, but there was good knowledge of mosquito behavior however, this was not reflected in preventive practices.

Ordinioha's (2012) study in Rivers State, south –south Nigeria revealed that bed-nets ownership did not always translate into usage, which was as low as 20%. The bed-nets were predominantly and erroneously used for fishing nets and mosquito nuisance control, and not for malaria control.

KAP of Some Communities in Other West African Regions

Owusu et al. (2018) reported inadequate KAP about malaria among symptomatic outpatient in some hospitals in Ghana. According to Diallo et al., (2017) who conducted a study in Greater Accra, Ghana, the use of herbs to cure malaria was very popular among mobile populations because people believed the herbs put fear in the malaria illness.

Nyavor et al. (2017) reported in another study that the use of bed-nets was not popular in Hohoe Municipality, Ghana. The malaria operational plan (2019) in Cote D' Ivoire, reported that even individuals with sound knowledge of malaria resulted to self-medication and also use local herbs. It was also reported that mosquito bed-nets were known but only few people slept under bed-nets despite the availability while some regarded bed-nets as expensive and scarce in the local market. There were also local beliefs hindering the use of ITNs. Mosquito coils and insect sprays were preferred because they were available and cheaper despite the potential side effects.

KAP of Some Communities in the East African Region

In Ugandan, a KAP study by Musoke et al. (2015) reported that participants had low knowledge of malaria prevention methods and knowledge was associated with age, income and level of education. They also reported that bed-nets ownership increased with household income. Mazigo et al. (2010) and Sumari et al. (2016) in two different studies reported significant differences between educational level and the knowledge and transmission of malaria in Tanzania, East Africa. Mazigo et al. (2010) also corroborated the fact that the uses of bed- nets were associated with high educational level.

In Ethiopia, North Eastern Africa, knowledge and awareness of malaria and the control was quite high. The symptoms of malaria were well recognized but only 25% of the communities use bed-nets even though they all had bed-nets. The misuse of available bed-nets was also observed in a study in Ethiopia by Ashton et al. (2011).

In another study in Ethiopia, houseflies were mistaken by students to be involved in transmission of malaria (Amir & Beyene, 2018).

The Malawi malaria indicator report (2017) noted that rurality and lack of education accounted for more exposure and incidence of malaria in some communities in Malawi. About 82% of households own at least one insecticide treated net but 7% use the nets for other reasons such as fencing and fishing. In another study in Malawi, it was reported that the KAP of malaria among some selected school pupils in Malawi, South Eastern Africa was encouraging. However, of 2,667 school children studied by the researchers, only 32.4% slept under mosquito bed-nets. The study showed low to moderate level of practice of malaria prevention ranging from 32.4% in Malawi to 67.9% in Kenyan school children (Umwangange et al., 2018). In Rwanda, misconceptions about the cause and transmission of malaria among school children still persist. However, as at 2018, no study had been conducted in Rwanda regarding school children's KAP towards malaria (Umwangange et al., 2018).

KAP of Some Communities in the Southern African Region

The potential contribution of KAP studies to malaria research and control has not received much attention in most Southern African countries. In a Namibian university, Jacob & Nuuyoma (2019) reported that 95% of the students know that mosquito transmit malaria and but 80% believed that the disease is preventable. However, the students believed that only children and pregnant women should avoid mosquito bites. The students had a sound knowledge of malaria with few misconceptions, but the knowledge did not reflect in their practices.

A study which was conducted among grade three school children, aged 8-10 years in Zimbabwe, south- central Africa revealed that low knowledge of malaria caused low treatment seeking. Only 19.2% of school children knew the cause of malaria and most of them (75%) had no idea about its prevention (Umwangange et al., 2018). In a study in Swaziland, Southern Africa, a substantial number of research participants showed reasonable knowledge of malaria, including correct association between malaria and mosquito bites, its potentially fatal consequences and correct treatment practices. However, bed- nets ownership was low at 38% (Khumbulani et al., 2009)

SOLUTIONS AND RECOMMENDATIONS

- The low fraction of people using bed-nets or ITNS and the moderate ownership of these nets which was observed in most studies call for continued health education, evaluation of the distribution, availability and affordability of these nets in affected communities of SSA.

- Education and awareness programmes for people in endemic communities and the introduction of curricula- based malaria courses and among school children is strongly advocated. These calls for urgent need to revisit the course-based curriculum and make the necessary changes so that the school children will be able to assimilate and comprehend correctly the right KAP about malaria.
- Radio, television and social media are the best-known means of health education that can be exploited to inform students and the general populace on malaria. Television and radio could intensify health advertisements on malaria, which gives information to the common man.

FUTURE RESEARCH DIRECTIONS

- There is need for targeted and sustainable health educational programs to increase the communities' efforts to develop desirable attitude and practices regarding malaria and the communities' participation for malaria control. Zero malaria starts with everyone in the community (Tambo, 2019)
- There should be social enlightenment programs for understanding who already knows about malaria and its prevention, who has adopted malaria prevention and mosquito avoidance practices, and who is at risk of malaria infection. This is a necessary precursor to identifying and targeting vulnerable populations and ensuring successful implementation and sustainability of the efforts to control malaria

DISSCUSION

Most of the studies analyzed in this chapter, revealed a significant link between low education and low KAP of malaria. It is therefore true that misconceptions about the cause and transmission of malaria still exist widely in SSA. On the contrary, knowledge about preventive measures does not necessarily translate into improvement in practices as researchers observed in some of the communities. The continued prevalence of malaria in SSA is largely due to sociocultural factors which are often at variance with standard control measures (Jombo et al., 2010). However, taking preventive measures is related to ones knowledge of a disease. Wrong knowledge and misconceptions about malaria will lead to wrong attitudes and wrong practices. This leads to a rising increase in the incidence and prevalence of malaria, which ultimately impacts on the prevention, control and elimination (Khumbulani et al., 2009).

Okwa et al. (2012a, 2012b) reiterated the fact that malaria is everybody's business, no matter the educational level and status. Education for health begins with people and motivates them with whatever interests they may have in improving their living conditions. The aim is to develop in the masses a sense of responsibility for health conditions for themselves as individuals, members of families, and communities. In infectious disease control, health education commonly includes an appraisal of what is known by a population about a disease, an assessment of habits and attitudes of the people as they relate to spread and frequency of the disease, and the presentation of specific means to remedy observed deficiencies (WHO, 2017).

CONCLUSION

The World Health Organization defined health education as "comprising of consciously constructed opportunities for learning involving some form of communication designed to improve health literacy, including improving knowledge, and developing life skills which are conducive to individual and community health (WHO, 2016). Health education is also an effective tool that helps improve health in developing nations. It not only teaches prevention and basic health knowledge but also conditions ideas that re-shape everyday habits of people with unhealthy lifestyles in developing countries (NCDC, 2016).

This type of conditioning not only affects the immediate recipients of such education but also future generations will benefit from improved and properly cultivated ideas about health which will eventually be ingrained. Suffice to say that, without a rational concept of the nature of a disease, it is impossible to visualize a management procedure. A sound local and adequate understanding of malaria and its proper recognition and awareness tailored to the need of a community, preventive measures, home management and health seeking behavior are crucial for the control of malaria. Considering all the issues above can be an important step towards developing strategies which are aimed at controlling malaria.

REFERENCES

Adedotun, A. A., Morenikeji, O. A., & Odaibo, A. B. (2010). Knowledge, attitudes and practices about malaria in an urban community in south-western Nigeria. *Journal of Vector Borne Diseases*, *47*(3), 155–159. PubMed

Amir, A., & Beyene, P. (2018). Knowledge, attitudes and practices of malaria transmission and preventive measures in Woreta town, Northwest Ethiopia. Bio Medical Central Research Notes, 11, 491. doi:10.118613104-018-3607-z

Ashton, R. A., Kefyalew, T., Tesfaye, G., Pullan, R. L., Yadeta, D., Reinthinger, R., & Brooker, S. (2011). School-based surveys of malaria in Oromia regional State, Ethiopia: A rapid survey method for malaria in low transmission settings. *Malaria Journal*, *10*(1), 25. doi:10.1186/1475-2875-10-25 PubMed

Atulomah, E. T., Farotimi, A. A., & Atulomah, N. O. (2014). Knowledge, attitudes and practices of malaria prevention among expectant mothers attending antenatal clinic at OOUTH, Sagamu, Ogun State, Nigeria. *Acta Satech*, *5*(1), 9–25.

Awolola, T. S. (2017). *Malaria, Mosquitoes and Man: The Battle Continues* (7th ed.). Nigerian Institute of Medical Research.

Centre for Disease Control (CDC). 2019). Saving lives, protecting people: Malaria impact worldwide (Social and Economic toll). Retrieved from https://www.cdc.gov/parasites/malaria/index.html

Deaton, A. S., & Tortora, R. (2014). People in sub-Saharan Africa rate their health and health care among lowest in the world. *Health Affairs (Project Hope)*, *34*(3), 519–527. doi:10.1377/hlthaff.2014.0798 PubMed

Deida, J., Tahar, R., Khalef, Y. O., Khadijetou, M. L., Hmeyade, A., Khairu, M. L., & Boukhary, A. (2019). Oasis malaria in North Mauritania. *Emerging Infectious Diseases*, *25*(2), 282–289. doi:10.3201/eid2502.180732 PubMed

Diallo, N., Akweongo, P., Maya, E., Aikins, M., & Safo, B. (2017). Burden of malaria in mobile populations in the Greater Accra region, Ghana: A cross- sectional study. *Malaria Journal*, *16*(1), 109. doi:10.1186/s12936-017-1751-x PubMed

Diiro, G. M., Hippolyte, D., Affognon, B. W., Muriithi, S. K., Mbogo, W. C., & Clifford, M. (2016). The role of gender on malaria preventive behaviour among rural households in Kenya. *Malaria Journal*, *15*, 14. doi:10.118612936-015-1039y

Ernst, K. C., Hayden, M. H., Olsen, H., Cavanaugh, J. L., Ruberto, I., Agawo, M., & Munga, S. (2016). Comparing ownership and use of bed nets at two sites with differential malaria transmission in western Kenya. *Malaria Journal*, *15*(1), 217. doi:10.1186/s12936-016-1262-1 PubMed

Federal Ministry of Health, Nigeria. (2015). FMoHN document: National Guidelines for Diagnosis and Treatment of Malaria, 2015.

Jacob, V., & Nuuyoma, V. (2019). Knowledge, attitudes and practices of University students on Malaria prevention in Kavango, East, Namibia. *Global Journal of Health Science*, *11*(2), 102–109. doi:10.5539/gjhs.v11n2p102

Jombo, G. T., Mbaawuagu, E. M., Denen, A., Alao, O. O., Peters, E. J., Utsulo, S. J., & Etukumana, E. A. (2010). Sociocultural factors influencing the control of malaria in an endemic city in north central, Nigeria. *International Journal of Biological and Medical Research*, *1*(4), 277–282.

Kampala, L. T. (2019). Explaining the World daily: What is sub-Saharan Africa? The Economist explains. Retrieved from http://www.economist.com

Khumbulani, W. H., Musawenkosi, L. H., Mabaso, S. K., Dayanandan, G., & Rajendra, M. (2009). Community knowledge, attitudes and practices (KAP) on malaria in Swaziland, a country earmarked for malaria elimination. *Malaria Journal*, *8*(1), 29–36. doi:10.1186/1475-2875-8-29 PubMed

Malawi Malaria Indicator Survey. (2017). MMIS document: Ministry of health. National Malaria Control Program. Retrieved from https://dhsprogram.com/pubs/pdf/mis28/pdf

Mazigo, H. D., Obasy, E., Mauka, W., Manyiri, P., Zinga, M., Kweka, E. J., & Henkelbach, J. (2010). Knowledge, attitude and practices about malaria and its control in rural North West Tanzania. *Malaria Research and Treatment*, *10*, 1–9. doi:10.4061/2010/794261 PubMed

Musoke, D., Karani, G., Ssempebwa, J. C., Etajak, S., Guwatudde, D., & Musoke, B. M. (2015). Knowledge and practices on malaria prevention in two rural communities in Wakiss District, Ugandan. *African Health Sciences*, *15*(2), 401–412. doi:10.4314/ahs.v15i2.13 PubMed

Nigeria Federal Ministry of Health, Nigeria (2014). FMoHN and NMEP document: National Malaria Elimination Programme (NMEP, Nigeria) and the National Malaria Strategic Plan, 2014-2020.

Nigerian Centre for Diseases. (2016). NCDC document on Malaria: Protecting the health of Nigerians.

Nyavor, K., Kweku, M., Agbemafle, I., Takramah, W., Norman, I., Tarkang, E., & Binka, F. (2017). Assessing the ownership, usage and knowledge of Insecticide Treated Nets (ITNs) in Malaria Prevention in the Hohoe-Municipality, Ghana. *The Pan African Medical Journal*, *28*, 67. doi:10.11604/pamj.2017.28.67.9934

Okafor, F. U., & Oko-Ose, J. N. (2012). Prevalence of malaria infections among children aged 6 months -11 years in a tertiary institution in Benin City, Nigeria. *Global Advanced Research Journal of Medicine and Medical Sciences*, *1*(10), 273–279.

Okafor, I. P., Ezekwe, C., Oluwole, E. O., & Onogbogi, O. O. (2019). A community based study on the knowledge, perception and prevention among Nigerian women. *Journal of Family Medicine and Primary Health Care*, *8*(40), 1359–1364.

Okwa, O. O. (2019). Nipping the malaria vectors in the bud: Focus on Nigeria: In Malaria. In-Tech Publishers. doi:10.5772.83554

Okwa, O. O., Akinmolayan, F. I., Carter, V., & Hurd, H. (2009). Transmission dynamics of malaria in four selected ecological zones of Nigeria in the rainy season. *Annals of African Medicine*, *8*(1), 1–9. Retrieved from http://www.ajol.info

Okwa, O. O., Bello, B. A., & Olundegun, S. A. (2011). Social Aspects of Malaria among Students in Two Tertiary Institutions in Lagos, Nigeria. Sierra Leone Journal Biomedical Research, 3(2), 97- 103. Retrieved from **Error! Hyperlink reference not valid.**www.sljbr.com

Okwa, O. O., & Ibidapo, C. A. (2010). Malaria situation, perception of cause and treatment in a Nigerian University. *Journal of Medicine and Medical Sciences*, *1*(6), 213–222.

Okwa, O. O., Sanyaolu, L. O., & Olatokunbo, A. F. (2012a). Malaria and working performance of academic staff in a Nigerian University. *Research Journal of Biology*, *2*(5), 151–156.

Okwa, O. O., & Savage, A. (2018). Oviposition and breeding water sites preferences of mosquitoes within Ojo Area, Lagos State, Nigeria. *Biomedical Journal of Scientific and Technical Research*, *7*(5), 1–7. doi:10.26717/BJSTR.07.001565

Okwa, O. O., Soremekun, B. M., Adeseko, O., & Raheem, A. M. (2012b). Artisans and traders knowledge, attitude and practices of malaria in selected areas of Lagos, Nigeria. Global Advanced Research Journal of Medicine and Medical Sciences, 1(3), 68-74. Retrieved from http://garj.org/garjmms/index.htm

Oladimeji, K. E., Tsoka-Gwegweni, J. M., Ojewole, E., & Yunga, S. T. (2019). Knowledge of malaria prevention among pregnant and non-pregnant mothers of children aged under 5 years in Ibadan, South West Nigeria. *Malaria Journal*, *18*(92), 92. doi:10.1186/s12936-019-2706-1 PubMed

Onah, I. E., Adesina, F. P., Uweh, P. O., & Anumba, J. U. (2017). Challenges of malaria elimination in Nigeria (A Review). *International Journal of Infectious Diseases and Therapy*, *2*(4), 79–85. doi:10.11648/j.ijidt.20170204.14

Ordinioha, B. (2012). The use and misuse of mass distributed free insecticide treated nets in a semi urban community in Rivers State, Nigeria. *Annals of African Medicine*, *11*(3), 163–168. doi:10.4103/1596-3519.96879 PubMed

Owusu, D. A., Cremer, A. L., Brown, C. A., & Grosbusch, M. (2018). Knowledge, attitudes and practices regarding malaria in people living with HIV in rural and urban Ghana. *Acta Tropica*, *181*, 16–20. doi:10.1016/j.actatropica.2018.01.016 PubMed

Oyedeji, O. A., Elemile, P. O., Adepoju, A. A., & Oyedeji, G. A. (2009). An evaluation of the use of ITNs among children presenting with malaria at a Nigerian health facility. *International Journal of Medical and Medical Sciences*, *1*(11), 501–504.

PMI. (2019). MOP document: CDC, USAID & United State Presidents Malaria initiative FY 2018 and FY 2019. Retrieved from https://www.pmi.gov/docs/default-source/default-document-library/malaria-operational-plan

Salomon, J. A. (2014) Disability-Adjusted Life Years (DALY). In Encyclopedia of Health Economics Science Direct (pp. 200-203). Academic Press. doi:10.1016/B978-0-12-375678-7.00511-3

Singh, R., Musa, J., Singh, S., & Ukatu, V. E. (2014). Knowledge, attitudes and practices of malaria in Aleiro, Kebbi State, Northern Nigeria. *Journal of Family Medicine and Primary Care*, *3*(1), 39–44. doi:10.4103/2249-4863.130271 PubMed

Sumari, D., Dillip, A., Ndume, V., Mugasa, J. P., & Gwakisa, P. S. (2016). Knowledge, attitudes and practices on malaria in relation to its transmission among primary school children in Bagamoyo district, Tanzania. *MalariaWorld Journal*, *7*(2), 1–7.

Tambo, E. (2019). World Malaria Day, April 25th 2019: Zero malaria starts with me. Bio Med Central. Retrieved from http://blogs.biomedcentral.com/onhealth/2019/04/25/zero-malaria-starts-with-me-practice

Umwangange, M. L., Chironda, G., & Mukeshimana, M. (2018). Knowledge, Attitude and Practice towards malaria prevention among school children aged 5 -14 years in sub-Saharan Africa - A review of literature. *Rwanda Journal of Medicine and Health Sciences*, *1*(1), 22–30. doi:10.4314/rjmhs.v1i1.4

UNICEF. (2018). Malaria: Malaria mortality as a cause of death in children under five. Child Health. *Database*.

World Health Organization. (2016). World Malaria Report 2016. Retrieved from https://www.who.int/malaria/publications/world-malaria-report-2016/report/en/

World Health Organization. (2017). World Malaria Report 2017. Retrieved from https://www.who.int/malaria/publications/world-malaria-report-2017/en/

World Health Organization. (2018) World Malaria Report 2018. Retrieved from https://www.who.int/malaria/publications/world-malaria-report-2018/en/

World Health Organization. (2019). Bulletin on the African Health Report. *The Health of the People*, *§§§*, 97.

Yalewayler, T., Ashmelash, D., Anibachew, S., Eschetie, S., Addisu, A., & Zelek, A. J. (2019). The Prevalence of Malaria among pregnant women in Ethiopia: A systematic review and data analysis. *Journal of Parasitology Research*. doi:10.1155/2019/8390091

ADDITIONAL READING

Agomo, C. O., & Oyibo, W. A. (2013) Factors associated with risk of malaria infection among pregnant women in Lagos, Nigeria. *Infectious Diseases of Poverty*, *2*(19). doi:10.1186/2049-9957-2-19

Chukwuocha, U. M. (2012). Malaria Control in Nigeria. *Primary Health Care: Open Access*, *2*, 118. doi:10.4172/2167-1079.1000118

Malaria Operational Plan. (2019). MOP document: CDC, USAID & United State Presidents Malaria initiative Nigeria-FY-2019. Retrieved from https://www.pmi.gov/docs/default-source/default-document-library/malaria-operational-plan

Manana, P. N., Kuonza, L., Musekiwa, A., Mpangane, H. D., & Koekemoer, L. L. (2018). Knowledge, attitudes and practices on malaria transmission in Mamfene, KwaZulu-Natal Province, South Africa 2015. *BMC Public Health*, *18*(1), 41. doi:10.118612889-017-4583-2 PMID:28728572

Munisi, D. Z., Nyundo, A. A., & Mpondo, B. C. (2019). Knowledge, attitude and practice towards malaria among symptomatic patients attending Tumbi Referral Hospital: A cross-sectional study. *PLoS One*, *14*(8), e0220501. doi:10.1371/journal.pone.0220501 PMID:31381600

Okoli, C. A., & Enna, M. (2014). A cross-sectional study on knowledge of, attitudes towards and practice of malaria prevention and control measures in central Nigeria. *The Southern African Journal of Epidemiology & Infection*, *29*(1), 37–42. doi:10.1080/23120053.2014.11441565

Saha, A., Sarker, M., Kabir, M., Lu, G., & Müller, O. (2019). Knowledge, attitudes, and practices regarding malaria control among the slash and burn cultivators in Rangamati Hill tracts of Bangladesh. *Malaria Journal*, *18*(1), 216. doi:10.118612936-019-2849-0 PMID:31238990

Severe Malaria Observatory. (2019). Severe malaria facts in Democratic Republic of Congo: Knowledge sharing for severe malaria. Retrieved from https://www.severemalaria.org/countries/democratic-republic-of-congo

Sheet, M. F. (2019). *United States embassy in Nigeria*. US Embassy. Retrieved from http://nigeria.usembassy.gov

KEY TERMS AND DEFINITIONS

Burden: The load or weight of a disease in a particular place at a given time.

Disability Adjusted Life Years (DALYS): This is a measure of overall disease burden, expressed as the number of years lost due to ill-health, disability or early death.

Endemicity: The common and widespread presence of a disease in a particular place or region.

Etiology: The cause or origin of a disease or illness.

Holoendemic: The intense transmission of a disease throughout the seasons or all year round.

Incidence: The number of times or rates at which something happens at a given time.

Morbidity: A diseased state or a state of ill health.

Mortality: The number of deaths occurring in a place and time.

Prevalence: The percentage of a population that is infected with a particular disease at a given time.

Risk: A possibility of being infected with a disease.

Section 3

HIV/AIDS

Chapter 4
Importance of HIV Care Continuum

Simon George Taukeni
University of Namibia, Rundu Campus, Namibia

Eveline Ndinelao Kalomo
Wichita State University, USA

ABSTRACT

This chapter seeks to create further awareness and public health education on the importance of the human immunodeficiency virus (HIV) care continuum as one of the key policy focal areas to significantly reduce the HIV epidemic. Specific efforts were directed into the need to implement comprehensive HIV care continuum. The chapter argues that rolling out HIV counseling and testing, enrolled and linked patients to care, prescribing antiretroviral therapy, viral load testing and monitoring are key to achieve viral load suppression. Recommendations and future research direction have put much emphasis on an effort to address psychosocial factors such as stigma, inadequate healthcare facilities, laboratory testing equipment, social and cultural barriers to testing and treatment, to improve access and overall implementation of HIV care continuum.

INTRODUCTION

Interventions to end Immunodeficiency Syndrome (AIDS) cannot be more effective if they do not include the implementation and assess of human immunodeficiency virus (HIV) care continuum programs among populations of people with HIV (Jose et al., 2018). This chapter places great emphasis on the most effective and efficient

DOI: 10.4018/978-1-7998-2139-7.ch004

implementation of HIV care continuum in order to end AIDS. The chapter elaborates in more detail the importance of what HIV entails and illustrated step by step the HIV care continuum with the overall goal to help achieve viral load suppression among people living with HIV. In general, the importance of HIV care continuum is an important measuring instrument to determine the success or failure of national HIV programs and strategies.

BACKGROUND

Human immunodeficiency virus (HIV) is the virus that causes Acquired Immunodeficiency Syndrome (AIDS). AIDS is a serious, life-threatening illness that has a variety of symptoms (Stevens, Lynm, & Golub, 2012). Additionally, Stevens et al. (2012) assert that HIV infection can be treated with medication to make people living with HIV feel better and to prolong their lives. However, there is no cure for HIV infections or AIDS. Globally, 37.9 million people are living with HIV worldwide (WHO, 2018). The past three decades, human immunodeficiency virus (HIV) has united the international community in an unprecedented fashion. For example, in sub-Saharan Africa, the region with the highest incidence of HIV in the world (UNICEF, 2017).

Global epidemiology reports show that 90% (i.e., approximately 3 million) children and adolescents in sub-Saharan Africa live with HIV (UNICEF, 2017). In 2016, an estimated 80 000 new infections among children and adolescents were reported in Eastern and Southern Africa. In addition, adolescent girls (aged 15-19 accounted for approximately two-thirds of new HIV infections among young people (UNAIDS, 2015). With the advent of pediatric antiretroviral therapy (ART) and viral load suppression (Davies & Pinto, 2015; Ojikutu et al., 2014) efforts grassroots groups have mobilized policy makers, researchers, civil society and donor agencies from both developed and developing nations to respond to the epidemic (Webb, Cluver & Luo, 2018). The literature is replete with studies that have shown the significant progress that has been made with ART (Kline, 2006; Meyers et al., 2007; Ojikutu et al., 2014). For example, a systematic review of pediatric ART adherence research studies from middle and low-income countries, found that estimates of ART among this vulnerable population ranged from 49% to 76% of the studies reporting greater than 75% adherence (Vreeman et al., 2008).

Elimination of HIV epidemic by 2030 continues to be a global priority (WHO, 2014). The Joint United Nations Program on HIV/AIDS (UNAIDS) launched 90-90-90 targets to end AIDS by 2030. This simply means that 90% of people with HIV will be diagnosed, 90% of those diagnosed will be on antiretroviral therapy (ART), and 90% of those on ART will achieve viral suppression (Davies & Pinto,

2015). Even though achieving 90-90-90 targets should be done comprehensively and inclusively of each target, authors are stressing the easy access of HIV viral load testing and monitoring in order to achieve viral load suppression. According to WHO guidelines revised in 2010, they recommended the use of HIV viral load to detect or confirm treatment failure and to inform decisions about switching to second-line regime (WHO, 2010).

Major breakthroughs in the prevention of HIV have been noted in recent research. Of those breakthroughs, include the introduction of antiretroviral for the prevention of Mother-to- Child transmission (Kak et al., 2011) as a key intervention to reduce AIDS related deaths and new HIV transmission. PMTCT covers: antenatal HIV counseling and testing, avoiding unintended pregnancy, provision of appropriate antiretroviral regime for mothers and newborns and support for safer infant feeding options and practices (Kak et al., 2011).Voluntary Male Medical Circumcision (VMMC) has been yet another intervention yielding positive results in the prevention and infection of HIV (Auvert, et al., 2005).With the support of donor funding in low-income and middle-income countries in the past years nearly eight million people were recorded receiving ART in 2011 (UNAIDS, 2012). Despite the efforts of on-going interventions to support people living with HIV to be on ART, there have been some noticeable challenges. Stigma and discrimination have been persistent challenges in HIV prevention and new infection (Kalichman & Simbayi, 2003; Kalomo, 2017).

There has been no doubt that the last decade has witnessed an unprecedented growth in coverage of HIV care and treatment programs globally (Achwoka, Waruru, Chen et al., 2019). Even though recent research posited specific interventions and prevention programs to eliminate the spread of HIV epidemic, a gap in terms of a framework was identified. Therefore, Gardener and colleagues developed HIV care continuum framework to fill that existing gap. The importance of HIV care continuum has been given considerable recognition globally. The framework represents HIV care as a progression from testing to engagement in treatment care, antiretroviral therapy (ART) and ultimately, suppression of the virus (Gardner, McLees, Steiner et al., 2011). Centers for Disease Control and Prevention (2017) argue that research findings estimate that in the United States, 85% of people living with HIV are diagnosed, 62% are linked to care, and only 49% achieve HIV viral suppression. It is imperative to acknowledge the importance of HIV care continuum as a tool to monitor the progress attained in addressing HIV in terms of diagnosis, enrollment and linkage to care, retention, treatment with ART and achievement of HIV viral suppression (Korthuis & Edelman, 2018).

Importantly, this chapter has a unique relevance to the theme of the book since the implementation of HIV care continuum has direct significant effects on communicable and non-communicable diseases (NCDs). In their study in Kenya, Achwoka et al. (2019) conclude that people living with HIV (PLHIV) have a high prevalence of

NCD diagnoses. In the absence of systematic, effective screening, NCD burden is likely underestimated in this population. Systematic screening and treatment for NCDs using standard guidelines should be integrated into HIV care and treatment programs in sub-Saharan Africa. World Health Organization (WHO, 2018) estimated about 41 million NCD-related deaths annually, where low and middle-income countries being the most affected. The four major NCDs that contribute largely to both morbidity and mortality are: cardiovascular diseases, cancers, diabetes and chronic lung diseases (WHO, 2013). In 2016, over three quarters of NCD deaths, 31.5 million occurred in low and middle-income countries with about 46% of deaths occurring before the age of 70 in these countries (WHO, 2018). Many researchers highlighted the importance of the integration of HIV and primary care systems to facilitate routine monitoring for non-communicable diseases in HIV-infected patients (George, McGrath & Oni, 2019). For instance, Mendenhall and Norris (2015) affirm that low-income communities in South Africa had experienced a higher prevalence of NCDs and the highest burden of HIV resulting in concurrent epidemics. It was established that people living with HIV (PLWHIV) are at a significantly higher risk for cardiovascular diseases than HIV-negative persons. Sadly, older people living with HIV over 49 years of age have 60% higher risk of cardiovascular diseases than HIV-negative adults of the same age (Mascolini, 2010).

Yang, Su, Zhao et al. (2016) had studied the prevalence and mortality of cancer among HIV-infected inpatients in Beiging, China. In their study, they concluded that the prevalence of cancer concurrence among hospitalized HIV-infected patients was 7.7%. Concurrent cancer also increased mortality among HIV-infected patients. Their results showed the importance of promoting cancer screening and early ART initiation among HIV-infected patients (Yang et al., 2016). Also, research shows that HIV increases a woman's risk of cervical cancer (Newcomb-Fernandez, 2003).

Research confirmed that people living with HIV/AIDS are at higher risk of developing concurrent cancer as a result of weakened immune system (Biggar, Chaturvedi, Goedert et al., 2007; Pinzone, Fiorica, Di Rosa et al., 2012). Other risk factors for developing cancer among HIV-infected people may include co-infection with other viruses, alcohol consumption, cigarette smoking and old age. Alcohol consumption for example, Cook et al. cited in Korthuis and Edelman (2018) assert that people with HIV who report heavy drinking experienced increased odds of failing to achieve sustained HIV viral suppression.

According to Es and Boyle (2002), there have been many complex psychosocial factors to the disproportionate impact of HIV in resource-poor settings namely: stigma, poverty, cultural and social barriers to testing and treatment, insufficient healthcare infrastructure to support the large patient pool and lack of health literacy. Inadequate medical equipment, scarcity of manpower to distribute healthcare throughout the region and inadequate laboratory facilities (Es & Boyle, 2002) were also noted.

Previous research studies emphasize that a person's lifestyle on HIV does not necessarily start after diagnosis with the virus but the combined effects of psychosocial and biological risk factors occurring in early life should be considered (Hertzman, Power, Matthew & Manor, 2001). For example, research shows that people living with HIV, depression can lead to accelerated disease progression, increased mortality and poor adherence to ART (Starace, Ammassari, Trotta et al., 2002). However, there is a significant recognition of important interactions between different diseases and useful synergies and benefits that can be gained from exploiting overlapping treatments and strategies (Harries, Kumar, Satyanarayan et al., 2015). For example, a strong association between HIV and tuberculosis (TB). HIV exacerbates the risk of TB, including recurrent disease and increase morbidity and mortality in those with TB. Also, TB is one of the most significant opportunistic infections and the cause of death in many persons living with HIV (Harries et al., 2015). Meanwhile, the most effective treatment for preventing TB in people living with HIV is ART (Suthar, Lawn, del Amor et al., 2012) and ART is also the most effective treatment for reducing mortality in people living with HIV and TB as well as treatment of other opportunistic infections (Maartens, Celum, & Lewin, 2014).

In the next section, authors present the HIV care continuum which comprises what steps need to be followed in order to eliminate HIV and AIDS epidemic. Hogg (2018) assured that HIV care continuum is an important tool that can provide crucial insights into the HIV care within and across countries.

HIV Care Continuum

The HIV care continuum is a framework that models the five steps of HIV treatment care. The continuum consists of five main steps which, at the population level, are depicted cross-sectional as the HIV treatment cascade (Kay, Batey, & Mugavero, 2016). These steps include (1) Diagnosis, (2) linkage to care, (3) retention in care, (4) adherence to antiretroviral therapy and (5) viral suppression (Kay, Batey, & Mugavero, 2016). These steps are essential to effectively treat and prevent the spread of HIV (Korthuis & Edelman, 2018). As a model developed by Gardner, McLees, Steiner, del Rio and Burman, HIV care continuum has become internationally recognized and gained visibility in the United States of America in 2013 (Office of National AIDS Policy, 2013). Figure 1 illustrates HIV care continuum.

Figure 1. HIV care continuum

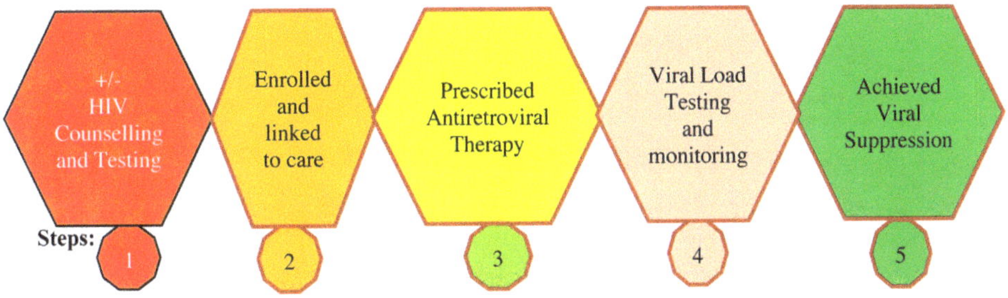

Step 1: HIV Counseling and Testing

The importance of HIV Counseling and Testing (HCT) cannot be overemphasized. It contributes to early screening and detection which results into one knowing his or her HIV status. An HCT is used to determine if one has been infected with the human immunodeficiency virus (HIV), commonly performed on a blood sample (Boskey, 2019). Simon, Ho and Abdool (2006) advise that early identification and treatment are crucial to reduce transmission of the virus, but many people remain unaware of their HIV status during the crucial early months of infection when transmission risk is high and secondary to elevated levels of viraemia. In most cases, infected people only go for HIV testing when they get sick.

Stevens et al. (2012) warn that individuals with HIV infection may not feel sick at first because HIV infection is often accompanied by a variety of symptoms which vary from person to person and how long the person has been infected. Symptoms tend to increase in severity depending on how long the virus has been in the body and if the individual remains undiagnosed. This simply implies that early HCT is very important. HCT involves three steps: pre-test counseling, the HIV test and post-test counseling. The process can take 30 to 45 minutes (Boskey, 2019). HIV tests are available at both private and public health facilities, including hospitals, clinics, mobile testing sites and drug and alcohol treatment centers (Boskey, 2019). There have been some factors noted that appeared to influence the testing behavior, more so among adolescents. Of those factors, Helleringer et al. (2009) identified a distance to an HIV testing facility, knowledge and understanding of HIV and treatment, previous testing experience, cost involved to go for the test, number of sexual partners and antenatal care visits. Figure 2 shows different HIV testing options.

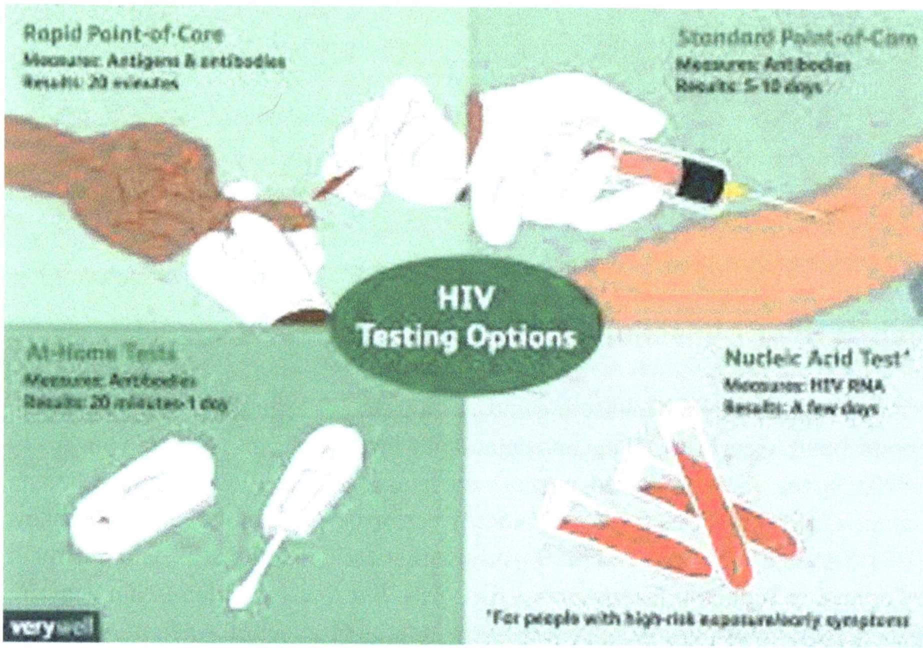

Figure 2. HIV counseling and testing options
Source: Verywell Health illustrated by Boskey (2019)

Step 2: Enrolled and Linked to Care

Kay, Batey and Mugavero (2016) assured that linkage to care is the second step in the HIV care continuum. This is usually a period of three months or less between documentation of diagnosis and initiation of medical treatment with an HIV care provider (Institute of Medicine, 2012). Enrollment and linking people diagnosed with HIV should be done promptly without any delay. Lee and Hazra (2015) support that services need to link HIV-testing and diagnosis with prevention and treatment services, address other adolescent health needs, especially sexual and reproductive health. In sub-Saharan Africa for example, the rollout of ART across general populations has dramatically increased the life expectancy of those initiated on ART (George, McGrath & Oni, 2019).

Step 3: Prescribed Antiretroviral Therapy

The second 90 target envisioned that 90% of people living with HIV should receive antiretroviral therapy (Staveteig, 2017). It has been more than thirty years of the HIV epidemic and still there is no cure; however, there have been major advances in treating

HIV (Lundgren et al. 2015). The availability and rapid scale up of antiretroviral therapy (ART) has transformed what was inevitably a fatal disease to a chronic, manageable condition leading to notable decline in the worldwide rates of AIDS related deaths and new infections (Kharsany & Karim, 2016). Global scale-up of ART has been the primary contributor to a 48% decline in deaths from AIDS-related causes from a peak of 1.9 million (1.7 million - 2.2 million) in 2005 to 1.0 million (830 000 -1.2 million) in 2016 (UNAIDS, 2017). HIV treatment, also called antiretroviral therapy (ART) works by controlling the replication of HIV in the body to reduce HIV's ability to make copies of itself. When replication is controlled, the viral load in the blood and bodily fluids decreases (Arkell & Harrigan, 2018). Since its inception in 1996, ART has led to dramatic reduction in morbidity and mortality (Marston et al., 2012). ART usually consists of a combination of at least three antiretroviral drugs taken daily. Newer HIV treatments are safer, simpler and more effective than when ART was first introduced (Arkell & Harrigan, 2018). When successful treatment lowers the viral load to undetectable levels, this can greatly reduce and eliminate the risk of HIV transmission (Arkell & Harrigan, 2018).

Step 4: Viral Load Testing and Monitoring

The third 90 target call for 90% of people living with HIV (PLHIV) on antiretroviral therapy to achieve viral suppression by the year 2020 (Staveteig, 2017). In this respect, lack of access to routine viral load monitoring in many settings is a major obstacle both to achieving 90% suppression (Davies & Pinto, 2015). Gilks et al. (2006) noted a widespread of ART which has been supported by the initiation and monitoring of ART based on clinical criteria. Viral load testing and monitoring play important role of identifying HIV-infected individuals at high risk for morbidity and mortality (Colebunders, Moses, Laurence et al., 2006). CD4+ T Cells and plasma HIV viral load are commonly used laboratory measurements to establish a patient's degree of immuno suppression and to monitor the virus progression (Weinberg & Kovarik, 2010). However, the cost of viral load monitoring, has been a prohibitive factor (Trinh et al., 2011). Researchers suggest that in order to improve the cost-effectiveness of laboratory monitoring, market barriers need to be overcome to bring about a large reduction in the cost of viral load testing and monitoring (Boyer, et al., 2013). Figure 3 shows the viral load testing and monitoring instruments.

Figure 3. Viral load testing and monitoring
Source: The Body Pro (2016)

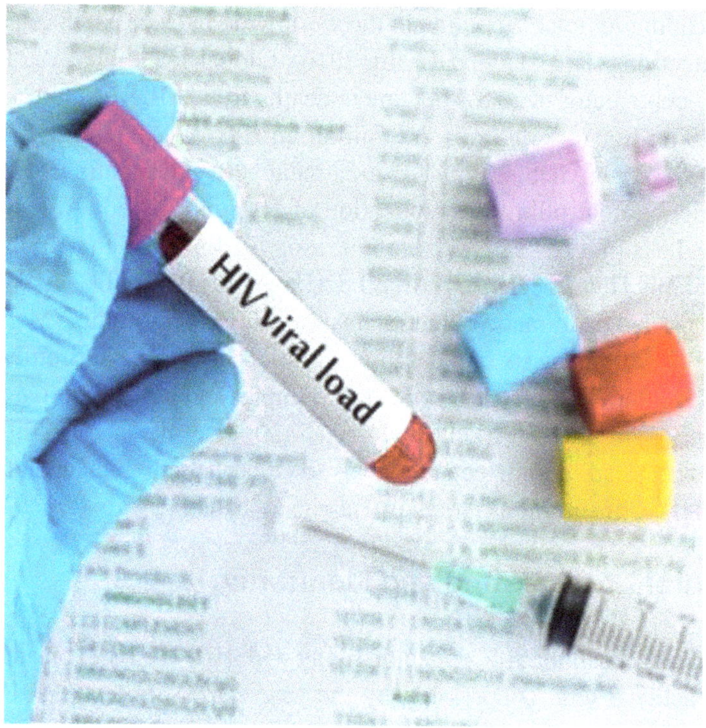

Step 5: Achieved Viral Load Suppression

The final step in the HIV care continuum is also the primary goal of HIV treatment and public health interventions-viral suppression through ART. Sustained viral suppression is the key to optimal health outcomes at both the individual and population levels, and treatment does serve as prevention (Kay, Batey, & Mugavero, 2016). Trinh et al. (2011) assert that virologic suppression is the measure of successful antiretroviral therapy. Many studies reported that achieving viral load suppression was not linked to HIV transmission. A study of nearly 58000 sexual engagement without using condoms among HIV-discordant couples, there were no reports of HIV transmissions (LeMessurier et al., 2018). It is therefore important that people living with HIV should take their ART as prescribed in order to achieve viral load suppression (Eisinger, Dieffenbach, & Fauci, 2019). Even though, lack of adherence with ART has been noted as a great barrier to achieving viral load suppression. Eisinger, Dieffenbach, and Fauci (2019) cited lack of adherence with ART due to many factors such as lack of accessibility of quality health care. Social-economic and psychological factors such as poverty, stigma and discrimination could also lead to lack of adherence. Figure 4 illustrates viral load suppression.

Figure 4. Viral suppression
Source: Kampala Dispatch (2017)

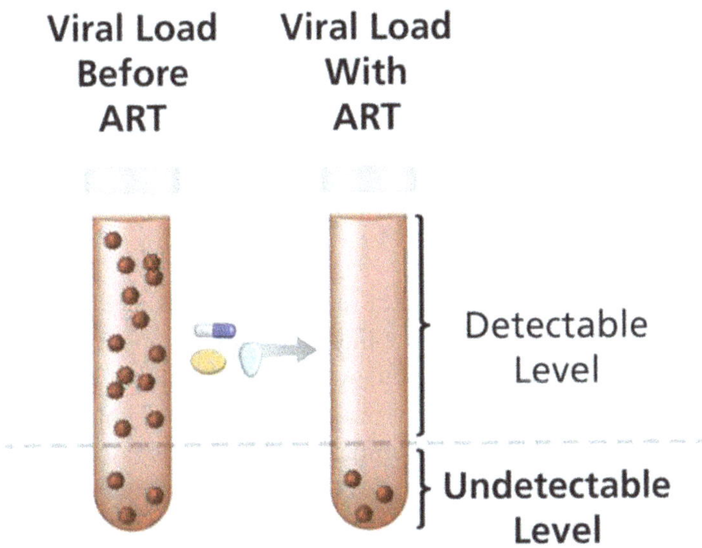

SOLUTIONS AND RECOMMENDATIONS

Boyer et al. (2013) findings suggest that effort should focus on overcoming market barriers and providing tests that are low cost and easy to use to improve the cost-effectiveness of laboratory monitoring in the near future. HIV intervention and prevention measures should focus on getting people to go for HIV counseling and testing, enroll and put those diagnosed with HIV on ART and monitor and evaluate those on ART their viral load in order to address bottlenecks on time. Even though the focus of this chapter is on the call to increase HIV viral load testing and monitoring, it is important to take into account that the authors are basically recommending the implementation of HIV care continuum. A call for concerted collaboration among policymakers, HIV providers and other key stakeholders is paramount for improving better health outcomes at each step of the HIV care continuum at the population level (Kay, Batey, & Mugavero, 2016).

FUTURE RESEARCH DIRECTIONS

Future research should look into psychosocial factors such as inadequate healthcare facilities, laboratory equipment social and cultural barriers to testing and treatment to improve access and implementation of HIV care continuum. Also, future research direction should look into the roll out of HIV viral load testing and monitoring in public health facilities and centers in terms of efficacy and costs. Every person on ART should have an easy access to know his or her viral load as a motivation to adhere to treatment, to determine if the treatment is working and or to change the regimen.

CONCLUSION

Ending AIDS requires consistent health services to increase HIV care continuum including HIV counseling and testing, linked to care, prescribed ART, viral load monitoring and viral load suppression. Achieving viral load suppression would only be possible with more viral load testing machines in public health facilities and setting up one stop HIV care facilities and equipment. Achieving viral load suppression by 2030 is possible but a well-defined and targeted monitoring and evaluation policy should be considered as one of the key intervention in achieving viral load suppression. What also came out clear in this chapter, was the fact that HIV interventions and prevention strategies have great potential to contribute to the overall better health outcome for other associated diseases such as TB, cancer, hypertension, cardiovascular disease, tuberculosis and other Non-Communicable Diseases (NCDs).

REFERENCES

Achwoka, D., Waruru, A., Chen, T.-H., Masamaro, K., Ngugi, E., Kimani, M., ... De Cock, K. M. (2019). Noncommunicable disease burden among HIV patients in care: A national retrospective longitudinal analysis of HIV-treatment outcomes in Kenya, 2003-2013. *BMC Public Health*, *19*(1), 372. doi:10.118612889-019-6716-2 PMID:30943975

Suthar, A. B., Lawn, S. D., Del Amo, J., Getahun, H., Dye, C., Sculier, D., ... & Granich, R. M. (2012). Antiretroviral therapy for prevention of HIV-associated tuberculosis in developing countries: A systematic review and meta-analysis. *PLoS Medicine*, *9*. doi:10.1371/journal.pmed.1001270

Arkell, C., & Harrigan, M. (2018). *HIV treatment and an undetectable viral load to prevent HIV transmission.* Retrieved from https://www.catie.ca/en/factsheets/transmission/hiv-viral-load-hiv-treatment-and-sexual-hiv-transmission

Auvert, B., Taljaard, D., Lagarde, E., Sobngwi-Tambekou, J., Sitta, R., & Puren, A. (2005). Randomized controlled intervention trial of male circumcision for reduction of HIV infection risk: The ANRS 1265 Trial. *PLoS Medicine, 2*(11), e298. doi:10.1371/journal.pmed.0020298 PMID:16231970

Biggar, R. J., Chaturvedi, A. K., Goedert, J. J., & Engels, E. A. (2007). AIDS-related cancer and severity of immunosuppression in persons with AIDS. *Journal of the National Cancer Institute, 99*(12), 962–972. doi:10.1093/jnci/djm010 PMID:17565153

Boskey, E. (2019). What is an HIV test?: What to expect when undergoing this test. Verywell Health. Retrieved from https://www.verywellhealth.com/everything-you-need-to-know-about-getting-an-hiv-test-3132731

Boyer, S., March, L., Kouanfack, C., Laborde-Balen, G., Marino, P., Aghokeng, A. F., ... Moatti, J.-P. (2013). Monitoring of HIV viral load, CD4 cell count, and clinical assessment versus clinical monitoring alone for antiretroviral therapy in low-resource settings (Stratall ANRS 12110/ESTHER): A cost-effectiveness analysis. *The Lancet. Infectious Diseases, 13*(7), 577–586. doi:10.1016/S1473-3099(13)70073-2 PMID:23602084

Centers for Disease Control and Prevention. (2017). Understanding the HIV care continuum. Retrieved from https://www.cdc.gov/hiv/pdf/library/factsheets/cdc-hiv-care-continuum.pdf

Davies, M. A., & Pinto, J. (2015). Targeting 90-90-90 – don't leave children and adolescents behind. *Journal of the International AIDS Society, 18*(7 Suppl. 6), 20745. doi:10.7448/IAS.18.7.20745 PMID:26639121

Eisinger, R.W., Dieffenbach, C.W., & Fauci, A.S. (2019). HIV viral load and transmissibility of HIV infection: Undetectable equals untrasmittable. *Journal of American Association*, E1-E2.

Es, M., & Boyle, B. (2002). Excess and access: The continuing controversy regarding HIV and health care in Africa. *The AIDS Reader, 12*(7), 288–292. PMID:12161849

Garner, E. M., McLees, M. P., Steiner, J. F., del Rio, C., & Burman, W. J. (2011). The spectrum of engagement in HIV care and its relevance to test and treat strategies for prevention of HIV infection. *Clinical Infectious Diseases, 52*(6), 793–800. doi:10.1093/cid/ciq243 PMID:21367734

George, S., McGrath, N., & Oni, T. (2019). The association between a detectable HIV viral load and non-communicable diseases comorbidity in HIV positive adults on antiretroviral therapy in Western Cape, South Africa. *BMC Infectious Diseases, 19*(1), 348. doi:10.118612879-019-3956-9 PMID:31029087

Gilks, C. F., Crowley, S., Ekpini, R., Gove, S., Perriens, J., Souteyrand, Y., ... De Cock, K. (2006). The WHO public-health approach to antiretroviral treatment against HIV in resource-limited settings. *Lancet, 368*(9534), 505–510. doi:10.1016/S0140-6736(06)69158-7 PMID:16890837

Helleringer, S., Kohler, H. P., Frimpong, J. A., & Mkandawire, J. (2009). Increasing uptake of HIV testing and counseling among the poorest in sub-Saharan countries through home-based service provision. *Journal of Acquired Immune Deficiency Syndromes, 51*(2), 185–193. doi:10.1097/QAI.0b013e31819c1726 PMID:19352202

Hertzman, C., Power, C., Matthew, S., & Manor, O. (2001). Using an interactive framework of society and lifecourse to explain self-rated health in early adulthood. *Social Science & Medicine, 53*(12), 1575–1585. doi:10.1016/S0277-9536(00)00437-8 PMID:11762884

Hogg, R. (2018). Understanding the HIV care continuum. *The Lancet. HIV, 3018*(18), 30102–30104. PMID:29893238

Institute of Medicine. (2012). *Monitoring HIV care in the United States: Indicators and data systems*. Washington, DC: National Academies Press.

Jose, S., Delpech, V., Howarth, A., Burns, F., Hill, T., Porter, K., ... Walsh, J.UK CHIC Study Steering Committee. (2018). A continuum of HIV care describing mortality and loss to follow-up: A longitudinal cohort study. *The Lancet. HIV, 5*(6), e301–e308. doi:10.1016/S2352-3018(18)30048-1 PMID:29893243

Kak, L., Chitsike, I., Luo, C., & Rollins, N. (2011). *Prevention of Mother-To-Child Transmission of HIV/AIDS programs, opportunities for Africa's newborns: Practical data, policy and programmatic support for newborn care in Africa.* Retrieved from www.who.int/pmnch/media/publications/oanfullreport.pdf

Kalichman, S. C., & Simbayi, L. C. (2003). HIV testing attitudes, AIDS stigma and voluntary HIV counseling and testing in a black township in Cape Town, South Africa. *Sexually Transmitted Infections, 79*(6), 442–447. doi:10.1136ti.79.6.442 PMID:14663117

Kalomo, E. N. (2017). Associations between HIV-related stigma, self-esteem, social support, and depressive symptoms in Namibia. *Aging & Mental Health*. PMID:29019412

Kampala Dispatch. (2017). *Low HIV load suppression worries Kabarole medics.* Available online:http://dispatch.ug/2017/11/21/low-hiv-viral-load-suppression-worries-kabarole-medics/

Kay, E. S., Batey, D. S., & Mugavero, M. J. (2016). The HIV treatment cascade and care continuum: Updates, goals, and recommendations for the future. *AIDS Research and Therapy, 13*(1), 35. doi:10.118612981-016-0120-0 PMID:27826353

Keulder, C. (2011). *Positive vibes. HIV/AIDS and stigma in Namibia: Results of a qualitative study among support group members.* Retrieved from https://www.positivevibes.org/02_Stigma%20report.pdf

Kharsany, A. B. M., & Karim, Q. A. (2016). HIV infection and AIDS in sub-Saharan Africa: Current status, challenges and opportunities. *The Open AIDS Journal, 10*(1), 34–48. doi:10.2174/1874613601610010034 PMID:27347270

Kline, M. W. (2006). Perspective on the pediatric HIV/AIDS pandemic: Catalyzing access of children to care and treatment. *Pediatrics, 117*(4), 1388–1393. doi:10.1542/peds.2005-1348 PMID:16585337

Korthuis, P. T., & Edelman, E. J. (2018). Substance use and the HIV care continuum: Important advances. *Addiction Science & Clinical Practice, 13*(1), 13. doi:10.118613722-018-0114-4 PMID:29530080

Lundgren, J. D., Babiker, A. G., Gordin, F., Emery, S., & Grund, B. (2015). INSIGHT Start Study Group. Initiation of antiretroviral therapy in early asymptomatic HIV infection. *The New England Journal of Medicine, 373*(9), 795–807. doi:10.1056/NEJMoa1506816 PMID:26192873

Maartens, G., Celum, C., & Lewin, S. R. (2014). HIV infection: Epidemiology, pathogenesis, treatment and prevention. *Lancet, 384*(9939), 258–271. doi:10.1016/S0140-6736(14)60164-1 PMID:24907868

Marston, M., Michael, D., Wringe, A., Isingo, R., Clark, B. D., Jonas, A., ... Urassa, M. (2012). The impact of antiretroviral therapy on adult mortality in rural Tanzania. *Tropical Medicine & International Health, 17*(8), 58–65. doi:10.1111/j.1365-3156.2011.02924.x PMID:22943380

Mascolini, M. (2010). HIV raises heart disease risk 60% in people over 49. In *Proceedings of the XVIII International AIDS Conference*. Academic Press.

Médecins Sans Frontières. (2012). *Undetectable-how viral load monitoring can improve HIV treatment in developing countries*. Geneva: Médecins Sans Frontières.

Mendenhall, E., & Norris, S. A. (2015). When HIV is ordinary and diabetes new: Remaking suffering in a South African township. *Global Public Health: An International Journal for Research, Policy and Practice*, *10*(4), 449–462. doi:10.1080/17441692.2014.998698 PMID:25643001

Meyers, T., Moulrie, H., Naidoo, K., Cotton, M., Eley, B., & ... (2007). Challenges to pediatric HIV care and treatment in South Africa. *The Journal of Infectious Diseases*, *196*(3), 474–481. doi:10.1086/521116 PMID:18181697

Newcomb-Fernandez, J. (2003). Cancer in the HIV-infected population. *Research Initiative, Treatment Action*, *9*(1), 5–13. PMID:14971360

Ojikutu, B., Higgins-Biddle, M., Greeson, D., Phelps, B. R., Amzel, A., Okechukwu, E., ... Hirschhorn, L. R. (2014). The association between quality of HIV care, loss to follow-up and mortality in pediatric and adolescent patients receiving antiretroviral therapy in Nigeria. *PLoS One*, *9*(7), e100039. doi:10.1371/journal.pone.0100039 PMID:25075742

openPr. (2018). Antiviral drugs market: New investments expected to boost the demand with rising awareness regarding vast benefits to drive market. Retrieved from https://www.openpr.com/news/990905/Antiviral-Drugs-Market-New-Investments-Expected-to-boost-the-Demand-with-Rising-Awareness-Regarding-Vast-Benefits-to-Drive-Market.html

Pinzone, M. R., Fiorica, F., Di Rosa, M., Malaguarnera, G., Malaguarnera, L., Cacopardo, B., & ... . (2012). Non-AIDS-defining cancers among HIV-infected people. *European Review for Medical and Pharmacological Sciences*, *16*(10), 1377–1388. PMID:23104654

LeMessurier, J., Traversy, G., Varsaneux, O., Weekes, M., Avey, M. T., Niragira, O., ... & Rodin, R. (2018). Risk of sexual transmission of human immunodeficiency viral load and condom use: A systematic review. *Canadian Medical Association Journal*, *190*(46), E1350–E1360. doi:10.1503/cmaj.180311 PMID:30455270

Simon, V., Ho, D. D., & Abdool, K. Q. (2006). HIV/AIDS epidemiology, pathogenesis, prevention and treatment. *Lancet*, *368*(9534), 489–504. doi:10.1016/S0140-6736(06)69157-5 PMID:16890836

Starace, F., Ammassari, A., Trotta, M. P., Murri, R., De Longis, P., Izzo, C., ... Antinori, A. (2002). Depression is a risk factor for suboptimal adherence to highly active antiretroviral therapy. *JAIDS Journal of Acquired Immune Deficiency Syndromes*, *31*(3), 136–139. doi:10.1097/00126334-200212153-00010 PMID:12562037

Staveteig, S., Croft, T. N., Kampa, K. T., & Head, S. K. (2017). Reaching the 'first 90': Gaps in coverage of HIV testing among people living with HIV in 16 African countries. *PLoS One*, *12*(10), e0186316. doi:10.1371/journal.pone.0186316 PMID:29023510

Stevens, L. M., Lynm, C., & Golub, R. M. (2012). HIV infection: The basics. *Journal of the American Medical Association*, *308*(4), 419. doi:10.1001/jama.2012.4079 PMID:22820800

The Body Pro. (2016). Virological response without routine viral load monitoring in children: Results from the ARROW Trial. Retrieved from https://www.thebodypro.com/content/78528/virological-response-without-routine-viral-load-mo.html

Trinh, T. T., Montague, B. T., Flanigan, T. P., & Gerard, H. M. (2011). HIV suppression among patients on treatment in Vietnam: A review of HIV viral load testing in a public urban clinic in Ho Chi Minh City. *AIDS Research and Treatment*. doi:10.1155/2011/230953 PMID:21490776

UNAIDS. (2012). *Global report: UNAIDS report on the global AIDS epidemic*. Geneva: UNAIDS.

UNAIDS. (2015). *How AIDS changed everything*. Retrieved from https://www.unaids.org/sites/default/files/media_asset/MDG6Report_en.pdf

UNAIDS. (2017). State of the AIDS epidemic: UNAIDS data 2017. Retrieved from www.unaids.org/sites/default/files/media_asset/20170720_Data_book_2017_en.pdf

UNICEF. (2011). *Children and HIV & AIDS in Namibia*. Windhoek: UNICEF.

Vreeman, R. C., Wiehe, S. E., Pearce, E. C., & Winstone, N. M. (2008). A systematic review of pediatric adherence to antiretroviral therapy in low and middle-income countries. *The Pediatric Infectious Disease Journal*, *27*(8), 686–691. doi:10.1097/INF.0b013e31816dd325 PMID:18574439

Webb, D., Cluver, L., & Luo, C. (2018). Evolution or extinction? Pediatric and adolescent HIV responses in the Agenda 2030 era. *Journal of the International AIDS Society*, *21*(S1), 1–3. doi:10.1002/jia2.25071 PMID:29485744

Weinberg, J. L., & Kovarik, C. L. (2010). The WHO clinical staging system for HIV/AIDS. *The Virtual Mentor*, *12*(3), 202–206. PMID:23140869

WHO. (2010). *Antiretroviral therapy for HIV infection in adults and adolescents: recommendations for a public health approach (2010 revision)*. Geneva: WHO.

WHO. (2013). Global Action Plan for the prevention and control of noncommunicable diseases 2013-2020. Retrieved from https://www.who.int/nmh/events/ncd_action_plan/en/

WHO. (2018). Global health observatory data. NCD mortality and morbidity. Retrieved from https://www.who.int/gho/ncd/mortality_morbidity/en/

Yang, J., Su, S., Zhao, H., Wang, D., Wang, J., Zhang, F., & Zhao, Y. (2016). Prevalence and mortality of cancer among HIV-infected inpatients in Beijing, China. *BMC Infectious Diseases*, *16*(1), 82. doi:10.118612879-016-1416-3 PMID:26883427

ADDITIONAL READING

Bruton, J., Rai, T., Day, S., & Ward, H. (2014). Patient perspective on the HIV continuum of care in London: A qualitative study of people diagnosed between 1986 and 2014. *BMJ Open*, *8*(3), e020208. doi:10.1136/bmjopen-2017-020208 PMID:29602851

Chkhartishvili, N., Sharavdze, L., Chokoshvili, O., DeHovitz, J. A., del Rio, C., & Tsertsvadze, T. (2015). The cascade of care in the Eastern European country of Georgia. *HIV Medicine*, *16*(1), 62–66. doi:10.1111/hiv.12172 PMID:24919923

Juma, K., Reid, M., Roy, M., Vorkoper, S., Temu, T. M., Levitt, N. S., ... Yonga, G. (2018). From HIV prevention to non-communicable disease health promotion efforts in sub-Saharan Africa: A narrative Review. *AIDS (London, England)*, *32*, S63–S73. doi:10.1097/QAD.0000000000001879 PMID:29952792

Marston, M., Michael, D., Wringe, A., Isingo, R., Clark, B. D., Jonas, A., ... Urassa, M. (2012). The impact of antiretroviral therapy on adult mortality in rural Tanzania. *Tropical Medicine & International Health*, *17*(8), 58–65. doi:10.1111/j.1365-3156.2011.02924.x PMID:22943380

Penazzato, M., Bendaud, V., Nelson, L., Stover, J., & Mahy, M. (2014). Estimating future trends in pediatric HIV. *AIDS (London, England)*, *28*(4), 445–451. doi:10.1097/QAD.0000000000000481

Taukeni, S. (2019). *A study of adolescents diagnosed with HIV in 2013 in the Oshakati Health District* [Dissertation of Master of Public Health]. University of Fort Hare, East London.

Wakeman, S. E. (2017). Medications for addiction treatment: Changing language to improve care. *Journal of Addiction Medicine*, *11*(1), 1–2. doi:10.1097/ADM.0000000000000275 PMID:27898497

KEY TERMS AND DEFINITIONS

Antiretroviral Therapy: ART stands for a combination of drugs that suppress the human immunodeficiency virus (HIV) in order to reduce mortality and morbidity rates among HIV-infected people and to improve their quality of life.

HIV Care Continuum: A framework that guides the sequential steps of treatment care that people with HIV should go through from diagnosis and achieving sustained viral load suppression.

HIV Counseling and Testing: A public health intervention whereby individuals, family members, couples and community members receive HIV counseling and testing for prevention, treatment and support purposes. It is very important for each member of society to know his or her HIV status in order to prevent HIV transmission, to receive treatment on time, to receive care and support.

Poor HIV Adherence: When HIV patients are missing their appointments and skipping their medicines which increases the chances of HIV to multiply and destroy their immune system. Poor adherence also contributes to high risk of drug resistance and treatment failure.

Viraemia: The presence of viruses in the blood.

Viral Load: This is the level of HIV in one's blood. The main function of ART is to lower the viral load to levels below <40-75 copies/ml. Lower viral load means lower amounts of HIV function in the body.

Viral Load Tests: These tests are used to diagnose HIV infection in a blood sample and guide treatment choices.

Viral Suppression: This is when antiretroviral therapy (ART) lowers an infected person's viral load to an undetectable level, which means that the amount of HIV in one's blood is very low. HIV-infected people with viral suppression are healthy and they can live longer.

Chapter 5
Elderly Grandparents as Caregivers of Children Affected or Infected by HIV and AIDS in Namibia

Eveline N. Kalomo
Wichita State University, USA

Simon George Taukeni
University of Namibia, Rundu Campus, Namibia

ABSTRACT

Kinship care is one of the most prevalent forms of placement that is used for children affected and/or infected by HIV and AIDS in Namibia. However, the literature lacks a systematic theory-informed understanding with respect to what is currently known about caregivers generally and specifically, elderly caregivers of orphans, and vulnerable children (OVC) in sub-Saharan Africa. This foundational chapter attempts to provide readers with content to assist in their understanding of the characteristics, role, and experiences of kinship elderly caregivers of children affected and/or infected by HIV and AIDS. In addition, the chapter highlights what is known about children living with HIV in Namibia. Finally, the chapter offers suggestions for policy and practice.

DOI: 10.4018/978-1-7998-2139-7.ch005

INTRODUCTION

Elderly grandparent caregivers "*Omufilishisho*" have always played a key role in the lives of their grandchildren, great grandchildren and other vulnerable children. However, in recent years this role has amplified in intensity, as increasing numbers of grandparents, especially grandmothers have become the primary caregivers of orphans and vulnerable (OVC) (AVERT, 2015). Namibia is one of the countries most affected by the HIV epidemic in southern Africa. HIV is acquired primarily through heterosexual transmission (UNAIDS, 2014). Studies show that the country's HIV prevalence was 12.6% among adults aged 15-64 in 2017(NAMPHIA, 2017).

Recent data shows that 53,000 children aged 0-17 live in grandparent-headed households (UNAIDS, 2014). The United Nations defines an 'orphan' as a child who has lost one or both parents (UNAIDS, 2014). Globally, by 2015 it was estimated that 13.4 million children and adolescents between the ages of 0-17 years had lost one or both parents to AIDS. Moreover, well over 80% of these children (10.9 million) disproportionally live in sub-Saharan Africa (UNICEF, 2016). For example, in some AIDS endemic countries such as Zimbabwe (74%) and South Africa (63%), a large proportion of all orphaned children are orphaned due to AIDS (World Health Organization [WHO], 2014). Scholars report remarkable gains in mitigating the economic and social impact of HIV and AIDS on the well-being of children and their caregivers over the past decade (UNICEF, 2016). Studies show that AIDS orphans including those who are themselves HIV-infected, are predominately living to aging elder caregivers (UNAIDS, 2014), Furthermore, the literature is replete pointing to the increased risk of physical, social, and emotional outcomes of children affected by HIV and AIDS compared with other children in sub-Saharan Africa (UNICEF, 2016). In addition, the caregivers of these children, in many instances are kinship caregivers (i.e., elderly grandmothers), although well-intentioned are from economically impoverished backgrounds themselves and suffer inadequacies in similar areas of well-being as the children they are attempting to care and support. Despite the large numbers of elderly women who are primary caregivers of OVC, the current literature in much of southern Africa, including Namibia, has predominately focused on the needs of OVC and paid less attention to the myriad challenges primary caregivers of children affected by HIV and AIDS face on a daily basis. This chapter puts forth a literature review of issues that elderly caregivers of OVC in Namibia might face. The primary objective of this is to provide readers with content to assist in their understanding about elderly caregivers of children affected and/or infected by HIV and AIDS. The chapter highlights who are caregivers of children orphaned by HIV/AIDS in sub-Saharan Africa; what is known about caregivers' physical and psychological well-being; their ability to care for children in their care. Finally, the chapter offers suggestions for economic empowerment practice approach for social work practitioners and other gerontological professionals working with culturally diverse elderly caregivers. The issues addressed in this chapter, although they may not be new to practitioners working with elderly caregivers, point to the importance of working from a strength-based paradigm.

BACKGROUND

African culture is known for its unique large kin group that transcends the nuclear family (Kayongo-Male & Onyango, 1984). Ethnographic scholars assert that African elders are an integral part of providing social support for its members who are connected together by virtue of reciprocal support obligations and responsibilities (Kayongo-Male & Onyango, 1984). Elders play an important role of passing on traditional practices, imparting knowledge and wisdom and serving as conflict mediators. Conversely, adult children have a traditional responsibility to provide support to their aging parents, grandparents, siblings, and their children (Isiugo-Abanihe, 1985). This philosophy continues to be practiced today and is entrenched in cultural norms values. For example, the Ondonga tribe in Namibia have a proverb that says: *Otunaokukwathelaaakuluntuyetu, shaashinayooyetuwathela.* A literal translation in English means: "We have to help our parents/elders because they helped us." Historically, "*Oku tekula*" which means fostering or raising a child or children by next of kin or someone else other than the child's biological parents is a common practice in African communities (Kuyini, Alhassan, Tollerud, Weld, & Haruna, 2009). Traditionally, African children are viewed as a precious gift from God and the entire clan has a responsibility to bring up that child. The African proverb: "it takes a village to raise a child" is embedded in this practice philosophy. Consequently, children are often given to extended family such as grandparents and other kin not just to be cared for, but to be part and parcel of the that family (Isiugo-Abanihe, 1985).

Today however, fosterage or caregiving is being contested in the literature. Scholars Patel and colleagues (2017); Lekalakala-Mokgele (2011); and Njororai & Njororai (2012) contend that the "informal" caregiving social safety net is not a "social sponge" with limitless capacity to absorb caregiving demands. Scholars argue that the AIDS epidemic has compounded the already severely strained family resources and adding enormous caregiving demands for the extended family to care and support AIDS affected kin in their homes (Kalomo & Lao, 2018; Kalomo & Besthorn, 2018). Thus, caregiving in the era of HIV and AIDS is changing the contours of the African family structure and its capacity to care for OVC in southern Africa. East and southern Africa is the region most affected by the AIDS epidemic (UNCEF, 2016). Compared to the rest of the world, nations in this region have witnessed a disproportional increase in the number of AIDS-orphans (UNICEF, 2016). Elderly caregiving is more prevalent among other nations in sub-Saharan Africa, such as Botswana, Cameroon, Tanzania, Malawi, Lesotho, Swaziland, Namibia, South Africa, Zambia, and Zimbabwe, that are grappling with the AIDS-epidemic (UNICEF, 2016).

The survival rates of prenatally human immunodeficiency virus (HIV) on children in sub-Saharan Africa have significantly improved with the advent of antiretroviral therapy (ART). However, it has simultaneously, created an unprecedented orphan crisis particularly in southern Africa, including Namibia. For the purpose of this chapter the term 'orphan' will be defined as a child under the age of 18 whose biological mother or father has died or who has lost both biological parents. Namibia has one of the highest HIV prevalence rates and highest or orphanhood in the world (AVERT, 2015, UNAIDS, 2014). In general, like in many African communities orphaned children are cared for by extended family members after the death of one or both parents and in some cases when the whereabouts of the remaining parent is unknown (Breckenridge, Black-Hughes, Rautenbach, & McKinley, 2019).

CARING FOR ORPHANS AND VULNERABLE CHILDREN

Who is Caring for Orphans and Vulnerable Children?

The elderly is at the heart of the caregiving in sub-Saharan Africa. Researchers have identified that grandparents were providing care and support to OVC (Njororai & Njororai, 2012). This trend of grandparents raising OVC was documented in studies conducted South Africa (Breckenridge, Black-Hughes, Rautenbach, & McKinley, 2019; Govender, 2012; Kuo & Operario, 2011), Malawi (Littrell, Murphy, Kumwenda, & Macintyre, 2012), Uganda (Ssengonzi, 2009) Togo (Moore, 2007-2008), Kenya (Chepngeno-Langat, Falking, Madise, & Evandrou, 2010), Zimbabwe (Mhaka-Mutepfa, Mpofu, & Cumming, 2014), the Democratic Republic of Congo (Kipp, Matukala, Laing, & Jhangri, 2006), and Tanzania (Dayton & Ainsworth, 2004). In Namibia over 60% of children affected by HIV and AIDS are being care for by aging, often impoverished, elderly grandparents (AVERT, 2015).

Studies in this review also showed the gendered patterns of caregiving (Kipp et al., 2006; Njororai & Njororai, 2012), particulary grandmothers (Boon et al., 2010; Kamya & Poindexter, 2009; Ice, Zidron, & Juma, 2008; Ogunmefun, Gilbert, & Schatz, 2011). For example, Beegle and colleague's study in rural South Africa found that over 50% of grandmothers were caregivers to AIDS-orphans (Beegle, Filmer, Strokes, Tiererova, 2008). Similarly, the first *"Situational Analysis of Orphans in Namibia"* conducted in 2002 found that many AIDS orphans live with relatives before the biological parents die, and that a grandmother may be caring for and raising several sets of orphans from different families at one time (SIAPAC,2002). Furthermore, the northern region of Namibia (Ovamboland) is governed by a matrilineal system (Brown, 2011).

In patrilineal societies, the primary responsibility of a man is to support his mother, siblings, and other next of kin rather than his wife and children. In matrilineal systems, children essentially belong to the mother's side of the family (Brown, 2011). It is not uncommon for patrilineal systems to take the property of the deceased member such as clothes, cattle, land, houses, money, or cars, among others (Kayono-Male & Onyango, 1984), often with little consideration of the welfare of the children and remaining family members (Kayono-Male & Onyango, 1984). For Ruiz-Casares's (2009) study in northern Namibia specifically in the Caprivi, Kavango and Omusati regions revealed that after the death of biological parents, some children and youth experienced property loss at the hands of their paternal relatives, leaving children and their elderly caregivers with only basic kitchen utensils, clothes, and small personal items from their deceased parents (Ruiz-Casares, 2009).

Physical and Psychological Well-Being of Elderly Caregivers

Previous scholars have examined the mental well-being of elder caregivers Researchers have examined how caregiving responsibilities impact caregiver well-being (Boon et al., 2010; Govender et al., 2012; Kagotho & Ssewamala, 2012). Kamya &Poindexter, 2009; Ssengonzi, 2007; Kipp et al., 2006). A phenomenological study on the lived experiences of caregivers who lost an adult child due to AIDS in Togo, West Africa found that elderly women were bearing a heavy caregiver burden (Moore & Henry, 2005) making them susceptible to multiple vulnerabilities such as emotional stress, depression, financial burdens, displacements, high unemployment levels, and untreated personal illnesses (Chazan, 2008). A study by Kalomo and colleagues's (2017) in rural northern Namibia examined the mental well-being among older caregivers raising children impacted by HIV/AIDS found elevated levels of depressive symptomotology among this vulnerable population. Further, scholars assert that mental well-being of elderly caregivers is highly associated with child rearing practices and child well-being outcomes (Lyons-Ruth, Wolfe, & Lyubchik, 2000). Research on caregiver-child relationship for instance has found that caregivers who experienced depressive symptoms are more likely to present negative parenting practices (Bronte-Tinkew, Moore, Matthews, & Carrano, 2007; Kelly, Whitley, & Campos, 2013).

Scholars have also noted that elderly caregivers including those caring for a HIV-infeceted and/or affected child experienced increased levels of isolation and loneliness (Boon et al., 2010; Casale, Wild, Cluver, & Kuo, 2015), reported high levels of emotional distress (Oburu & Palmerus, 2005), had higher levels of chronic illness and poorer general health (Kipp et al., 2006). Furthermore, other researchers have found that elderly caregivers reported symptoms of posttraumatic stress disorder to various degrees (Kuo & Operario, 2011), revealed a heighted sense of being overwhelmed by the magnitude of their new caregiving demands (Govender et al., 2012). Moreover, caregivers also experienced increased levels of HIV-related social stigma as compared to caregivers who were not caring for a child affected by HIV and AIDS (Hejoaka, 2009).Lindsey and colleagues (2003) found that families affected by HIV/AIDS more often than not experienced HIV-related stigma because they had a family member who had either died due to AIDS or was ill. Stigma can manifest in the form of gossip from neighbors and/or the community, blame or abandonment from family or friends, children skipping school from the fear of being ridiculed for having a family member who was HIV-positive, and finger pointing (Demmer, 2011; Lindsey et al., 2003; Ogunmefun et al., 2011). Thus, it is critical that social work and gerontological practitioners understand the association between HIV/AIDS caregiving and mental well-being as it relates to elder caregivers in HIV endemic communities. Such an understandings assists practitioners to identify, address and design targeted culturally appropriate interventions that address the overall well-being of caregivers.

The Ability of Elderly Caregivers to Care for HIV Affected Children

Researchers have examined the ability of elderly kin caregivers to continue caring for OVC (Boon et al., 2012; Abebe & Aase, 2007; Dayton & Ainsworth, 2004; Foster, 2000). Empirical research suggests that caregiving responsibilities have the potential to add to the over-burdened and stretched extended familiy support systems, especially in resource-poor settings, as a result of pre-existing economic challenges weakening social support networks (Abebe & Aase, 2007). Although scholars have applauded the resilience of the elderly African caregivers (Ankrah, 1993; Foster, 2000), scholars contend that what was previously believed to be an "impermeable traditional extended family network" (Miller et al., 2006, p. 1430) is continually being eroded by the AIDS epidemic. The devastating impact of AIDS-related morbidity and mortality is trickling down to the family structure and affecting household income, household food consumption patterns security, and the quality of care to those infected and affected, including OVC (Chimwaza & Watkins, 2004; Lightfoot & Kalomo, 2010).

In addition,the caregiving duties create complex challenges for caregivers such higher demands on household chores (Dayton &Ainsworth, 2004), increased physical ailments among the elderly (Ssengonzi, 2007) and increased financial demands (Schatz & Ogunmefun, 2007),

In Namibia, child social grants follow the child and are intended to provide for the basic needs of the child (e.g., medical care, food, clothing, shelter). The government subsidy does not include income allocated for a caregiver whose caregiving duties may at times remove her from the labor market. Many of these elderly caregivers have spent their lives providing unpaid care and support for their families, often compromising their own physical and mental well-being (Boon et al., 2012; Hai, 2003). Additionally, studies have shown that Namibian caregivers experience an array of challenges when accessing social grants on behalf of the childen in their care (Project Hope, 2006; Taukeni, 2011; Yamano & Jayne, 2004). For example, some caregivers were unable to access these social grants because they did not possess the official identification documentation, birth certificates and/or death certificates (Taukeni, 2011). Consequently, orphaned children were not attending school because caregivers lacked money to pay for school fees and school uniforms (Project Hope, 2006; Taukeni, 2011).

A review of 32 studies on survival strategies employed by HIV/AIDS affected households found that many caregivers reported having to sell their assets, including land and property, or using their savings to support OVC in their care (Naidu & Harris, 2005). The lack of free treatment and affordable, accessible medication adds to caregivers' financial burden (Mathambo & Gibbs, 2009). It is not uncommon for grandparents to depend primarily on their government-funded pensions. Studies have shown that the elderly often have no choice but to use their monthly state pension to supplement household income to buy food, clothing, shelter, pay school fees, and provide transportation as well cover funeral costs and medical expenses (Moore, 2007-2008; Schatz & Ogunmefun, 2007). Due to pre-existing conditions of poverty and extremely high rates of unemployment, common in much of southern Africa, the elders' pension is often the most stable and reliable income for many households (Ogunmefu & Schatz, 2009). Thus, pensions are an important safety net in southern Africa, serving to mitigate the many consequences that elderly could suffer when their adult child dies and leaves behind OVC (Ardington et al., 2010). However, living with limited financial income means poor caregivers and the children in their care are more likely to experience food insecurity.

For the purpose of this paper the term food security refers to the availability and access to food. The advent of HIV/AIDS in Namibia has claimed the lives of many young productive able-bodied individuals thereby reducing labor availability and food security in HIV affected households headed by the elderly. In rural Namibia, majority of families' main livelihood is subsistence farming with livestock rearing supplementing crop production. A study by Schroeder and Nichola (2006) examined whether low income families that adopted AIDS orphans in Ingwavuma rural South

Africa had a high prevalence of being food insecure compared to with families who had not adopted AIDS orphans. The findings of the study showed that households that adopted children orphaned by HIV and AIDS tend to have high dependency ratios. Further, the study revealed that food insecurity increased with orphan adoption, number of family members and loss of food production. Other scholars contend that another factor that accounts for food insecurity in households of the elderly raising OVC was the diminishing cash remittance and social support from extended family and kin (Bohman, Vasuthevan, van Wyk, & Ekman, 2007). Studies have consistently shown that decreasing cash remittance have significantly reduced food availability due to widespread unemployment and HIV/AIDS-related mortality (Madhavan, Schatz, Gomes-Olive, & Collinson, 2017). Consequently, elderly caregivers are left to fend for themselves and their dependents with little or no cash remittance. Taken together these precarious situations have potential to exacerbate the vulnerability of elderly caregivers to food insecurity and psychological distress (Muga & Onyango-Ouma, 2009).

SOLUTIONS AND RECOMMENDATIONS

Given that sub-Saharan Africa is one of the most economically deprived regions in the world and the epicenter of the AIDS epidemic. It is critical that research should explore the economic stress facing elderly caregivers (Freeman & Nkomo, 2006). There is a need for community development practitioners to design culturally appropriate evidence-based economic empowerment interventions, specifically those that target caregivers and children and are focused on economic strengthening. In brief, economic strengthening is defined as "approaches to strengthen the capacity of caregivers and communities to address the financial issues to ensure vulnerable children are able to access essential services, including safety, healthcare, education, and other basic needs" (USAID, 2008, p. 11). There is a need for service providers to develop various economic opportunities for elderly caregivers. Scholars have shown how income-generating projects, microfinance, and cash transfer projects (Adato & Bassett, 2009; Ssewamala, Neilands, Waldfogel, & Ismayilova, 2012;) may buffer the economic shocks of households affected by HIV and AIDS. in developing countries. Other researchers contend that cash transfers show the strongest evidence, particularly in programs in developing countries (Adato & Bassett, 2009). Furthermore, other economic empowerment interventions that can act as safety nets include, among others, community-based capital cash transfers (Skovdal, Mwasiaji, Webale, & Tomkins, 2011) and child support grants and youth saving accounts (Ssewamala, 2007). Economic empowerment initiative such as these have the potential to drastically and rapidly improve outcomes of children and families in poverty stricken and AIDS-endemic communities (Plagerson et al., 2011).

FUTURE RESEARCH DIRECTIONS

Authors are of the idea that the future research directions should dig deeper to unearth the coping mechanisms of elderly caregivers in the context of HIV/AIDS. Further research should also focus on community evidence-based economic empowerment interventions that seek to capacitate elderly caregivers and their children. Specifically, interventions should aim to strengthen the capacity of caregivers in accessing essential services such as: healthcare, education, and other basic needs (USAID, 2008, p. 11).

CONCLUSION

This chapter reviewed several trends among caregivers of children orphaned by AIDS in sub-Saharan Africa. Firstly, grandparents, particularly maternal grandmothers have become primary caregivers of children who have lost on or both parents due to AIDS. Secondly, there is compelling evidence that the AIDS epidemic has changed the household living arrangements of the African family. Thirdly, the gendered pattern of caregiving was explicated. Fourthly, the literature revealed the myriad challenges that elderly caregivers experience in their caregiving role including poor physical and mental health outcomes, HIV-related stigma, food insecurity, and financial burden. Finally, this review showed that there is a compelling need for an economic empowerment practice model to mitigate the financial burden of elderly caregivers. It is well known that the child welfare system depends heavily on this vulnerable population as a means to provide familiar continuity for OVC, it is imperative for service providers to intentionally redress the needs of elderly caregivers in order to safeguard their service needs.

REFERENCES

Adato, M., & Bassett, L. (2009). Social protection to support vulnerable children and families: The potential of cash transfers to protect, health and nutrition. *AIDS Care*, *21*(1), 60–75. doi:10.1080/09540120903112351 PMID:22380980

Ankrah, E. (1993). The impact of HIV/AIDS on the family and other significant relationships: The African clan revisited. *AIDS Care*, *5*(1), 5–22. doi:10.1080/09540129308258580 PMID:8461361

Ardington, C. A., Case, A., Islam, M., Lam, D., Leibbrandt, M., Menendez, A., & Olgiati, A. (2010). The impact of AIDS on intergenerational support in South Africa: Evidence form the Cape Area Panel Study. *Research on Aging*, *32*(1), 91–121. doi:10.1177/0164027509348143 PMID:20161477

AVERT. (2015). *Children and HIV/AIDS*. Sussex, Brighton: AVERT.

Beegle, K., Filmer, D., Strokes, A., & Tiererova, L. (2008). *Orphanhood and living arrangements of children in sub-Saharan Africa*. New York, NY: World Bank.

Bohman, D. M., Vasuthevan, S., van Wyk, N. C., & Ekman, L. (2007). "We clean our houses, prepare for weddings and go to funerals": Daily lives of elderly Africans in Majaneng, South Africa. *Journal of Cross-Cultural Gerontology*, *22*(4), 323–337. doi:10.100710823-007-9040-8 PMID:17616794

Boon, H., James, S., Ruiter, R. A. C., van den Borne, B., Williams, E., & Reddy, P. (2010). Explaining the perceived ability among older people to provide care as a result of HIV and AIDS in South Africa. *AIDS Care*, *22*(4), 399–408. doi:10.1080/09540120903202921 PMID:20140795

Breckenridge, T.N., Black-Hughes, C., Rautenbach, J., & McKinley, M. (2019). HIV/AIDS orphans in South Africa: NGO interventions supporting transitions to alternative care. *International Social Work, 62*(2), 502, 517.

Bronte-Tinkew, J., Moore, K. A., Matthews, G., & Carrano, J. (2007). Symptoms of Major Depression in a Sample of Fathers of Infants. *Journal of Family Issues*, *28*(1), 61–99. doi:10.1177/0192513X06293609

Casale, M., Wild, L., Cluver, L., & Kuo, C. (2015). Social support as a protective factor for depression among women caring for children in HIV-endemic South Africa. *Journal of Behavioral Medicine*, *38*(1), 17–27. doi:10.100710865-014-9556-7 PMID:24510353

Chazan, M. (2008). Seven 'deadly' assumptions: Unraveling implications of HIV/AIDS among grandmothers in South Africa and beyond. *Aging and Society*, *28*(7), 935–958. doi:10.1017/S0144686X08007265

Chepngeno-Langat, G., Falking, J., Madise, N. J., & Evandrou, M. (2010). Socioeconomic differentials between HIV caregivers and non-caregivers: Is there a selection effect? A case of older people living in Nairobi city slums. *Research on Aging*, *32*(1), 67–96. doi:10.1177/0164027509348116 PMID:21552461

Chimwaza, A. F., & Watkins, S. C. (2004). Giving care to people with symptoms of AIDS in rural sub-Saharan Africa. *AIDS Care*, *16*(7), 795–807. doi:10.1080/09540120412331290211 PMID:15385234

Dayton, J., & Ainsworth, M. (2004). The elderly and AIDS: Coping with the impact of adult death in Tanzania. *Social Science & Medicine*, *59*(10), 2161–2172. doi:10.1016/j.socscimed.2004.03.013 PMID:15351481

Demmer, C. (2011). Experiences of families caring for HIV-infected child in KwaZulu-Natal, South Africa. *AIDS Care*, *23*(7), 873–879. doi:10.1080/09540121.2010.542123 PMID:21400305

Foster, G. (2000). The capacity of the extended family safety net for orphans in Africa. *Psychology & Health*, *346*, 1907–1910.

Freeman, M., & Nkomo, N. (2006). Guardianship of orphans and vulnerable children: A survey of current and prospective South African caregivers. *AIDS Care*, *18*(4), 302–310. doi:10.1080/09540120500359009 PMID:16809107

Govender, K., Penning, S., George, G., & Quilan, T. (2012). Weighing up the burden of care on caregivers of orphan children: The Amajuba District Child Health and Wellbeing Project, South Africa. *AIDS Care Psychological and Socio-Medical Aspects of HIV/AIDS*, *24*(6), 712-721.

HelpAge International (HAI). (2003). *Forgotten families: Older people as carers of orphans and vulnerable children.* London: Help Age International.

Ice, G. H., Zidron, A., & Juma, E. (2008). Health and health perceptions among Kenyan grandmothers. *Journal of Cross-Cultural Gerontology*, *23*(2), 111–129. doi:10.100710823-008-9063-9 PMID:18437546

Isiugo-Abanihe, U. (1985). Child fosterage in West Africa. *Aging and Development*, 53-73.

Kagotho, N., & Ssewamala, F. M. (2012). Correlates of depression among caregivers of children affected by HIV/AIDS in Uganda: Findings from the Suubi-Maka family study. *AIDS Care*, *24*(10), 1226–1232. doi:10.1080/09540121.2012.658754 PMID:22375826

Kalomo, E.N., & Besthorn, F.H. (2018). Elderly grandmothers raising orphans and vulnerable children affected by HIV/AIDS in sub-Saharan Africa: A literature review and emerging efforts in Namibia. *GrandFamilies: The Contemporary Journal of Research, Practice and Policy, 5*(1).

Kalomo, E. N., Kyoung, H. L., & Besthorn, F. H. (2017). Depressive symptoms among older, female caregivers raising children affected by HIV/AIDS in the Omusati Region of Namibia. *Health Care for Women International, 38*(12), 1327–1343. doi:10.1080/07399332.2017.1368514 PMID:28850326

Kalomo, E. N., & Liao, M. (2018). Burden of care among caregivers of persons living with HIV/AIDS in rural Namibia. *Social Work in Public Health, 33*(1), 70–84. doi:10.1080/19371918.2017.1415180 PMID:29297790

Kamya, H., & Poindexter, C. C. (2009). Mama Jaja: The stresses and strengths of HIV-affected Ugandan grandmothers. *Social Work in Public Health, 24*(1-2), 4–21. doi:10.1080/19371910802569294 PMID:19229769

Kayono-Male, H., & Onyango, P. (1984). *The sociology of the African family.* London: Longman.

Kelly, S. J., Whitley, D. M., & Campos, P. E. (2013). Psychological distress in African American grandmothers raising grandchildren: The contribution of child behavior problems, physical health, and family resources. *Research in Nursing & Health, 36*(4), 373–385. doi:10.1002/nur.21542 PMID:23606233

Kiggundu, E., & Oldewage-Theron, W. (2009). Coping: A challenge for guardians of children orphaned by HIV/AIDS in a South African Township. *Development Southern Africa, 26*(3), 383–397. doi:10.1080/03768350903086754

Kipp, W., Matukala, T., Laing, L., & Jhangri, G. S. (2006). Care burden and self-reported health status of informal women caregivers of HIV/AIDS patients in Kinshasa, Democratic Republic of Congo. *AIDS Care, 18*(7), 694–697. doi:10.1080/13548500500294401 PMID:16971277

Kuo, C., & Operario, D. (2011). Health of adults caring for orphaned children in an HIV-endemic community in South Africa. *AIDS Care, 23*(9), 1128–1135. doi: 10.1080/09540121.2011.554527 PMID:21480009

Kuyini, A. B., Alhassan, A. R., Tollerud, I., Weld, H., & Haruna, I. (2009). Traditional experiences and views of children and carers and adults in Tamle. *Child & Family Social Work, 14*, 440–449. doi:10.1111/j.1365-2206.2009.00616.x

Lightfoot, E., & Kalomo, E. N. (2010). The interplay of population aging and HIV/AIDS on social development in Southern Africa: The case of Namibia. *Social Development Issues*, *32*(1), 1–15.

Lindsey, E., Hirschfeld, M., Tlou, S., & Ncube, M. (2003). Home-based care in Botswana: Experiences of older women and young girls. *Health Care for Women International*, *24*(6), 486–501. doi:10.1080/07399330390199384 PMID:12851169

Littrell, M., Murphy, L., Kumwenda, M., & Macintyre, K. (2012). Gogo Care and protection of vulnerable children in rural Malawi: Changing responsibilities, capacity to provide, and implications for well-being in the era of HIV and AIDS. *Journal of Cross-Cultural Gerontology*, *27*(4), 335–355. doi:10.100710823-012-9174-1 PMID:22869344

Lyons-Ruth, K., Wolfe, R., & Lyubchik, A. (2000). Depression and parenting of young children: Making the case for early preventative mental health services. *Harvard Review of Psychiatry*, *8*(3), 148–153. doi:10.1080/hrp_8.3.148 PMID:10973939

Madhavan, S., Schatz, E., Gomes-Olive, F. X., & Collinson, W. (2017). Social positioning of older persons in rural South Africa. *Change or Stability or Journal of South African Studies*, *43*(6), 1293–1307. doi:10.1080/03057070.2017.1365522 PMID:30686854

Mhaka-Mutepfa, M., Mpofu, E., & Cumming, R. (2014). Impact of protective factors on resilience of grandparent carers fostering orphans and non-orphans in Zimbabwe. *Journal of Aging and Health*, *27*(3), 454–479. doi:10.1177/0898264314551333 PMID:25260649

Miller, C., Gruskin, S., Subramanian, S., Rajaraman, D., & Heymann, J. (2006). Orphan care in Botswana's working households: Growing responsibilities in the absence of adequate support. *American Journal of Public Health*, *96*(8), 1429–1435. doi:10.2105/AJPH.2005.072280 PMID:16809585

Moore, A. R. (2007-2008). Older poor parents who lost an adult child to AIDS in Togo, West Africa: A Qualitative study. *Omega*, *56*(3), 289–304. doi:10.2190/OM.56.3.e PMID:18300652

Muga, G. O., & Onyango-Ouma, W. (2009). Changing household composition and food security among the elderly caretakers in rural Western Kenya. *Journal of Cross-Cultural Gerontology*, *24*(3), 259–272. doi:10.100710823-008-9090-6 PMID:19137419

Namibia Population-Based HIV Impact Assessment (NAMPHIA). (2018). Summary Sheet: Preliminary Findings.

Njororai, F., &Njororai, W. W. S. (2012). Older adult caregivers to people with HIV/AIDS in sub-Saharan Africa: A review of literature and policy implications for change. *International Journal of Health Promotion and Education*. iFirst.

Ogunmefun, C., Gilbert, L., & Schatz, E. (2011). Older female caregivers and HIV/AIDS-related secondary stigma in rural South Africa. *Journal of Cross-Cultural Gerontology*. *Journal of Cross-Cultural Gerontology*, *27*(1), 85–102. doi:10.100710823-010-9129-3 PMID:20957421

Palattiyil, G., & Chakrabarti, M. (2008). Coping strategies of families in HIV/AIDS care: Some exploratory data from two developmental contexts. *AIDS Care*, *20*(7), 881–885. doi:10.1080/09540120701767166 PMID:18608058

Patel, L., Knijn, T., Gorman-Smith, D., Hochfeld, T., Isserow, M., Garthe, R., & Kgaohola, I. (2017). *Families, the child support grant, and child well-being outcomes*. Johannesburg: Centre for Social Development in Africa.

Plagerson, S., Patel, V., Harpham, T., Kielmann, K., & Mathee, A. (2011). Does money matter for mental health? Evidence from the child support grants in Johannesburg. *Global Public Health: An International Journal for Research, Policy and Practice*, *6*(7), 760–776. doi:10.1080/17441692.2010.516267 PMID:20938853

Retrieved fromhttp://www.unaids.org/en/regionscountries/countries/namibia

Schatz, E., & Ogunmefun, C. (2007). Caring and Contributing: The role of older women in rural South Africa multi-generational households in the HIV/AIDS era. *World Development*, *35*(8), 1390–1403. doi:10.1016/j.worlddev.2007.04.004

Schroeder, E., & Nichola, T. (2006). The adoption of HIV/AIDS orphans and food security in rural Ingwavuma, South Africa. *International Journal of Technology Management & Sustainable Development*, *5*(2), 173–187. doi:10.1386/ijtm.5.2.173_1

Skovdal, M., Mwasiaji, W., Webale, A., & Tomkins, A. (2011). Building orphan competent communities: Experiences from a community-based capital cash transfer initiative in Kenya. *Health Policy and Planning*, *16*(3), 233–241. doi:10.1093/heapol/czq039 PMID:20805235

Social Impact Assessment and Policy Analysis Corporation (SIAPAC). (2002). *Situational analysis of orphan children in Namibia*. Windhoek, Namibia: Ministry of Health and Social Services.

Ssengonzi, R. (2007). The plight of older persons as caregivers to people infected/affected by HIV/AIDS: Evidence from Uganda. *Journal of Cross-Cultural Gerontology*, *22*(4), 339–353. doi:10.100710823-007-9043-5 PMID:17694427

Ssewamala, F. M., Neilands, T. B., Waldfogel, J., & Ismayilova, L. (2012). The impact of a comprehensive microfinance intervention on depression levels of AIDS-orphaned children in Uganda. *The Journal of Adolescent Health, 50*(4), 346–352. doi:10.1016/j.jadohealth.2011.08.008 PMID:22443837

UNICEF. (2016). Seventh Stocktaking Report on Children & AIDS, 2016.

United Nations Programme on HIV/AIDS (UNAIDS). (2014).

United States Agency for International Development (UNAIDS). (2008). *Third annual report on orphans and vulnerable children in developing countries*. Washington, DC: USAID. Retrieved from www.healthpolicyinitiative.com/Publications/Documents/1346

World Health Organization (WHO). (2014). Worlds AIDS Day: Business Unusual: Time to end the AIDS epidemic.

ADDITIONAL READING

Kalomo, E. N., Lee, K. H., Lightfoot, E., & Freeman, R. (2018). Resilience among older caregivers in rural Namibia: The role of financial status, social support and health. *Journal of Gerontological Social Work, 61*(6), 605–622. doi:10.1080/01634372.2018.1467524 PMID:29683784

Kalomo, E. N., & Liao, M. (2018). Burden of care among caregivers of persons living with HIV/AIDS in rural Namibia. *Social Work in Public Health, 33*(1), 70–84. doi:10.1080/19371918.2017.1415180 PMID:29297790

Ramona, W. D. (2016). *Kinship care: Increasing child well-being through practice, policy, and research*. New York, NY: Springer Publishing Company.

Taukeni, S. (2015). Orphan adolescents' life-worlds on school-based psychosocial support. *Health Psychology and Behavioural Medicine: An Open Access Journal, 3*(1), 12–24. doi:10.1080/21642850.2014.987778

Taukeni, S. G., & Ferreira, R. (2016). HIV/AIDS awareness among adolescent children in an at-risk South African rural community. *Southern African Journal of HIV Medicine, 17*(1), 1–7. doi:10.4102ajhivmed.v17i1.418 PMID:29568602

KEY TERMS AND DEFINITIONS

Caregiver: An individual who is taking care of OVC. These individuals are eligible to receive supports on behalf of the children in their care

Elderly Parent: An individual who is 60 and above years of older taking a responsibility of providing care and support to children.

Kinship Care: Refers to the care and support of OVC by extended family members or relatives.

Orphan Children: Children under the age of 18 years who lost one or both biological parents due to death or permanently abandoned or whose parents are unknown.

Psychological Well-Being: A state of mind when an Individual has a positive rewarding relationship with other people, a feeling of purpose in life and opportunity for personal growth and development.

Safety Net: A safeguard against possible hardship or adversity.

Vulnerable Children: Children under the age of 18 years who are at high risk of lacking adequate care and basic support such as clothing, food, shelter, love, belonging and safety.

Section 4
Smoking

Chapter 6
Smoking:
A Biopsychosocial Perspective

Daniel Ashipala
University of Namibia, Rundu Campus, Namibia

Nestor Tomas
University of Namibia, Rundu Campus, Namibia

Joel M. H. Medusalem
https://orcid.org/0000-0003-3886-0367
University of Namibia, Rundu Campus, Namibia

ABSTRACT

Smoking involves inhaling, exhaling, holding or otherwise having control over an ignited tobacco product. This practice remains a global budden and deaths caused by smoking-related conditions is believed to have escalated. Many countries in the world have policies in place that regulate the production, transportation, handling and utilization of tobacco products in order to compact this budden of smoking. Despite these effort, various contributing factors of smoking amongst which peer-pressure forms part, are believed to be cause of an increase in the number of new smokers. Nicotine is one of the constituents of tobacco smoke which causes a pleasant feelings which in return contributes to addiction. Cigarette smoke contains thousands of chemicals with some known to be carcinogens. Smoking during pregnancy poses danger to a pregnant mother and her unborn babe as they exchange blood. The public needs to be educated on the danger of smoking, and exposure to second-hand smoke as well as on strategies that one can follow to quit smoking.

DOI: 10.4018/978-1-7998-2139-7.ch006

INTRODUCTION

West (2017) defined tobacco smoking as smoking that consists of drawing into the mouth, and usually the lungs, smoke from burning tobacco. About 4 million people die each year from tobacco smoking related conditions, with the number projected to reach 10 million by the year 2030 (Amakali, Haoses-Gorases, & Taukuheke, 2013). The use of tobacco, challenges associated with addictions and morbidity trajectory have moved from being the challenges of developed countries to that of low and middle income countries, similar to tobacco marketing efforts. Sub-sahara Africa is relatively new to dealing with the challenges associated with tobacco epidemic. The consumption of tobacco products in Sub-sahara Africa is estimated to record the highest growth in the world (Siddiqi, 2019). Smoking habits are believed to be associated with an increased global morbidity which are non-communicable diseases related (Naikaku, 2018).

In an effort to control smoking, Namibia signed a Convention for Tobbacco Control (CFTC) in 2010 and enacted a Tobacco Control Act, nearly 20 years after independence without a piece of legislature that prohibit public smoking, adverstising and sales of tobacco products (Tam & Van Walbeek, 2013). The legislative on tobacco control is seen as a tool to control the use of tobacco, particulary in youth population.

This chapter will discuss the factors contributing to smoking, dangers, challenges and strategies to quiting smoking and the effects of smoking on the body.

BACKGROUND

Namibia is classified as a middle income country with peaceful political environment that has attracted many investors to compete for investment opportunities. However, the world economic down turn has also negatively affect the country with youth unployment rate standing at 46.1% (Trading Econmics, 2019). Amid to economic challenges, tobacco companies continue to take advantage of weak tobacco control legislations in Namibia to aggressively promote tobacco products underthe presence of creating jobs opportunities. Namibian Cambinet has approved acontrovential tobacco plantation in Zambezi region, on the Eastern part of the country, despite the call from the affected communities, civil societies, some governmental and non-governmental organizations who had objected the approval of the environmental clearance in 2014. The project is seen to be a health hazard and inconflict with its' 2005 WHO ratification framework on tobacco control in Namibia (Kahiurika, 2019). According World Health Organization's Global Tobacco Survey of 2011, it was discovered that children in Namibia starts smoking as young as nine, with about 16% of children smoking cigarette. With the youth currently making up 60%

of the Namibian population, it is estimated that about 50% of youth in Namibia smoke cigarettes (Amakali et al., 2013). In India about 28.6% of children were smoking cigarettes in 2016 (Thomas, 2018). In South Africa the use of tobacco use among adolescent stood at 44%, while adults stood at 17.6% (Reddy, Zuma, Shisana, Jonas, & Sewpaul, 2015; Morojele, Brook, & Brook, 2016). To curb the prevalence of smoking-related mortality, Namibia has added legislative measures to the 1997 smoking ban through the Tobacco Product Control Act, Act No.1 of 2010. In terms of the Act, the Ministry of Health and Social Services (MoHSS) enforces standards for the manufacturing, advertising, promotion, sponsorship, packaging and labelling of cigarettes and the restriction of smoking in public places, while simultaneously promoting campaigns targeted towards stopping smoking".. As a result of the dependence causing agent, e.g. nicotine, most smokers in Namibia are likely to face challenges associated with quitting smoking, owing to accessibility tobacco products and the lack of critical information relevant to cessation. Although Namibia implemented the tobacco control act, most people continue to disregard the use of tobacco products on free zones, hence the increase in exposure to tobacco products in general. This chapter discusses critical issues that peer educators must consider in supporting smoking cessation campaigns at schools in the country.

MAIN FOCUS OF THE CHAPTER

This chapter focusses on smoking, its biopsychosocial contributory factors as well as negative health issues consequent to tobacco smoking. This chapter further speaks to addiction, contributory factors related to and strategies to be employed if one opts to quit smoking.

Issues, Controversies, and Problems

Authorities in different countries across the globe established smoking policies in an attempt to regulate the use of different tobacco agents as well as that of other smoking agents. Namibia established tobacco products control act, Act No. 1 of 2010 with objectives to provide the established Tobacco Products Control Committee with powers, duties and functions as well as to create a reduction in the demand and supply of tobacco products. On contrary, the approval of tobacco plantation in Namibia remain a controvential issue that needs further public deliberation. In addition, the act sought to safeguard citizens from exposure to tobacco smoke (Tobacco Control Act, 2010). Despite this effort, smoking has not declined as its increase remain notable world-wide particularly in low income countries (Da Silva, De Araújo, De Queiroz, Sales, Castellano, &Comissão de Tabagismo da SBPT,

2016). It can be projected that, peer-pressure could be a root cause of an increased smoking prevalence rate among citizens specifically teenagers not only in Namibia but whole at large (Jafari, Zamani & Alizadeh, 2011).

BIOPSYCHOSOCIAL FACTORS RELATED TO SMOKING

Biological Factors

Nicotine triggers reward circuits, mainly in the midbrain. The habenulo interpeduncular (MHb-IPN) pathway has been suggested as a new critical crossroad that influences the brain response to nicotine" because of its richness in nicotinic acetylcholine receptors (Antolin-Fontes, Ables, & Ibanez-Tallon, 2014). It is involved in various reward-related circuits, designating the MHb-IPN as a convergent track for cholinergic, serotoninergic and dopaminergic signals (Antolin-Fontes et al., 2014).A change in the density of nerve tissue in the anterior cingulate cortex and nucleus accumbency, as a result of antenatal nicotine, has also been discovered. This, together with exposure to nicotine in the childhood stage and second-hand, passive smoking, is believed to be a contributing factor to the development of smoking behaviours (Mychasiuk, Muhammad, Carroll, & Kolb, 2013).Cigarette smoke contains more than 4,000 chemicals including nicotine and carbonmonoxide which enter fetal blood circulation and causes teratogenic effects that include low birth weight, premature birth and stillbirths (MacArthur, Knox & Lancashire, 2001; Burguetet, al. 2004; Siu, 2015). Therefore, smoking during pregnancy poses an increased risk of 47% to stillbirth with the risk much higher in cigarette consumption(Marufu, Ahankari, Coleman & Lewis, 2015).

Psychological Factors

Nicotine substitution may not be experienced as being satisfactory as smoking (Perkins, Conklin, & Levine, 2008). While smoking may please the smoker emotionally on a short-term basis, its awful consequences appear as smoking progresses. Lack of awareness of the dangers of smoking is a major concern, especially in regions with a low literacy rate (Stoll, 2015). However, even in more affluent societies, it is believed that the youth may still underestimate the risk of smoking dependency, including its negative long-term consequences (Stoll, 2015). In addition, smokers often pay more attention to false knowledge despite being in possession of correct information on the dangers of smoking, as well as smoking cessation. Smokers may also experience challenges in withstanding the pressures of not smoking (Festinger, 1962). According to Hagger et al. (2013), smokers' self-control resources are exhausted by smoking-related stimuli. Sustained smoking behaviour can result from a failure to observe one's cognitive habits, limiting available coping strategies. On the other hand, nicotine plays a role in stimulating the brain's reward circuits, therefore a history of other addictions and substance abuse has to be taken into consideration (Stoll, 2015). Smokers use smoking as a coping strategy for prior trauma; even so, it is unclear whether smoking behaviour intensifies or alleviates the specific trauma (Perkins et al., 2008).

Social Factors

Smoking sometimes emanates from social reasoning. Social ideologies that portray smoking behaviours as positive have been found to be a primary driving force for smoking. In the second half of the 20th century, smoking was portrayed as an activity for men only; as a result,the majority of smokers were male. However, nowadays women often smoke to convey a certain image (Laureate, 2014). Smoking behaviour may become a ritual between partners or friends. As a result, youngsters consider parents and older siblings who smoke to be role models. Non-smokers exposed to second-hand smoke "conciliate the link between parental smoking and students smoking," which poses considerable risk for smoking behaviour in children (Wang, Ho, & Lam, 2011).

CAUSES OF SMOKING ADDICTION

Cigarettes are made from the tobacco plant. Tobacco leaves and stems contain high amounts of nicotine. The inhaled nicotine from cigarettes is raised further by the addition of ammonia to tobacco. The over 4000 chemical compounds found in cigarettes include carbon monoxide, nitrogen oxide, hydrogen cyanide, ammonia and other toxic irritants (German Technical Cooperation, 2009; The Royal Australian College of General Practitioners, 2011).

The nicotine obtained by smoking causes the release of dopamine which results in a pleasant feeling. The effects of a cigarette depend on how long someone has been smoking usually about thirty minutes. Once the levels of dopamine and acetylcholine drop, the person will feel the craving for another cigarette to boost the mood chemical levels. Eventually, the body starts to become resistant to the nicotine (it releases less dopamine each time you smoke) so higher quantities of nicotine are needed more frequently to have the same effect. This is known as tolerance.

DANGER OF PASSIVE SMOKING

Side-stream smoke may be even more dangerous than the mainstream smoke inhaled by a smoker, as cigarettes are designed to draw smoke through a cooling filtering mechanism on its way into the lungs. About two-thirds of this smoke is not inhaled by the smoker but may find its way into the surrounding air where it enters a non-smoker's lungs. Such unfiltered smoke may contain as many as 50 chemicals identified as cancer-causing agents (German Technical Cooperation, 2009). Children are at particular risk from second-hand smoke and tend to develop respiratory illnesses such as asthma, bronchitis and heart disease due to their immature bodies. Further, studies have linked side-stream smoke not only to lung cancer but also to heart disease and cancers of the sinuses, brain, breast, uterus and cervix (Benjamin, 2010; Sui, 2015).

SIGNS AND SYMPTOMS OF NICOTINE ADDICTION

Nicotine takes less than eight seconds after smoking to reach the brain and causes the following signs and symptoms German Technical Cooperation (2009):

1. Decreased fatigue
2. Increased alertness
3. Reduced anxiety
4. Mental alertness

The effects of nicotine on the body cause dependence on smoking and that makes an individual person to feel alert, energise and happy. In the absence of smoking, the smoker will feel unhappy and weak until such time that the person have smoked.

STRATEGIES TO STOP SMOKING

Stopping smoking may require additional support from doctors, loved ones or work. The choice is for an individual to identify the support needed once a decision to stop smoking is made.Such support may include:

1. **Exercise Every Day**: Exercise cuts stress and makes you feel relaxed and happy. It also makes you feel better about yourself. The more you accept and love yourself, the less you will need to "hide" behind smoke (World Health Organization 2001; Hammond, 2005).

2. **Eat Healthy Food**: Most ex-smokers do gain weight. This happens because your appetite improves without nicotine. Your taste buds heal, so food tastes delicious (World Health Organization 2001; Hammond, 2005).
3. **Drink Lots of Water:** Water will flush the chemicals from cigarettes out of your body. Many people find that a glass of water can flush away a craving for a cigarette too. Drinking water is also a way to keep your hand and mouth busy without having a cigarette. Carry a water bottle with you instead of a pack of smokes. Try drinking from a straw or sucking on a water bottle with a pop-up spout(World Health Organization 2001; Sui, 2015).
4. **Cut Down on Tea, Coffee, Fizzy Drinks and Alcohol:** First because these drinks often act as a "trigger" to make you crave a cigarette. When you see, taste or smell tea, coffee or alcohol, you may suddenly crave a cigarette. The caffeine in coffee and tea may cause bad headaches thus exacerbating the withdrawal symptoms.
5. **Sleep More**: If you can, sleep more than usual for the first week or two when you quit. Take a nap in the afternoon if possible and give yourself an extra hour or two of sleep each night.
6. **Chemical Aid (Patch, Gum, Pill or Oral Spray)**: These products can increase your chances of quitting; however, there are issues to consider before deciding which one to use. Nicotine-replacement products work by supplying your body with just enough nicotine to keep the craving under control, thereby helping you fight the urge to smoke. Of the three types available, the gum and the spray offer a blast of nicotine similar to what you experience when you light up a cigarette. The patch works in a slightly different way; it supplies a low but steady stream of nicotine that helps fight cravings around the clock. The replacement products have side effects worth noting, including headaches, dizziness, blurred vision, itchy skin, muscle weakness, upset stomach and diarrhoea. Sprays may also cause nasal irritation and coughing (RACGP, 2011; World Health Organization 2001).

The replacement regime should be continued for 10 to 12 weeks with a gradual withdrawal over this period. If you do not stop smoking within three months, you should review the regimen with a doctor. If you use the patch, nicotine goes through your skin all day long. It is therefore really important not to smoke while the patch is on your skin, as you could get an overdose of nicotine, and consequently get really sick or even die.

Furthermore, The World Health Organization (2001) outlined five useful behavioural tips to remember and practise when confronted with the urge to smoke while trying to quit as follow: delay even for a short while, drink water, deep breathing, do something different and discuss the craving with another person (Sui, 2015).

7. **Rehabilitation**: Most cases of severe of tobacco or addictions of other drugs in Namibia are referred to the available rehabilitation centers.While many cases recover, others takes long to recover depending on the severity and compliance to treatment guidelines (New Era article, 2014). However, the country is still faced with a shortage of rehabilitation centers of substance abuse specifically. Some of the rehabilitative services offered at the available rehabilitation centers include, support groups as well as smoking programs and classes(Ministry of Health and Social Services, 2010). This will help in dealing with relapse tendency and in restoring normal daily being and function (MoHSS, 2010).

CHALLENGESRELATED TO QUITTING

Smoking is a crutch which relaxes and soothes smokers which makes quitting smoking a terrifying experience. It acts as an appetite suppressant and a stimulant. Withdrawal and cravings are not pleasant, and the smoker knows this. Some of the challenges drawn from World Health Organization (2001) & German Technical Cooperation (2009) are as follow:

1. **Withdrawal:** The lowered levels of nicotine can lead to a variety of symptoms, including irritability, depression, cigarette cravings, headaches, nervousness, insomnia and difficulty concentrating. Withdrawal effects peak at about 48 hours and then start to diminish. All withdrawal symptoms will be gone after about one month. This is the hardest time for the quitter and mental preparation and support is needed during this period (German Technical Cooperation (2009).
2. **Cravings:** No onequits without having cravings. These are an intense desire to smoke. Cravings feel as though they last a lifetime but in reality, it lasts not more than a few minutes. One may experience cravings but if you can overcome each craving, the feeling will go away.
3. **Weight Gain:** Many people will not quit smoking as they are afraid of gaining weight. The typical scenario leading to weight gain is someone who gives up smoking and replaces their smoking habit with an eating habit. Reaching for a snack every time you have a nicotine craving will lead to weight gain. However, healthy snacking and moderate exercise can easily combat possible weight gain when quitting.
4. **Stress Management:** Smoking relaxes the smoker. When a smoker feels stressed or anxious, they reach for a cigarette. When they quit, smokers no longer have this crutch. If you are quitting you need to find alternative ways to handle stress. Go for a quick stroll, sip on water, take deep breaths or punch a

pillow – whatever it takes. Exercise is very useful in helping quitters cope with some of their pent-up frustrations (German Technical Cooperation, 2009).

5. **Substance Use (Alcohol and Other Drugs):** Alcohol and drugs alter the normal functioning of the brain leading to smoking relapse.
6. **Living With Other Smokers:** Quitting while living with other smokers can be challenging, as seeing them smoke may increase the urge to smoke (German Technical Cooperation, 2009).
7. **Circumstances That Result in the Smoker Giving Quitting a Low Priority, such as Poverty and Social Isolation:** Loneliness may tempt the person to engage inhigh-risk activities such as smoking or taking alcohol, while poverty reduces the person's buying power and increases feelings of hopelessness. According to American Lung Association (2019) challenges associated with quiting smoking includes trouble sleeping, inability to contrite, restlessness, inpatient with one self and unable to control the strong urges to smoke.
8. **Nicotine Replacement Therapy and Bupropion/Varenicline:** (antidepressant medications) can help reduce the number of cravings. Bupropion and varenicline are considered to have favourable effect but due to an escallated number of psychiatric comorbidity in smoking addicts, such patients nee to be closely monitored for potential neuropsychiatric symptoms(Aubin, Luquiens& Berlin, 2013). However, majority of smokers often relapse after an attempt to quit therefore there is a need for alternative pharmacotherapies boost cessation rates and to prevent relapses (Pollock, Koustova Hoffman, Shurtleff &Volkow, 2009). During the first period of quitting, it is advisable to avoid the places and people with which smoking was associated. The cravings are very strong under these circumstances. As time passes (usually within a month), a quitter can gradually begin exposing themselves. However, although cravings lessen with time, they can still arise years after quitting (Aubin, Luquiens& Berlin, 2013; RACGP, 2011).

TOBACCO CONTROL POLICIES IN NAMIBIA

In 2006, Namibia joined the World Health Organization (WHO) Framework Convention on Tobacco Control. The implementation of the Convention on Tobacco Control has four important focus areas, namely:

Smoke-Free Zones

The Minister may prohibit the smoking of any tobacco product in any prescribed outdoor public place, or such portion of an outdoor public place as may be prescribed, if persons are likely to congregate within close proximity of one another or where smoking may pose a fire or other hazard. Smoking is prohibited in all indoor public places or within two metres of public places, in all indoor workplaces and in all public transport. Further, no smoking is allowed in private areas used for childcare activities or schooling (Tobacco Control Act, No. 1 of 2010).

Tobacco Advertising, Promotion and Sponsorship

The policy prohibits all activities related to advertising or promoting tobacco products in public and discourages tobacco sponsorship and publicity for such sponsorships.

Tobacco Packaging and Labelling

All tobacco products are required to have warning text and pictures taking up 50% of the front and 60% ofthe back of the package. All information that may entice clients to think that tobacco products are less harmful is prohibited and all emission yields of all substances in tobacco must be displayed on the package.

Tobacco Taxation and Prices

Despite WHO recommendationsthat tobacco products should be taxed at 70% of the retail price, Namibia places only 30% levies on tobacco products, hence below the recommendations.

Enforcing the Tobacco Product Control Act

The Tobacco Product Control Act No. 1 of (2010) provides for the appointment of inspectors appointed by the MoHSS to inspect and give fines to corporate organizations or individual found to contravene the act on advertising andthe sale of counterfeit and contraband products. In addition, the Act allows any member of the public to lay charges in writing against any person who smokes in public places,leading to investigation and prosecution. This practice is supported by many countries namely Australia and India (van der Sterren, Greenhalgh, Knoche, &Winstanley, 2019).

Dangerous Chemicals in Tobacco Smoke

Hazardous chemical components in tobacco smoke include the following:

1. **Tar**: This is a sticky brown, solid particle in the cigarette smoke containing chemicals which include carcinogens. It is one of the main causes of lung cancer (Better Health Channel, 2019).
2. **Carbon Monoxide**: This isa colourless, odourless poisonous gas. When inhaled in large amounts,carbon monoxide can cause death as it replaces oxygen particles in the blood, leading to cyanosis.
3. **Oxidising Chemicals**: These are highly reactive chemicals capable of damaging the smoker's heart muscles and blood vessels. Their reaction with cholesterol can cause fatty material to build up in the arterial walls, leading to heart disease, stroke and diseases of the blood vessels.
4. **Metals**: Tobacco smoke contains metals such as arsenic, beryllium, cadmium, chromium, cobalt, lead and nickel, which have the potential to cause cancer.
5. **Radioactive Compounds:** These compounds are known to be carcinogens (Better Health Channel, 2019).

EFFECTS OF SMOKING ON THE BODY

The inhalation of cigarette/tobacco smoke damages many organs and systems in the body.

Effects of Smoking on the Respiratory System

Continuous smoking destroys the tiny, brush-like cells called "cilia" lining the airways, which are responsible for sweeping out mucous and dirt, thus keeping the lungs clear (Benjamin, 2010). This explains why smokers usually cough frequently. Other damage include the following:

1. **Reduction of Lung Function and Lack of Breath as a Result of Swelling**: The narrowing of the airways of the lung and excessive mucous.
2. **Malfunctioning of the Clearance System of the Lungs**: This leads to the accumulation of poisonous substances, causing irritation and damage to the lungs.
3. **An Increase in the Risk of Lung Infections and Cancer**: Tobacco smoke causes damage to the DNA, leading to abnormal growth of lung cells which results in cancerous tumours.
4. **Smoking Causes Lung Diseases which Include:**
    a. Chronic obstructive pulmonary disease (COPD)
    b. Emphysema,which is characterised by a loss of ability of the walls between the alveoli in the lungs to stretch and shrink back.

c. Chronic bronchitis, which refers to the inflammation of the inner layer of the bronchial tubes, resulting in a low flow of air to and from the lungs (Benjamin, 2010).

Figure 1. Effects of smoking on the respiratory system
Source: CDC (2019)

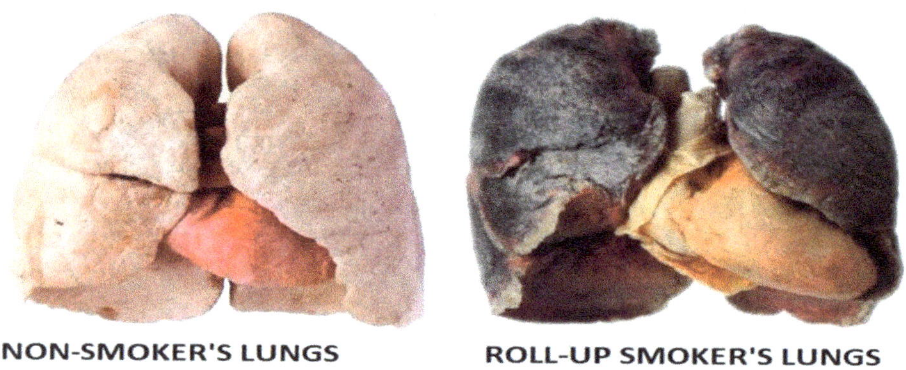

Effects of Smoking on the Cardiovascular System

Inhaling tobacco smoke is likely to alter the blood chemistry, resulting in damage to the blood vessels. After inhaling tobacco smoke, the cells lining the blood vessels in the body react to the poisonous tobacco smoke. As a result, the smoker's heart rate and blood pressure increase because the blood vessels thicken and grow narrower (Benjamin, 2010). Further related cardiovascular problems resulting from smoking include:

1. Vasocontraction of blood vessels in the skin, leading to a drop-in skin temperature.
2. Low oxygen carried by the blood during exercise.
3. Reduced blood flow to the extremities.
4. Increased risk of stroke and heart attack as a result of blockages of the blood supply (Better Health Channel, 2019).

Effects of Smoking on the Gastrointestinal System

Smoking is believed to increase the smoker's risk of cancers of the mouth, oesophagus, stomach and pancreas. Additionally, researchers have suggested that smoking may also enhance the risk of liver cancer, colon cancer and cancer of the rectum.

Figure 2. Heart effect of smoking
Source: CDC (2019)

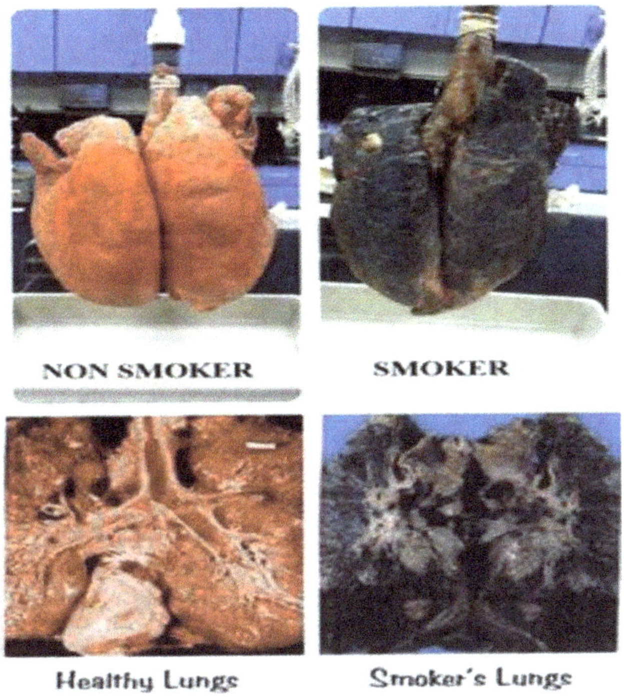

Figure 3. Oral effects of smoking
Source: CDC (2019)

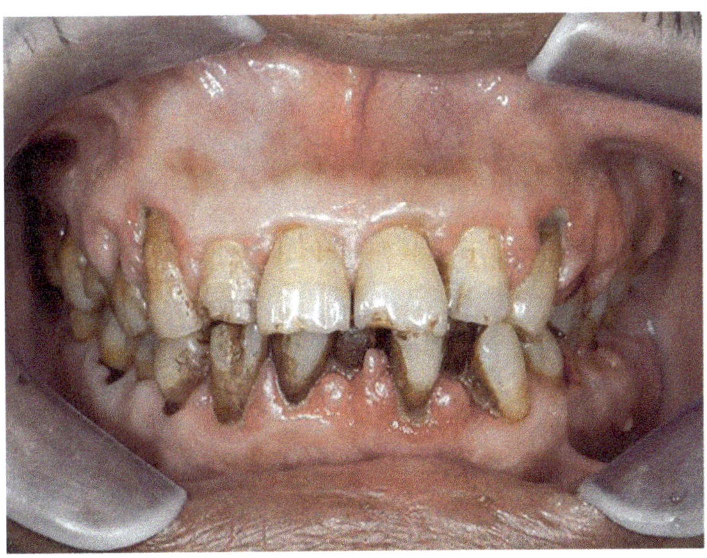

1. Smoking causes irritation (resulting in peptic ulcers) and inflammation of the stomach and the intestines (Li at al., 2014).
2. Minimises the ability to smell and taste.
3. Increases the risk of gum disease (Better Health Channel, 2019).

Effects of Smoking on the Immune System

1. Smoking increases the susceptibility to infections, e.g. pneumonia and influenza.
2. Causes more severe and longer-lasting infection.
3. Decreases the level of protective antioxidants (e.g. vitamin C) in the blood (Better Health Channel, 2019).

Effects of Smoking on the Musculoskeletal System

1. Smoking causes the tightening of certain muscles in the body.
2. Reduces bone density (Better Health Channel, 2019).

Effects of Smoking on the Male Sexual Organs

1. Smoking causes low sperm count in men which may lead to reduced fertility.
2. Results in increased percentage of deformed sperm.
3. Causes genetic damage to sperm (Better Health Channel, 2019).

Effects of Smoking on the Female Sexual Organs

Smoking can make it harder for a woman to become pregnant. It can also affect the baby's health before and after birth. In addition, tobacco smoke endangers the tissues of the unborn baby's growing brain and lungs. When a pregnant mother smokes, there are believed to be challenges to placental growth thus increasing the risk of:

1. Preterm (early) delivery
2. Stillbirth (death of the baby before birth)
3. Low birth weight
4. Cleft palate and cleft lip
5. Sudden infant death syndrome (known as SIDS or crib death)
6. Ectopic pregnancy
7. Attention deficit hyperactivity disorder (ADHD) (US Department of Health and Human Services, 2010)

Smoking increases the risk of stroke and heart attacks in women over the age of 35 years and those taking oral contraceptive pills.

SOLUTIONS AND RECOMMENDATIONS

This chapter recommends that:

1. There is a need for more society education aiming to create more awareness on smoking in general as well as the physical and physiological effects of smoking on the body.
2. With an escalated risk of exposure to second-hand smoke, strict measures have to be employed to reinforce the rules and regulation on handling and utilization of tobacco smoking as per the Tobacco Product Control Act No.1 (2010).
3. Many Smokers need to be educated on the strategies they can employ to quit smoking as well as ways that they can follow in order to deal with addiction.

CONCLUSION

In this chapter, smoking was defined as the inhaling, exhaling and holding or otherwise having control over an ignited tobacco product. The nicotine in tobacco smoke causes the release of dopamine, which results in pleasant feelings, thus causing recurrent smoking behaviour which in turn contributes to addiction. Exposure to second-hand smoke may be even more dangerous than inhaling mainstream smoke.Tobacco smoke contains various harmful substances including carcinogens which affect almost every system in the body. Despite the difficulty associated with quitting smoking, there are several strategies that one can employ to quit smoking.The effectiveness of the strategies will depend on the availability of information to the population at risk.

REFERENCES

Amakali, K., Haoses-Gorases, L., & Taukuheke, L. (2013). Tobacco smoking among University of Namibia students: Behaviours, reasons, attitudes, awareness and knowledge of associated health risks. *Online Journal of Medicine and Medical Science Research*, *2*(3), 30–37.

American Lung Association. (2019). Be prepared for challenges when quiting smoking. Retrieved from https://www.lung.org/stop-smoking/i-want-to-quit/be-prepared-for-challenges.html

Antolin-Fontes, B., Ables, J. L., Görlich, A., & Ibañez-Tallon, I. (2015). *The habenulo-interpeduncular pathway in nicotine aversion and withdrawal*. Neuropharmacology, *96*(Pt. B), 213–222.

Ashalata, P. R., & Deepa, G. (2015). *Textbook of Anatomy and Physiology for Nurses* (4th ed.). New Delhi, India: Jaypee Brothers Medical Publishers.

Aubin, H. J., Luquiens, A., & Berlin, I. (2013). Pharmacotherapy for smoking cessation: Pharmacological principles and clinical practice. *British Journal of Clinical Pharmacology*, *77*(2), 324–336. doi:10.1111/bcp.12116 PMID:23488726

Benjamin, R. M. (2010). *A Report of the Surgeon General: How tobacco smoke causes disease*. CDC. Retrieved from https://www.cdc.gov/tobacco/data_statistics/sgr/2010/consumer_booklet/pdfs/consumer.pdf

Better Health Channel. (2019). *Smoking – effects on your body*. Retrieved from https://www.betterhealth.vic.gov.au/healthyliving/smoking-effects-onyour-body

Burguet, A., Kaminski, M., Abraham-Lerat, L., Schaal, J. P., Cambonie, G., Fresson, J., ... Larroque, B. (2004). The complex relationship between smoking in pregnancy and very preterm delivery. Results of the Epipage study. *BJOG*, *111*(3), 258–265. doi:10.1046/j.1471-0528.2003.00037.x PMID:14961888

Festinger, L. (1962). *A theory of cognitive dissonance*. Stanford, CA: Stanford University Press.

German Technical Cooperation. (2009). *Health and wellness: Peer educator handbook*.

Hagger, M. S., Leaver, E., Esser, K., Leung, C. M., Pas, N. T., Keatley, D. A., ... Chatzisarantis, N. L. D. (2013). Cue-induced urges deplete cigarette smoker's selfcontrol resources. *Annals of Behavioral Medicine*, *46*(3), 394–400. doi:10.100712160-013-9520-8 PMID:23720186

Hammond, M. (2005). First Nations of Quebec and Labrador Health and Social Services Commission. (2005). *Healing from smoking*. Retrieved from https://www.nicotinedependenceclinic.com/English/teach/SiteAssets/Pages/Special-Populations/Healing%20From%20Smoking.pdf

Kahiurika, N. (2019). *Tobacco plant approval draws criticism.* The Namibian Newspaper. Retrieved from https://www.namibian.com.na/189733/archive-read/Tobacco-plant-approval-draws-criticism

Laureate. (2014). *Smoking kills so why do people do it.* (Pt. 2).

Li, L. F., Chan, R. L. Y., Lu, L., Shen, J., Zhang, L., Wu, W. K. K., ... Cho, C. H. (2014). Cigarette smoking and gastrointestinal diseases: The causal relationship and underlying molecular mechanisms [Review]. *International Journal of Molecular Medicine, 34*(2), 372–380. doi:10.3892/ijmm.2014.1786 PMID:24859303

MacArthur, C., Knox, E. G., & Lancashire, R. J. (2001, January). Effects at age nine of maternal smoking in pregnancy: Experimental and observational findings. *BJOG, 108*(1), 67–73. doi:10.1111/j.1471-0528.2001.00006.x PMID:11213007

Marufu, C. T., Ahankari, A., Coleman, T., & Lewis, S. (2015). Maternal smoking and the risk of still birth: Systematic review and meta-analysis. *BMC Public Health, 15*(239), 1–15. doi:10.118612889-015-1552-5 PMID:25885887

Middleton, L., & Uys, L. (2014). *Mental Health Nursing: A South African Perspective* (6th ed.). Cape Town: Juta&Co.Ltd.

Ministry of Health and Social Services. (2010). *National policy for mental health.* Windhoek, Namibia.

Morojele, N. K., Brook, J. S., & Brook, D. W. (2016). Tobacco and Alcohol Use Among Adolescents in South Africa: Shared and Unshared Risks. *Journal of Child and Adolescent Mental Health, 28*(2), 139–152. doi:10.2989/17280583.2016.1200586 PMID:27562001

Mychasiuk, R., Muhammad, A., Carroll, C., & Kolb, B. (2013). Does prenatal nicotine exposure alter the brain's response to nicotine in adolescence? A neuroanatomical analysis. *The European Journal of Neuroscience, 38*(4), 2491–2503. doi:10.1111/ejn.12245 PMID:23679187

Naikaku.EN. (2018). *Knowledge, attitudes and practices of medical doctors on pharmacotherapy for smoking cessation in Khomas region, Namibia. Master in Public Health.* Windhoek: University of Namibia.

Namibia Tobacco Control Policies. (2006). Retrieved from https://www.tobaccocontrollaws.org/legislation/fakctsheet/policy_status/namibia

New Era Newspaper. (2015). Call for more alcoholism rehab Centres. Etrieved from https://neweralive.na/posts/calls-alcoholism-rehab-centres

Perkins, K. A., Conklin, C. A., & Levine, M. D. (2008). *Cognitive-behavioural therapy for smoking cessation:A practical guidebook to the most effective treatments*. New York, NY: Routledge.

Pollock, J. D., Koustova, E., Hoffman, A., Shurtleff, D., & Volkow, N. D. (2009). Treatments for nicotine addiction should be a top priority. *Lancet, 374*(9689), 513–514. doi:10.1016/S0140-6736(09)60352-4 PMID:19394686

Reddy, P., Zuma, K., Shisana, O., Jonas, K., & Sewpaul, R. (2015). Prevalence of tobacco use among adults in South Africa: Results from the first South African National Health and Nutrition Examination Survey. *SAMJ: South African Medical Journal., 105*(8), 648. doi:10.7196/SAMJnew.7932 PMID:26449697

Siddiqi, K. (2019). Tobacco Use in Sub-Saharan Africa: The Risks and Challenges. *Nicotine & Tobacco Research: Official Journal of the Society for Research on Nicotine and Tobacco, 21*(8), 1–4. doi:10.1093/ntr/ntz086 PMID:31112602

Silva, L. C. C. D., Araújo, A. J. D., Queiroz, Â. M. D. D., Sales, M. D. P. U., & Castellano, M. V. C. D. O. (2016). Smoking control: challenges and achievements. *Journal Brasilileiro de Pneumologia. 42*(4), 290-298. doi:10.1590/S1806-37562016000000145

Siu, A. L. (2015). Behavioral and Pharmacotherapy Interventions for Tobacco Smoking Cessation in Adults, Including Pregnant Women: U.S. Preventive Services Task Force Recommendation Statement. *Annals of Internal Medicine, 2015*(163), 622–634. doi:10.7326/M15-2023 PMID:26389730

Stead, L. F., Perera, R., Bullen, C., Mant, D., & Lancaster, T. (2008). *Nicotine replacement therapy for smoking cessation (Review)*. Oxford, UK: John Wiley & Sons; doi:10.1002/14651858

Stoll, D. J. (2015). *Running head: A biopsychosocial analysis of smoking*.

Tam, J., & van Walbeek, C. (2013). Tobacco control in namibia: The importance of government capacity, Media coverage and industry interference. *Tobacco Control, 23*. doi:10.1136/tobaccocontrol-2012-050725 PMID:23788605

The Royal Australian College of General Practitioners. (2011). *Supporting smoking cessation: A guide for health professionals*. Retrieved from https://www.racgp.org.au/download/documents/Guidelines/smoking-cessation.pdf

Thomas, M. 2018. Over half a million children in India are smoking cigarettes everyday. Retrieved from https://qz.com/india/1232112/indias-cigarette-smoking-epidemic-includes-over-600000-addicted-children/

Tobacco Product Control Act. (2010). Republic of Namibia. Government printer. Retrieved from https://www.tobaccocontrollaws.org/files/live/Namibia/Namibia%20-%20Tobacco%20Products%20Control%20-%20national.pdf

Trading Economics. (2019).Namibian unemployment rate. Retrieved from: https://tradingeconomics.com/namibia/youth-unemployment-rate

US Department of Health and Human Services. (2010). *How tobacco smoke causes disease: What It means to you. Atlanta: US Department of Health and Human Services, Centers for Disease Control and Prevention, National Center for Chronic Disease Prevention and Health Promotion, Office on Smoking and Health, 2010*. Retrieved from: https://www.ncbi.nlm.nih.gov/books/NBK53017/pdf/Bookshelf_NBK53017.pdf

van der Sterren, A., Greenhalgh, E. M., Knoche, D., & Winstanley, M. H. (2019). 8.13 Policies for advancing tobacco control programs among Aboriginal and Torres Strait Islander peoples. In M.M. Scollo & M.H. Winstanley (Eds.), *Tobacco in Australia: Facts and issues*. Melbourne: Cancer Council Victoria. Retrieved from https://www.tobaccoinaustralia.org.au/chapter-8-aptsi/8-13-policy-recommendations-for-advancing-tobacco-

Wang, M. P., Ho, S. Y., & Lam, T. H. (2011). Parental smoking, exposure to second-hand smoke at home, and smoking initiation among young children. *Nicotine & Tobacco Research: Official Journal of the Society for Research on Nicotine and Tobacco*, *13*(9), 827–832. doi:10.1093/ntr/ntr083 PMID:21525153

West, R. (2017). Tobacco smoking: Health impact, prevalence, correlates and interventions. *Psychology & Health*, *32*(8), 1018–1036. doi:10.1080/08870446.2017.1325890 PMID:28553727

World Health Organization. (2001). *Encouraging people to stop smoking*. Department of Mental Health and Substance Dependence. Retrieved from https://www.who.int/mental_health/evidence/stop_smoking_whomsdmdp01_4.pdf

World Health Organization. (2011). *Wolrd report on disability*. Geneva. USA. Retrived from https://www.who.int/disabilities/worldreport/2011/en/

ADDITIONAL READING

George, T. P. (2016). *Nicotine and tobacco.Goldman-Cecil Medicine* (L. Goldman & A. I. Schafer, Eds., 25th ed.). Philadelphia, PA: Elsevier Saunders.

Shi, M., Christensen, K., Weinberg, C. R., Romitti, P., Bathum, L., Lozada, A., ... Murray, J. C. (2007). Orofacial cleft risk is increased with maternal smoking and specific detoxification-gene variants. *American Journal of Human Genetics*, *80*(1), 76–90. doi:10.1086/510518 PMID:17160896

Yolton, K., Dietrich, K., Auinger, P., Lanphear, B. P., & Hornung, R. (2005). Exposure to environmental tobacco smoke and cognitive abilities among U.S. children and adolescents. *Environmental Health Perspectives*, *113*(1), 98–103. doi:10.1289/ehp.7210 PMID:15626655

KEY TERMS AND DEFINITIONS

Addiction: A special type of dependence in which people have compulsive need to use the substance no matter what consequences are.

Carcinogen: Any substance or agent that causes cancer.

Craving: Some of the subjective experience/behaviour experienced by individuals who abuse or are dependent on drugs, alcohol or smoking.

Nicotine Replacement Therapy (NRT): A smoking ceasation treatment in which nicotine from tobacco is replaced for a limited period by pharmaceutical nicotine.

Passive smoking: Inhaling other people's second-hand tobacco smoke.

Rehabilitation: A set of measures that aimed towards assisting individuals who is experiencing a negative life experience to achieve and maintain optimal function in interaction with the surrounding environment.

Vasoconstriction: Spasm or temporaly narrowing of blood vessels.

Withdrawal: The removal of nicotine from the body.

Section 5
Diabetes

Chapter 7
Diabetes:
Biopsychosocial Features Affecting Metabolic Control and Treatment Adherence

Fabian Miller
https://orcid.org/0000-0002-5821-1711
Faculty of Education, Mico University College, Jamaica

Melisa Anderson
Department of Pathology, Faculty of Medical Sciences, The University of the West Indies at Mona, Kingston, Jamaica

Dwayne Tucker
https://orcid.org/0000-0002-5241-6441
Department of Pathology, Faculty of Medical Sciences, The University of the West Indies at Mona, Kingston, Jamaica

Kurt Vaz
Department of Pathology, Faculty of Medical Sciences, The University of the West Indies at Mona, Kingston, Jamaica

Jabari Brown
Department of Pathology, Faculty of Medical Sciences, The University of the West Indies at Mona, Kingston, Jamaica

Lennox Anderson-Jackson
Department of Pathology, Faculty of Medical Sciences, The University of the West Indies at Mona, Kingston, Jamaica

Donovan Anthony McGrowder
Department of Pathology, Faculty of Medical Sciences, The University of the West Indies at Mona, Kingston, Jamaica

DOI: 10.4018/978-1-7998-2139-7.ch007

ABSTRACT

Worldwide diabetes mellitus affects millions of individuals. Diabetes mellitus presents biopsychosocial challenges for diabetic patients and their families. Psychological and sociocultural issues that affect individuals with Type 1 and Type 2 diabetic patients negatively impact self-management activities aimed at attaining metabolic control and prevents future diabetic complications such as retinopathy, nephropathy, and cerebrovascular diseases. There is increasing evidence that diabetes mellitus is associated with a number of psychological and psychiatric conditions. This review addresses the distinctive biological, psychological, and sociocultural factors such as social support, socioeconomic status and family interaction encountered by diabetic patients. Recommendations are provided that can enhance diabetic care and include improving current screening of psychological conditions as well as treatment practices. There is also the need for more support from family, friends and medical staff in addressing sociocultural issues that impede favorable diabetes management.

INTRODUCTION

According to the International Diabetes Federation statistics, the global prevalence of diabetes mellitus recorded in 2017 is 8.8% (95% confidence interval 7.2-11.3%) among adults in the age group 20 – 79 years (IDF, 2017). This is equivalent to 424.9 million of persons with diabetes mellitus globally. By the year 2045, the global prevalence of diabetes mellitus in the 20 – 79 age group is likely to further increase to 9.9% (95% CI 7.5-12.7%); equivalent to 628.6 million persons with diabetes mellitus globally (IDF, 2017; NCD Risk Factor Collaboration, 2016). In an earlier report the global age-standardized prevalence of diabetes mellitus in males increased from 4.3% in 1980 to 9.0% in 2014 in the 20 – 79 age group, and 5.0% to 7.9% in females (IDF, 2017). Further, the IDF Atlas approximates that globally another 352.1 million persons have impaired glucose tolerance (IGT) which is expected to increase to 531.6 million in 2045 (IDF, 2017; NCD Risk Factor Collaboration, 2016).

The prevalence of diabetes mellitus have increased faster in low- and middle-income countries compared with high-income countries with the greatest rise observed in the Eastern Mediterranean Region value of 13.7% (NCD Risk Factor Collaboration, 2016). The increase in prevalence of diabetes mellitus is due to a number of factors such as growth in population, ageing, and increased global obesity (Seshasai et al., 2011).

Diabetes mellitus has been recognized as a heterogeneous disorder associated with varying etiology and clinical manifestations. It encompasses pathogenic processes such as insulin deficiency attributable to autoimmune attack of pancreatic beta-cells, impaired insulin secretion and insulin resistance. The diagnostic classification of the disease is largely dependent on glycemic thresholds associated with microvascular complications (Punthakee et al., 2018). There are two main categories of diabetes: type 1 and type 2 diabetes mellitus.

Type 1diabetes mellitus is one of the most prevalent childhood diseases, although it can affect individuals across different age ranges. It encompasses T-cell mediated destruction of insulin producing pancreatic beta-cells resulting in deficient beta-cell mass, insulin deficiency and elevated blood glucose levels (Punthakee et al., 2018). The disease is also characterized by impaired pancreatic alpha-cell function and elevated peripheral glucagon which exacerbates the metabolic complications of insulin resistance (Ozougwu et al., 2013). Genetic, immunologic and environmental factors are the main etiological forces driving the disease (Mouri and Badireddy, 2019).

Type 2 diabetes mellitus is a progressive polygenic disorder characterized by diminished beta-cell insulin secretory capacity and impaired target tissue response to insulin (Lee and Halter, 2017). As such, insulin resistance and impaired beta-cell function are hallmarks of the disease. Type 2 diabetes mellitus often accounts for an estimated 90% of all diabetes cases and is typically manifested at later stages in life, even though there is evidence of increased occurrence in younger age groups (Bansal et al., 2017). It is well established that many genetic variants increase the risk for type 2 diabetes mellitus.

The chronic hyperglycemic milieu associated with diabetes mellitus results in long term adverse microvascular complications including peripheral neuropathy, nephropathy and retinopathy; and increases the risk for cardiovascular diseases (Punthakee et al., 2018).It was recently reported that a multifactorial treatment approach can be taken to circumvent deleterious complications in type 1 and type 2 diabetes (Imran et al, 2018). Notably, if there is stringent glycemic control with HbA1c values of $< 7.0\%$ alongside the prevention of hypoglycemia and glucose variability (Imran et al., 2018). The American and Canadian Diabetes Associations recommended less stringent glycemic target for diabetics with other co-morbidities and elderly patients (Coons et al., 2016). It is therefore reasonable to suggest that an individualized approach may be necessary to establish efficient glycemic control.

BACKGROUND

Diabetes mellitus is a chronic, multifaceted and demanding disease that causes serious psychological stress, which impede a patient's aptitude to adequately self-manage the condition. Psychological and other types of stress interrupts glycemic control by its effect on hormones such as cortisol and catecholamine (Hilliard et al., 2016). Further, the disease negatively affects the quality of life of patients as it dictates interaction in a multi-dimensional and recurring manner among biological, behavioral, psychological, social and cultural factors (Chew et al., 2014).

Diabetes mellitus has a negative impact on the physical health of patient, and it affects relationship with family and/or friends. Persons with diabetes mellitus require psychological support from the time of diagnosis to the remainder of their lives. Psychosocial seeks to report the emotional, psychological and/or mental, emotional and spiritual factors that influence health (Penckofer et al., 2014). The patient's ability to be engaged in self-management behaviors in a constant manner as well as gain in medical treatment will result in significant clinical outcomes as a result of improved and maintained glycemic control (Shrivastava et al., 2013). It is important that patients adhere to the prescribed therapies so as to maintain optimal control of the disease, prevention of diabetes-related problems and an acceptable quality of life, thus reducing the load on healthcare systems (Stetson et al., 2017).

The successful management of diabetes mellitus involves multiple factors and therefore a biopsychosocial approach to its management is critical in order to attaining improved and sustained patient health outcomes (Stolar, 2010). Research have shown that adherence to treatment leads to preserving tight blood glucose control which can prevent or delay the development of some of the severe long-term complications of diabetes mellitus (Borus and Laffel, 2910). However, even though the literature is clear concerning the benefits of treatment adherence, there is low rate of adherence to treatment resulting in significant economic challenges as well as compromised health status (Tiv et al., 2012).

Biopsychosocial variables comprise of social support, socioeconomic status, family interaction, job status, complications of diabetes mellitus, marital status, negative life events, anxiety, depression and other psychiatric conditions (Polonsky and Henry, 2016). The chapter will focus on the biopsychological aspects of how patients cope with diabetes mellitus particularly their emotional health, self-regulation, cognition, behavior and self-efficacy. Psychological aspects such as anxiety, depression, eating disorder, unhealthy behaviors in relation to glycemic control in patients diagnosed with type 1 and 2 diabetes mellitus will be explored. Relevant research findings on sociocultural factors including social support, socioeconomic, physical activity and family interaction are covered. The chapter concludes by citing future research where biopsychosocial models of diabetes mellitus can give further insight on how these factors affect individuals with the disease.

MAIN FOCUS OF THE CHAPTER

This section examines the main core issues of this chapter as mentioned in the introduction. In this section the psychological aspects such as anxiety, depression, eating disorder, unhealthy behaviors in relation to glycemic control in patients diagnosed with type 1 and 2 diabetes mellitus are explored and discussed at length. Sociocultural factors including social support, socioeconomic status, physical activity and family interaction and their impact on clinical outcomes and well-being of patients are also discussed.

PSYCHOLOGICAL ASPECT AND HOW THESE AFFECT GLYCAEMIC CONTROL AND CLINICAL OUTCOMES

Over the last two decades there is increased interest and evidence of the comorbidity of chronic health conditions such as diabetes mellitus and mental disorders. Compared with other chronic illnesses type 2 and type 1 diabetes mellitus are considered as two of the most psychologically challenging medical conditions in adult patients due to the pathophysiology of the disease, various etiology and different treatment regimens (Kruse et al., 2003). Increasingly diabetes mellitus is associated with psychosocial problems as the disease brings about changes in social functioning, changes in daily life routines, coping with recurrent symptoms, consistent taking of medication and economic cost related to managing the disease (Egede and Dismuke, 2012).

There are several disorders that affect the psychological faculties of diabetics and their ability to maintain optimal glycemic control. These include anxiety, depression, and eating disorders. These psychological challenges affect both type 1 and type 2 diabetics whether the age of disease onset is during childhood, adolescence, or adulthood (de Groot et al., 2016). Furthermore, Maia et al. reported a high prevalence of psychiatric disorders in both type 1 and type 2 diabetes mellitus from their study using the Mini International Neuropsychiatric Interview for the identification of psychiatric disorders. They found that 42.5% of diabetic patients experienced at least one psychiatric disorder which included anxiety, dysthymia, depression, panic disorder, social phobia, and risk of suicide (Maia et al., 2012).

Anxiety

Diabetes mellitus is more complicated with the coexistence of anxiety and depression which have been connected to increased somatic symptoms among persons with type 2 diabetes mellitus (Khan et al., 2019). Diabetic patients with anxiety disorders usually have poor outcomes compared with those without the psychiatric disorder

(Smith et al., 2013). In a meta-analysis of twelve studies of 12,626 adult subjects with diabetes mellitus, there was a 20% and 48% increased prevalence of anxiety disorders and anxiety symptoms respectively (Smith et al., 2013).

Diabetic patients with longer disease duration, of the female gender and other medical conditions are usually at higher risk of anxiety disorder. In a recent cross-sectional, observational study, the incidence of anxiety in type 2 diabetic patients was 50.7% and higher scores were statistically significant in individuals that were female, older, taking non-insulin treatment, longer duration of diabetes mellitus and those with nephropathy, neuropathy and foot ulcers (Khan et al., 2019). A lower prevalence of 16.0% was reported in a cross-sectional survey of 251 adult type 2 diabetic patients with females and individual with duration of diabetes greater than 5 years more likely to have anxiety (Zhao et al., 2018).

According to Grigsby and colleagues, the prevalence of elevated symptoms of anxiety is similar in both type I and type 2 diabetes (41.3% vs. 42.2%, $P = 0.80$), and higher in females compared to males (55.3% vs. 32.9%, $P < 0.0001$) (Grigsby et al., 2002). Furthermore, anxiety disorders are extremely persistent in individuals with diabetes mellitus as Fisher and colleagues found that for 506 type 2 diabetic patients assessed three times over 18 months, general anxiety disorder was 123% higher relative to community adults especially for younger adults and those of the female gender (Fisher et al., 2008).

Mental health illnesses such as anxiety and depression are prevalent in youth with type 1 diabetes, and the effects of anxiety symptoms are not well documented and understood. The prevalence of anxiety symptoms in youths with type 1 diabetes mellitus ranges from 13.0% to 21.3% with these individuals screened positive during childhood or adolescence (Rechenberg et al., 2018; Bernstein et al., 2013). Anxiety symptoms in patients with type 1 diabetes have been associated with decreased blood glucose monitoring rates, suboptimal glycemic control, conflict in family environment, increased diabetes related re-hospitalization and overall poorer quality of life (Bernstein et al., 2013). In a meta-analysis of 20 studies involving type 1 diabetic youths, anxiety symptoms have unfavorable effects on health outcomes and associated with worse self-management and coping behaviors, fear of hypoglycemia, reduced frequency of blood glucose monitoring and higher levels of glycosylated hemoglobin (HbA1c) (Rechenberg et al., 2017).

There are studies that have examined associations among anxiety and factors such as age, gender, quality of life and glycemic control in youths with type 1 diabetes mellitus. In one study of urban youth with poorly controlled type 1 diabetes, girls displayed greater anxiety than boys (Naar-King et al., 2006), while in another, girls exhibited worse metabolic control with average HbA1c levels 1.58% above that of boys (La Greca et al., 1995). Furthermore, girls diagnosed with trait anxiety were more likely to be concerned about hypoglycemic episodes than boys ($t = -2.45$,

$p < 0.02$) (Gonder-Frederick et al., 2006). In a study of adolescents with type 1 diabetes mellitus social anxiety was positively correlated with poor quality of life in both genders (girls, $r = 0.51$, $p < 0.01$; boys, $r = 0.54$, $p < 0.01$), reduced insulin adherence ($r = -0.39$, $p < 0.05$). The researchers suggested that the relationship between insulin adherence and social anxiety may be mediated by fear of hypoglycemia (Di Battista et al., 2009).

Research have found that fear of hypoglycemia suggests a history of hypoglycemic episodes. Also, fear of future episodes can contribute to heightened levels of stress and anxiety. Higher levels of problematic psychological functioning were linked with less frequent blood glucose monitoring and suboptimal glycemic control. Higher levels of anxiety symptoms contributed to deficient disease management and suboptimal glycemic outcomes (Herzer and Hood, 2010).

Other sources of anxiety include fear of self-care invasive procedures such as subcutaneous insulin infusion devices, finger pricks for glucose monitoring, and insulin needle injections. This subclinical symptom ultimately presents a barrier to continuous glycemic control in both type 1 and type 2 diabetics (de Groot et al., 2016). In their study of 150 children ranging from 6 to 17 years old, Cemeroglu and colleagues concluded that needle phobia is common in children with type 1 diabetes mellitus. The study further highlighted that "a more intense fear of needles was associated with higher HbA1c levels and less frequent glucose monitoring" (Cemeroglu et al., 2015).

Similarly, Bahrmann et al. states that fear of needles can also create a temporary barrier to continuous treatment compliance. This is especially evident in patients moving from oral to more self-invasive treatments, as well as in older adults with type 2 diabetes mellitus (Bahrmann et al., 2014). In their study, Bahrmann and colleagues emphasized that insulin-naive patients had higher psychological insulin resistance than patients who were already on insulin (Bahrmann et al., 2014). Therefore, this transitional period can facilitate a compromise in self-care behaviors which negatively impacts glycemic control (de Groot et al., 2016). The fear of needles may also impede site rotation. Diabetic patients on insulin treatment are usually advised to rotate injection sites to reduce subcutaneous scarring. Needle phobia may pose a hindrance to a smooth site rotation resulting in suboptimal insulin usage and diminished glycemic control (de Groot et al., 2016).

Depression

The burden of diabetes mellitus has serious psychological implications in patients, which ultimately affects how best they cope and self-manage the disease. This is highly due to the complex nature and the life-changing requirements that are important to successfully manage the disease long-term (Habtewold et al., 2016).

Furthermore, the encumbering life-changing requirements of living with diabetes mellitus can lead to depression and ultimately poor self-management of the disease (de Groot et al., 2016). It has being reported that epidemiologically 25% of patients with type 2 diabetes progresses to clinically significant depression (Semenkovich et al., 2015) and the prevalence is higher in females than males (Snoek et al., 2015).

A number of studies conducted mostly in developing countries have investigated the prevalence of depression in type 2 diabetic patients. There are reported prevalence values of 5.7% - 49.6% (Lee et al., 2017; Rodriquez et al., 2015; Zhang et al., 2015). Chew and colleagues investigated the prevalence of disease-related distress and depression among adults with type 2 diabetes in a primary care population in Malaysia. The prevalence of depression and depression-related disease in adults were 41.7% and 49.2% respectively. Patients with both disease-related distress and depression were four times more likely to be unemployed (OR 4.7, 95% CI: 1.02 - 21.20) while those with microvascular complications were more likely to be associated with depression (OR 1.4, 95% CI: 1.06 - 1.73) (Chew et al., 2016). The prevalence of depression was higher in a systematic randomized study conducted among 313 type 1 and type 2 patients in Ethiopia with 64.8% of type 2 and 62.6% of type 1 diagnosed with depression. The incidence of depression was higher in patients with the illness more than five years and lower than secondary school education (Erkie at al., 2003).

Researchers have examined the prevalence of depression among diabetic patients compared with the general populations. In a systematic review and meta-analysis of ten randomly controlled studies involving 51,331 persons, there was a prevalence of depression of 17.6% compared with 9.8% (OR = 17.6%, 95% CI: 1.2-2.0) (Ali et al., 2006). Similarly, in the meta-analysis of the European Depression in Diabetes (EDID) Research Consortium subjects with type 2 diabetes mellitus have an elevated risk of depression compared with those without the disease or with impaired glucose tolerance (OR 1.69, 95% CI: 1.37 - 2.08) (Nouwen et al., 2011). Furthermore, in a cohort study conducted in Taiwan of one million randomly selected persons, the incidence of depression in patients with diabetes mellitus was 1.80-times higher than in the non-diabetic subjects with a median follow-up of 6.5 years (Hsu et al., 2012).

Depressive symptoms are often connected to poor or inadequate glycemic control. There are studies that have examined the association between depression, glycemic control and psychosocial factors. In the study by Zhang and colleagues where the prevalence of depression in Chinese patients with type 2 diabetes mellitus was 5.7%, factors such as being single, low worth health insurance, low social support, high BMI and elevated HbA1c were associated with the presence of depression (Zhang et al., 2015).Conversely, in another study where the prevalence of depression was 16.8%, depression status was two or more times associated with infrequent inactivity (OR = 2.35, $p = 0.001$), lack of sleep (OR = 2.85, $p < 0.001$) and less frequent exercise (OR = 2.62, $p < 0.001$) (Lee et al., 2017). In a case control study of 109 type 2 diabetes patients and 91 healthy controls in a tertiary hospital, the prevalence of depression was 42.2% in the patients and 4.39% in the controls. The depression in the diabetic patients was strongly associated with poor glycemic control (Singh et al., 2014).

Several studies have reported an association between depressive symptoms and poorer glycemic control in both type 1 and type 2 diabetic patients (de Groot et al., 2016). The rates of depression are higher among type 2 diabetics with prescribed insulin compared to those using alternative medications or dietary and lifestyle interventions alone (de Groot et al., 2016). Depressed diabetics are less likely to adhere to therapeutic recommendations such as medical appointments, diet, exercise, and glucose monitoring, which lead to higher HbA1c levels due to a decline in proper self-management (de Groot et al., 2016). A study on Mexican-Americans showed that higher levels of depression and anxiety were found in diabetics than in most other chronic conditions. The study also reiterated the significant association between depression and anxiety with poorer self-management of the disease, and poorer glycemic control (Kendzor et al., 2014).

Depression is one of the most neglected symptoms in diabetic patients and is directly linked with lowering of quality of life (Zanoveli et al., 2016).A Cameroonian study using the Centre for Epidemiological Studies Depression Scale (CES-D) established that clinically significant depressive symptoms (CES-D>16) were found in 60% of patients with poorer glycemic scores (HbA1C >7.0%) (Hall et al., 2017). Moreover, the study highlighted that diabetic-related depressive symptoms had significant gender associations. Females with diabetes mellitus are more prone to depression than males. In this particular study, Cameroonian females experienced higher levels of depressive symptoms than their male counterparts (Hall et al., 2017). This finding corresponded with other studies such as one involving Hispanic Americans in which depression was more prevalent in female diabetics than in males (Kendzor et al., 2014). Nonetheless, in their meta-analysis, de Groot et al. adds that a long-term history of major depressive disorder continues to confer risk for worse outcomes years and even decades later including worse glycemic control and other physiological impairments (de Groot et al., 2016).

Knowledge of the diagnosis and the burden to manage the condition are associated with depressive symptoms(Holt et al., 2014). Gonzalez-Zacarias et al. (2016) shares a similar view that patients who know that they are diabetic have higher prevalence of depression compared to those that do not know.Studies have also shown that depressive states in diabetics hinder their problem-solving skills. Hills-Briggs and Gemmell reported consistent associations between problem solving and HbA1c levels in their 2007 report. The report highlighted that impaired problem solving skills is associated with poor metabolic control in persons with diabetes mellitus(Hill-Briggs and Gemmell, 2007). The outcome from this study also suggested that diabetic patients may benefit from intervention programs for depression as 50% of the studies reviewed in the meta-analysis showed improved HbA1c levels post-intervention (Hill-Briggs and Gemmell, 2007).

It is observed that a combination of diabetes mellitus and depression has been connected with diabetes-related morbidity and mortality (Zagarins et al., 2012). Almeida et al. demonstrated in a group of elderly men that the risk of developing depression progressively increased depending on the years that the patient becomes aware of the diagnosis (Almeida et al., 2016). Although it cannot be concluded that adjustment in diabetes-related distress is directly linked to the change in HbA1c, it was observed that a short-term decline in diabetes-related distress is associated with a sustained reduction in HbA1c (Zagarins et al., 2012).

Eating Disorder

Disordered eating behaviorsand eating disorders characterize a range of symptoms that may include distorted body image, constrained caloric intake, binge eating and/or purging behaviors such as vomiting, unnecessary exercise and the use of laxatives to lose weight (American Psychiatric Association, 2013). These behaviors correlate with decreased adherence to self-care behaviors and a negative impact on glycemic control (de Groot et al., 2016).The majority of studies usually involve women and adolescents (ages 15-35 years old) with type 1 diabetes mellitus at a period in their lives when there are weight concerns and when eating disorders and disordered eating behaviors are more likely to be prevalent (Mannucci et al., 2005). In the last two decades, there are reports of studies in the area involving male patients and those with type 2 diabetes mellitus (Mannucci et al., 2002).

Disordered eating behaviors and eating disorders are frequent among type 1and type 2 diabetics and are associated with worse metabolic and psychological outcomes (Young et al., 2013; Nicolau et al., 2015). Estimates of diagnosable disordered eating behaviorsand eating disorders in adolescent and young adult females with type 1 diabetes vary. Diagnostics interviews and self-reported questionnaires are used to determine the prevalence of disordered eating behaviors and eating disorders in individuals with type 1 and type 2 diabetes mellitus. In a meta-analysis of 13 studies of type 1 diabetic patients, there was a prevalence of 51.8% for

disordered eating behavior compared to 48.1% in non-diabetic peers, and as high as 6.4% for eating disorders using diabetes-adapted measures (Young et al., 2013). There were lower values observed in a large multisite case-controlled study where the prevalence of disordered eating behaviors (as defined by Diagnostic and Statistical Manual of Mental Disorders criteria) was 6.4% in type 2 diabetic patients compared to 3.0% in non-diabetes individuals using diabetes-adapted measures(Rodin et al., 2002).

Disordered eating behaviors and eating disorders are more prevalent among adolescent females who generally possess a greater concern regarding body size, weight and shape, and exhibit higher frequencies of global eating disorder psychopathologies. Therefore, eating disorders such as anorexia nervosa, bulimia nervosa, binge eating/ purging, excessive exercising, and starvation occur more often among adolescent girls with diabetes mellitus. Naturally, these girls are noted as having poorer glycemic control and a greater risk for comorbidities (Wisting et al., 2017). A four year follow-up study demonstrated that the presence of disordered eating behaviors is related to a threefold elevation in the risk of diabetic retinopathy, poor diabetes management and impaired family functioning (Rodin et al., 2002).

Body fat increases during puberty as self-consciousness which accompanies this developmental change raises the risk of disordered eating behaviors and eating disorders in females with type 1 diabetes mellitus and ultimately compromises their self-management of the disease (Young et al., 2013; Racicka & Brynska, 2015; Wisting et al., 2017). Insulin omission or under-administration is sometimes employed by these females in an effort to lose weight (Young et al., 2013). In addition to the risk of hyperglycemia in these instances, lowered or skipped insulin doses can result in diabetic ketoacidosis leading to coma and even death (de Groot et al., 2016). The result of poor glycemic control due to suboptimal insulin management also increases the risk for complications such as nephropathy, retinopathy and premature death (Racicka and Brynska, 2015).

There is less information in the literature on the association between type 2 diabetes and eating disorders as well as investigating the prevalence rates. The prevalence of binge eating disorder in 152 type 2 diabetic adult patients using a Structured Clinical Interview for DSM-IV Axis I Disorder, Clinical Version in terms of eating disorders was 5.6% (Celik et al., 2015). In another study Nicolau and colleagues investigate the frequency of positive screening for binge eating disorder in 320 type 2 diabetes subjects and reported prevalence of 14.0% (using Eating Attitudes Test-26) (Nicolau et al., 2015).

SOCIOCULTURAL FACTORS AND HOW THESE AFFECT GLYCAEMIC CONTROL AND CLINICAL OUTCOMES

Social Support and Family Interaction

The main support for patients with diabetes mellitus is family which assisted in ways such as emotional, information and instrumental. Social support from family can have a positive impact of diabetes self-management or act as barrier to disease management and glycemic control (Hu et al., 2013). Social support is a key prognosticator of outcomes in type 1 and type 2 diabetes mellitus (Strom and Egede, 2012). Social support from family, friends and healthcare providers is associated with increased physical activity and fitness (Keyserling et al., 2002); better metabolic control therefore lower HbA1c levels (Trento et al., 2001), better clinical outcomes (Strom and Egede, 2012), and lower diabetes-related distress (Baek et al., 2014). Walker and colleagues in using a structured equation modeling reported that higher social support ($r = 0.14$, $P = 0.01$) was significantly associated with diabetes self-care whilst lower social support ($r = 0.10$, $P = 0.02$) significantly correlated to lower glycemic control (Walker et al., 2015). However, studies have reported that social support was not related to metabolic control (Westaway et al., 2005; Trief et al., 1998).

Habtewold and colleagues examine possible underlying factors related biopsychosocial risk factors in type 2 diabetic patients who presented with depressive symptoms. Biopsychosocial variables such as diabetic complication, marital status, occupation, negative event in the last six months and poor social support considerably elevate the average depressive symptoms score (Habtewold et al., 2016). Others studies such as Zhang et al., 2015 reported the association of low social support and health insurance with the presence of depression (Zhang et al., 2015) and inverse association between depression and social support (OR 0.978; 95% CI: 0.963 - 0.993) in a prospective cohort study of 592 type 2 diabetic patients from the Madrid Diabetes Study (Salinero-Fort et al., 2018). In an earlier study conducted in Southern Taiwan, social support was negative correlated with depression (Wu, 2013). Furthermore, satisfaction with social support was a predictor for enhanced diabetes-specific quality of life and diabetes-related health behaviors among African Americans with type 2 diabetes mellitus ($r = -.579$, $P < .001$) (Tang et al., 2008).

There is a growing body of evidence which indicate that social support is vital to assist patients in coping with diabetes mellitus and improving treatment adherence (Ramkisson et al., 2017). In a cross-sectional study of 253 poorly controlled diabetic patients, those who had an informal caregiver and received social support were significantly more likely to indicate moderate or high medication adherence (OR = 1.93, 95% CI: 1.07-3.49, $p = 0.028$) (Bouldin et al., 2017). Support from family members has been instrumental as a major source of support and plays a critical part in disease management and lifestyle changes (Goetz et al., 2012). Low social support significantly influenced the observed low physical activity in type 2 diabetic patients. A study by Adeniyi and colleagues reported that patients with low social support were approximately four time more likely to display poor physical activity (OR=3.95, 95% CI: 3.13-5.24; Adeniyi et al., 2012). Therefore psychosocial supports through kind and empathetic family, friends, health care experts, and even other patients with diabetes mellitus could impart an optimistic outlook, sense of resilience and wellbeing in patients with diabetes mellitus.

Children with type 1 diabetes mellitus have a multi-faceted treatment regimen that comprises dietary requirements and insulin therapy. Ongoing family supervision and support as well as healthy collaborative interaction and communication between parent and type 1 diabetic children in the management of diabetic care are crucial as children transition into adolescence (Jaser, 2011). It is also important to emphasize that in this collaborative effort parents need psychological support in managing their own distress in order to continue this type of participation (Jaser, 2011).

Socioeconomic Status

Socioeconomic status is a multifaceted construct determined by a person's or group's comparative position in terms of social and economic factors in relation to others in a society (Galobardes et al., 2006). The social and economic position of the individual may result in health inequality. Social economic status is most frequently measured by indicators such as financial wealth, income, occupational social class and education (Pollack et al., 2007).

Epidemiologic studies using a diversity of social economic status measures have reliable demonstrated that lower status is associated with poor metabolic control, psychological distress and poor health outcomes in adults with diabetes mellitus (Pan et al., 1997). Secrest and colleagues reported that type 1 diabetes patients with lowest household income had the highest prevalence of diabetic complications such as neuropathy and retinopathy, and poor metabolic control as exhibited by being less likely to achieve HbA1c less than 7.0% (Secrest et al., 2011). Also note that in a recent population-based cohort study of Scottish type 2 diabetic patients, gender and socioeconomic status were related with decreased life cardiovascular risk factors and changes in glycemic control (Collier et al., 2015).

There is a paucity of evidence examining the association between low socioeconomic status and diabetes management particularly morbidity. In a systematic and meta-analysis of 33 studies low socioeconomic status was concomitant with higher levels of morbidity and mortality in adult type 1 diabetic patients (Scott et al., 2017). In another study conducted by Berham and colleagues, low social economic status increased the risk of mortality in patients (Berhan et al., 2016). The differences in socioeconomic status of diabetic patients associated with mortality may be due to cardiovascular-related deaths particular those with type 1 diabetes mellitus (Roper et al., 2001). It should be noted that there are other studies that have found little or no role of social economic status in the mortality of individuals with diabetes mellitus compared with the general population (Rope et al., 2001; Gnavi et al., 2004).

Young adults and older adolescents with type 1 diabetes mellitus who are socioeconomic disadvantages may experience poor glycemic conditions and diabetes-related complications (Zilioli et al., 2017). Similarly, low socioeconomic status and type 1 diabetic patients who resides in socially deprived areas are associated with a greater risk of diabetic ketoacidosis (Linder et al., 2019). In a study by Hassan and colleagues involving subjects 8 - 17 years-old with type 1diabetes mellitus, 9.5% of subjects who were poorly controlled were depressed. There was a 27% elevation in the prospect of depression per unit increase in HbA1c while higher socioeconomic status was related to improved quality of life and glycemic control (Hassan et al., 2006). More so in the GP-OSMOTIC study of 300 type 2 diabetic patients, greater socioeconomic status was associated with better attainment of glycemic target as seen by lower HbA1c levels (Tan et al., 2018).

Physical Activity

There is a worldwide tendency toward a rise in the incidence of diabetes mellitus, particularly type 2 diabetes. The main treatment regimen for glycemic control in diabetes mellitus is pharmacotherapy, diet treatment and exercise therapy. The American Diabetes Association recommend individuals with type 2 diabetes to be engaged in moderate to intensity aerobic physical activity at least 150 minutes per week (50 -70% of maximum heart rate) to maximize the effects of physical activity(Association AD, 2011).Consistent physical activity aids to regulate normal glucose uptake into peripheral tissues, and increases the number of insulin receptors and insulin sensitivity resulting in blood glucose control(Camacho et al., 2005). High-intensity aerobic interval training of 38 type 2 diabetic patients over 12 weeks resulted in a decrease in HbA1c by 0.58% points and reduced risk factors associated with diabetes mellitus (Stoa et al., 2017). Similarly, Boule and colleagues found that post-intervention aerobic or resistance training could significantly decrease HbA1c levels (exercise group vs control: 7.65% vs 8.31%) by 0.66% (Boule et al., 2001).

Exercise in an active lifestyle management practice for the deterrence of type 2 diabetes mellitus, and for the management of both types of the disease. Studies have reported that factors affecting physical activity in diabetes mellitus patients comprised gender, age, body mass index, psychosocial factors, as well as environmental factors that are life- and health-related (Delahanty et al., 2006). Effective interventions in exercise therapy requires dealing with barriers to physical activity and promoting psychosocial factors such as social support, self-efficacy and behavioral modification (Van Dyck et al., 2011).

Self-efficacy is one of the psychosocial constructs that may impact physical activity behavior. An integrative review of the literature by Allen, found that self-efficacy was prognostic of exercise initiation and maintenance over time (Allen,

2004). Similarly, Dutton and colleagues reported that self-efficacy mediated physical activity one-month post-intervention among type 2 diabetes (Dutton et al., 2009). Recently a cross-sectional study of type 2 diabetic patients found that diabetes management self-efficacy was significantly related with receiving health education thus improved knowledge, high level of academic education, adherence to self-care activities and glycemic control (Amer et al., 2018). The researchers suggested that implementation of appropriate interventions could empower diabetic patients with self-efficacy and adherence to self-care activities (Amer et al., 2018).

Yoga exercise is gradually used as an adjunctive treatment in the management of type 2 diabetes mellitus. In a two-arm randomized clinical trial comprising of Iyengar yoga and a supervised walking program, yoga significantly reduced HbA1c by 1.25% 6-months post-intervention with improvements in quality of life, diabetes self-care and reduced emotional stress (Bock et al., 2019). Similarly, a meta-analysis and systematic review of the literature of eight studies comprising of 842 participants found that yoga intervention has beneficial effects on glycemic control reducing HbA1c levels by 0.39% (Jayawardena et al., 2018). However, there are conflicting results when the effects of exercise training on psychological outcomes such as emotional well-being were evaluated (van der Heijden et al., 2013). Therefore, in order to achieve better insight into the role of exercise training high quality randomized clinical trials involving both type 1 and type 2 diabetes mellitus patients could be conducted.

SOLUTIONS AND RECOMMENDATIONS

Large proportions of diabetic patients may experience psychiatric disorders for which they are currently not receiving treatment or support. The resulting effect of this is a poor adherence to treatment, monitoring and control of glycemic state. Considering the increasing epidemic of diabetes mellitus, populations may benefit from psychiatric evaluations to clinically diagnose psychiatric disorders as part of healthcare policies in the future. In this manner professionals can have greater insight as to how best patients are adjusting to the struggle of managing their disease. Furthermore, psychiatric disorders can be diagnosed sooner, and an appropriate course of treatment recommended. It is evident that creating social support/intervention programs for type 1 and type 2 diabetic patients may help to nurture good adherence to treatment and lifestyle changes that foster improved glycemic control. However, it is also important that these programs satisfy the needs of both type 1 and type 2 diabetic patients. Notably, it is important to closely monitor females and males with type 1 diabetes to assess them for eating disorders and disordered eating behaviors that may lead to behaviors which threaten their willingness and capacity to properly maintain good glycemic control.

Family members are encouraged to be intimately and integrally involved in the management of patients with both types of diabetes mellitus as this has been constantly concomitant with improved outcomes. Family members who are caregivers especially of adolescents should supervised diabetes-related task such as medication adherence, assist the patient to improve problem-solving skills and independence, encourage engage in healthy lifestyle behaviors, reduce family conflicts and seek assistance from a professional behavioral health provider when problems arises that they are unable to solve on their own.

FUTURE RESEARCH DIRECTIONS

In order guarantee a satisfactory quality of life, a multidimensional approach to managing diabetic patients should take into consideration the mental health of these persons and identify those at risk of developing depression, anxiety, or eating disorders. There is the need for evidence-based intervention centering on these recognized biopsychosocial factors that are essential to prevent the development of psychiatric disorders and improve the outcomes of patients with diabetes mellitus. There is a need for more in-depth study and greater accuracy in our understanding of the co-occurrence and interaction among social and psychological disorders affecting persons with type 1 and type 2 diabetes mellitus. Future research could examine the use of comprehensive biopsychosocial models of diabetes mellitus and related conditions which could yield some insight into the multifaceted and multidimensional conduits between the biopsychosocial factors affecting patients with diabetes mellitus and their quality of life, wellbeing and clinical outcomes.

The chapter also examines the beneficial effects of physical exercise such as aerobic and resistance training as well as yoga on glycemic control. However, there is substantial heterogeneity among studies and so there is the need for well-designed and well-controlled randomized trials which will allow the scientific community to draw appropriate conclusions about the effectiveness of physical exercise on health outcomes of patients with diabetes mellitus.

CONCLUSION

Diabetes mellitus is a chronic and challenging metabolic disorder which necessitates management on a daily basis and stringent adherence to treatment, diet and exercise. It is designated as a lifetime psychological and social burden on the patient and his or her family. This chapter presented evidence that diabetes mellitus is associated with a number of psychiatric disorders including eating disorders, anxiety, depression and cognitive degeneration. The prevalence and diabetes-related risk factors that predispose to the development of these disorders is covered in this chapter.

On the basis of the literature presented which examines the association between biopsychosocial variables and outcomes of individuals with diabetes mellitus, lower socioeconomic status and poor social support, decreased physical activity and unhealthy family interaction are associated with poorer metabolic control and more diabetic complications.

The chapter concludes that type 1 and 2 diabetic patients may benefit from early diagnosis and appropriate treatment of psychiatric disorders with resulting better health outcomes. Future research investigating the use of biopsychosocial models of diabetes mellitus to gain insight into how the biopsychosocial factors affecting patients with diabetes mellitus is also given.

REFERENCES

Abuyassin, B., & Laher, I. (2015). Obesity-linked diabetes in the Arab world: A review. *Eastern Mediterranean Health Journal*, *21*(6), 420–439. doi:10.26719/2015.21.6.420

Adeniyi, A., Idowu, O., Ogwumike, O., & Adeniyi, C. (2012). Comparative influence of self-efficacy, social support and perceived barriers on low physical activity development in patients with type 2 diabetes, hypertension or stroke. *Ethiopian Journal of Health Sciences*, *22*(2), 113–119.

Ali, S., Stone, M. A., Peters, J. L., Davies, M. J., & Khunti, K. (2006). The prevalence of co-morbid depression in adults with type 2 diabetes: A systematic review and meta-analysis. *Diabetic Medicine*, *23*(11), 1165–1173. doi:10.1111/j.1464-5491.2006.01943.x

Allen, N. A. (2004). Social cognitive theory in diabetes exercise research: An integrative literature review. *The Diabetes Educator*, *30*(5), 805–819. doi:10.1177/014572170403000516

Almeida, O. P., McCaul, K., Hankey, G. J., Yeap, B. B., Golledge, J., Norman, P. E., & Flicker, L. (2016). Duration of diabetes and its association with depression in later life: The Health In Men Study (HIMS). *Maturitas*, *86*, 3–9. doi:10.1016/j.maturitas.2016.01.003

Amer, F. A., Mohamed, M. S., Elbur, A. I., Abdelaziz, S. I., & Elrayah, Z. A. (2018). Influence of self-efficacy management on adherence to self-care activities and treatment outcome among diabetes mellitus type 2. *Pharmacy Practice*, *16*(4), 1274. doi:10.18549/PharmPract.2018.04.1274

American Diabetes Association. (2018). Classification and diagnosis of diabetes: Standards of medical care in diabetes. *Diabetes Care*, *41*(Supplement 1), S13–S27. doi:10.2337/dc18-S002

American Psychiatric Association. (1994). Task Force on DSM-IV. Diagnostic and Statistical Manual of Mental Disorders: DSM-IV. American Psychiatric Association.

Babalola, E., Ross, N., & White, R. (2017). The biopsychosocial approach and global mental health: Synergies and opportunities. *Indian Journal of Social Psychiatry*, *33*(4), 291–296. doi:10.4103/ijsp.ijsp_13_17

Baek, R. N., Tanenbaum, M. L., & Gonzalez, J. S. (2014). Diabetes burden and diabetes distress: The buffering effect of social support. *Annals of Behavioral Medicine*, *48*(2), 145–155. doi:10.100712160-013-9585-4

Bahrmann, A., Abel, A., Zeyfang, A., Petrak, F., Kubiak, T., Hummel, J., & Bahrmann, P. (2014). Psychological insulin resistance in geriatric patients with diabetes mellitus. *Patient Education and Counseling*, *94*(3), 417–422. doi:10.1016/j.pec.2013.11.010

Bansal, V., Gassenhuber, J., Phillips, T., Oliveira, G., Harbaugh, R., Villarasa, N., ... Boehm, B. O. (2017). Spectrum of mutations in monogenic diabetes genes identified from high-throughput DNA sequencing of 6888 individuals. *BMC Medicine*, *15*(1), 213. doi:10.118612916-017-0977-3

Berhan, Y. T., Eliasson, M., Möllsten, A., Waernbaum, I., & Dahlquist, G. (2015). Swedish Childhood Diabetes Study Group 2013. Impact of parental socioeconomic status on excess mortality in a population-based cohort of subjects with childhood-onset type 1 diabetes. *Diabetes Care*, *38*(5), 827–832. doi:10.2337/dc14-1522

Bernstein, C. M., Stockwell, M. S., Gallagher, M. P., Rosenthal, S. L., & Soren, K. (2013). Mental health issues in adolescents and young adults with T1D prevalence and impact on glycemic control. *Clinical Pediatrics*, *52*, 10–15. doi:10.1177/0009922812459950

Bock, B. C., Thind, H., Fava, J. L., Dunsiger, S., Guthrie, K. M., Stroud, L., ... Wu, W. (2019). Feasibility of yoga as a complementary therapy for patients with type 2 diabetes: The Healthy Active and in Control (HA1C) study. *Complementary Therapies in Medicine*, *42*, 125–131. doi:10.1016/j.ctim.2018.09.019

Borus, J. S., & Laffel, L. (2010). Adherence challenges in the management of type 1 diabetes in adolescents: Prevention and intervention. *Current Opinion in Pediatrics*, *22*(4), 405–411. doi:10.1097/MOP.0b013e32833a46a7

Bouldin, E. D., Trivedi, R. B., Reiber, G. E., Rosland, A. M., Silverman, J. B., Krieger, J., & Nelson, K. M. (2017). Associations between having an informal caregiver, social support, and self-care among low-income adults with poorly controlled diabetes. *Chronic Illness*, *13*(4), 239–250. doi:10.1177/1742395317690032

Boulé, N. G., Haddad, E., Kenny, G. P., Wells, G. A., & Sigal, R. J. (2001). Effects of exercise on glycemic control and body mass in type 2 diabetes mellitus: A meta-analysis of controlled clinical trials. *Journal of the American Medical Association*, *286*(10), 1218–1227. doi:10.1001/jama.286.10.1218

Bursch, B. (2016). Pain and the biopsychosocial model. *Journal of the American Academy of Child and Adolescent Psychiatry*, *55*(10), S34. doi:10.1016/j.jaac.2016.07.565

Camacho, R. C., Galassetti, S. N., Davis, S. N., & Wasserman, D. H. (2005). Glucoregulation during and after exercise in health and insulin dependent diabetes. *Exercise and Sport Sciences Reviews*, *33*(1), 17–23.

Çelik, S., Kayar, Y., Önem Akçakaya, R., Türkyılmaz Uyar, E., Kalkan, K., Yazısız, V., ... Yücel, B. (2015). Correlation of binge eating disorder with level of depression and glycemic control in type 2 diabetes mellitus patients. *General Hospital Psychiatry*, *37*(2), 116–119. doi:10.1016/j.genhosppsych.2014.11.012

Cemeroglu, A., Can, A., Davis, A., Cemeroglu, O., Kleis, L., Daniel, M., & Koehler, T. (2015). Fear of needles in children with type 1 diabetes mellitus on multiple daily injections and continuous subcutaneous insulin infusion. *Endocrine Practice*, *21*(1), 46–53. doi:10.4158/EP14252.OR

Chew, B. H., Shariff-Ghazali, S., & Fernandez, A. (2014). Psychological aspects of diabetes care: Effecting behavioral change in patients. *World Journal of Diabetes*, *5*(6), 796–808. doi:10.4239/wjd.v5.i6.796

Chew, B. H., Vos, R., Mohd-Sidik, S., & Rutten, G. E. (2016). Diabetes-related distress, depression and distress-depression among adults with type 2 diabetes mellitus in Malaysia. *PLoS One*, *11*(3), e0152095. doi:10.1371/journal.pone.0152095

Coons, M. J., Greiver, M., Aliarzadeh, B., Meaney, C., Moineddin, R., Williamson, T., ... Kane, J. J. (2016). Is glycemia control in Canadians with diabetes individualized? A cross-sectional observational study. *BMJ Open Diabetes Research & Care*, *5*(1), e000316. doi:10.1136/bmjdrc-2016-000316 de Groot, M., Crick, K. A., Long, M., Saha, C., & Shubrook, J. H. (2016). Lifetime duration of depressive disorders in patients with type 2 diabetes. *Diabetes Care*, *39*(12), 2174–2181. doi:10.2337/dc16-1145

de Groot, M., Golden, S. H., & Wagner, J. (2016). Psychological conditions in adults with diabetes. *The American Psychologist*, *71*(7), 552–562. doi:10.1037/a0040408

Delahanty, L.M., Conroy, M.B., & Nathan, D.M. (2006). The diabetes prevention program research group psychological predictors of physical activity in the diabetes prevention program. *J. Am. Diabetic. Assoc.*, *l06*, 698-705.

Di Battista, A. M., Hart, T. A., Greco, L., & Gloizer, J. (2009). Type 1 diabetes mellitus among adolescents reduced diabetes self-care caused by social fear and fear of hypoglycemia. *The Diabetes Educator*, *35*, 465–475. doi:10.1177/0145721709333492

Dutton, G. R., Tan, F., Provost, B. C., Sorenson, J. L., Allen, B., & Smith, D. (2009). Relationship between self-efficacy and physical activity among patients with type 2 diabetes. *Journal of Behavioral Medicine*, *32*(3), 270–277. doi:10.100710865-009-9200-0

Egede, L. E., & Dismuke, C. E. (2012). Serious psychological distress and diabetes: A review of the literature. *Current Psychiatry Reports*, *14*(1), 15–22. doi:10.100711920-011-0240-0

Erkie, M., Feleke, Y., Desalegne, F., Anbessie, J., & Shibre, T. (2013). Magnitude, clinical and sociodemographic correlate of depression in diabetic patients, Addis Ababa, Ethiopia. *Ethiopian Medical Journal*, *51*(4), 249–259.

Fisher, L., Skaff, M. M., Mullan, J. T., Arean, P., Glasgow, R., & Masharani, U. (2008). A longitudinal study of affective and anxiety disorders, depressive affect and diabetes distress in adults with Type 2 diabetes. *Diabetic Medicine*, *25*(9), 1096–1101. doi:10.1111/j.1464-5491.2008.02533.x

Galobardes, B., Shaw, M., Lawlor, D. A., Lynch, J. W., & Davey Smith, G. (2006). Indicators of socioeconomic position (part 1). *Journal of Epidemiology and Community Health*, *60*(1), 7–12. doi:10.1136/jech.2004.023531

Gnavi, R., Petrelli, A., Demaria, M., Spadea, T., Carta, Q., & Costa, G. (2004). Mortality and educational level among diabetic and non-diabetic population in the Turin Longitudinal Study: A 9-year follow-up. *International Journal of Epidemiology*, *33*(4), 864–871. doi:10.1093/ije/dyh089

Goetz, K., Szecseny, J., Campbell, S., Rosemann, T., Rueter, G., Raum, E., ... Miksch, A. (2012). The importance of social support for people with type 2 diabetes: A qualitative study with general practitioners, practice nurses and patients. *Psycho-Social Medicine*, *9*, 1–9.

Gonder-Frederick, L. A., Fisher, C. D., Ritterband, L. M., Cox, D. J., Hou, L., DasGupta, A. A., & Clarke, W. L. (2006). Predictors of fear of hypoglycemia in adolescents with type 1 diabetes and their parents. *Pediatric Diabetes*, *7*(4), 215–222. doi:10.1111/j.1399-5448.2006.00182.x

Gonzalez-Zacarias, A. A., Mavarez-Martinez, A., Arias-Morales, C. E., Stoicea, N., & Rogers, B. (2016). Impact of demographic, socioeconomic, and psychological factors on glycemic self-management in adults with type 2 diabetes mellitus. *Frontiers in Public Health*, *4*. doi:10.3389/fpubh.2016.00195

Grigsby, A. B., Anderson, R. J., Freedland, K. E., Clouse, R. E., & Lustman, P. J. (2002). Prevalence of anxiety in adults with diabetes: A systematic review. *Journal of Psychosomatic Research*, *53*(6), 1053–1060. doi:10.1016/S0022-3999(02)00417-8

Habtewold, T. D., Islam, M. A., Radie, Y. T., & Tegegne, B. S. (2016). Comorbidity of depression and diabetes: An application of biopsychosocial model. *International Journal of Mental Health Systems*, *10*(1), 1–9. doi:10.118613033-016-0106-2

Hall, K. K., Tambekou, J., Penn, L., Camara, A., Balde, N. M., & Sobngwi, E. (2017). Association between depression, glycaemic control and the prevalence of diabetic retinopathy in a diabetic population in Cameroon. *South African Journal of Psychiatry*, *23*, 983. doi:10.4102ajpsychiatry.v23i0.983

Hassan, K., Loar, R., Anderson, B. J., & Heptulla, R. A. (2006). The role of socioeconomic status, depression, quality of life, and glycemic control in type 1 diabetes mellitus. *The Journal of Pediatrics*, *149*(4), 526–531. doi:10.1016/j.jpeds.2006.05.039

Herzer, M., & Hood, K. K. (2010). Anxiety symptoms in adolescents with Type 1 Diabetes: Association with blood glucose monitoring and glycemic control. *Journal of Pediatric Psychology*, *35*(4), 415–425. doi:10.1093/jpepsy/jsp063

Hill-Briggs, F., & Gemmell, L. (2007). Problem solving in diabetes self-management and control: A systematic review of the literature. *The Diabetes Educator*, *33*(6), 1032–1050. doi:10.1177/0145721707308412

Hilliard, M. E., Yi-Frazier, J. P., Hessler, D., Butler, A. M., Anderson, B. J., & Jaser, S. (2016). Stress and A1c Among People with Diabetes Across the Lifespan. *Current Diabetes Reports*, *16*(8), 67. doi:10.100711892-016-0761-3

Holt, R. I. G., de Groot, M., & Golden, S. H. (2014). Diabetes and Depression. *Current Diabetes Reports*, *14*(6), 491. doi:10.100711892-014-0491-3

Hsu, Y. M., Su, L. T., Chang, H. M., Sung, F. C., Lyu, S. Y., & Chen, P. C. (2012). Diabetes mellitus and risk of subsequent depression: A longitudinal study. *International Journal of Nursing Studies*, *49*(4), 437–444. doi:10.1016/j.ijnurstu.2011.09.019

Hu, J., Amirehsani, K., Wallace, D. C., & Letvak, S. (2013). Perceptions of barriers in managing diabetes: Perspectives of Hispanic immigrant patients and family members. *The Diabetes Educator*, *39*(4), 494–503. doi:10.1177/0145721713486200

Imran, S. A., Agarwal, G., Harpreet, S. B., & Ross, S. (2018). Targets for glycemic control. *Canadian Journal of Diabetes*, *42*, S42–S46. doi:10.1016/j.jcjd.2017.10.030

Jaser, S. S. (2011). Family interaction in pediatric diabetes. *Current Diabetes Reports*, *11*(6), 480–485. doi:10.100711892-011-0222-y

Jayawardena, R., Ranasinghe, P., Chathuranga, T., Atapattu, P. M., & Misra, A. (2018). The benefits of yoga practice compared to physical exercise in the management of type 2 Diabetes Mellitus: A systematic review and meta-analysis. *Diabetes & Metabolic Syndrome*, *12*(5), 795–805. doi:10.1016/j.dsx.2018.04.008

Kendzor, D. E., Chen, M., Reininger, B. M., Businelle, M. S., Stewart, D. W., Fisher-Hoch, S. P., & McCormick, J. B. (2014). The association of depression and anxiety with glycemic control among Mexican Americans with diabetes living near the U.S.-Mexico border. *BMC Public Health*, *14*(1), 176. doi:10.1186/1471-2458-14-176

Keyserling, T. C., Samuel-Hodge, C. D., Ammerman, A. S., Ainsworth, B. E., Henriquez-Roldan, C. F., Elasy, T. A., ... Bangdiwala, S. I. (2002). A randomized trial of an intervention to improve self-care behaviors of African-American women with type 2 diabetes: Impact on physical activity. *Diabetes Care*, *25*(9), 1576–1583. doi:10.2337/diacare.25.9.1576

Khan, P., Qayyum, N., Malik, F., Khan, T., Khan, M., & Tahir, A. (2019). Incidence of anxiety and depression among patients with type 2 diabetes and the predicting factors. *Cureus*, *11*(3), e4254. doi:10.7759/cureus.4254

Kruse, J., Schmitz, N., & Thefeld, W. (2003). German National Health Interview and Examination Survey On the association between diabetes and mental disorders in a community sample: Results from the German National Health Interview and Examination Survey. *Diabetes Care*, *26*(6), 1841–1846. doi:10.2337/diacare.26.6.1841

La Greca, A. M., Swales, T., Klemp, S., Madigan, S., & Skyler, J. (1995). Adolescents with diabetes: Gender differences in psychosocial functioning and glycemic control. *Children's Health Care*, *24*(1), 61–78. doi:10.120715326888chc2401_6

Lee, C. M., Chang, C. F., Pan, M. Y., Hsu, T. H., & Chen, M. Y. (2017). Depression and its associated factors among rural diabetic residents. *The Journal of Nursing Research*, *25*(1), 31–40. doi:10.1097/jnr.0000000000000143

Lee, P. G., & Halter, J. B. (2017). The pathophysiology of hyperglycemia in older adults: Clinical considerations. *Diabetes Care*, *40*(4), 444–452. doi:10.2337/dc16-1732

Lehman, B.J., David, D.M., & Gruber, J.A. (2017). Rethinking the biopsychosocial model of health: Understanding health as a dynamic system. *Social and Personality Psychology Compass, 11*, 8.

Lindner, L. M. E., Rathmann, W., & Rosenbauer, J. (2018). Inequalities in glycaemic control, hypoglycaemia and diabetic ketoacidosis according to socio-economic status and area-level deprivation in Type 1 diabetes mellitus: A systematic review. *Diabetic Medicine*, *35*(1), 12–32. doi:10.1111/dme.13519

Maia, A. C., Braga Ade, A., Brouwers, A., Nardi, A. E., & Oliveira e Silva, A. C. (2012). Prevalence of psychiatric disorders in patients with diabetes types 1 and 2. *Comprehensive Psychiatry*, *53*(8), 1169–1173. doi:10.1016/j.comppsych.2012.03.011

Mannucci, E., Rotella, F., Ricca, V., Moretti, S., Placidi, G. F., & Rotella, C. M. (2005). Eating disorders in patients with type 1 diabetes: A meta-analysis. *Journal of Endocrinological Investigation*, *28*(7), 417–419. doi:10.1007/BF03347221

Mouri, M. I., & Badireddy, M. (2019). *Hyperglycemia*. StatPearls Publishing. Retrieved from https://www.ncbi.nlm.nih.gov/books/NBK430900/

Nicolau, J., Simó, R., Sanchís, P., Ayala, L., Fortuny, R., Zubillaga, I., & Masmiquel, L. (2015). Eating disorders are frequent among Type 2 diabetic patients and are associated with worse metabolic and psychological outcomes: Results from a cross-sectional study in primary and secondary care settings. *Acta Diabetologica*, *52*(6), 1037–1044. doi:10.100700592-015-0742-z

Nouwen, A., Nefs, G., Caramlau, I., Connock, M., Winkley, K., Lloyd, C. E., ... Pouwer, F.European Depression in Diabetes Research Consortium. (2011). Prevalence of depression in individuals with impaired glucose metabolism or undiagnosed diabetes: A systematic review and meta-analysis of the European Depression in Diabetes (EDID) Research Consortium. *Diabetes Care*, *34*(3), 752–762. doi:10.2337/dc10-1414

Ozougwu, J. C., Obimba, K., Belonwu, C. D., & Unakalamba, C. B. (2013). The pathogenesis and pathophysiology of type 1 and type 2 diabetes mellitus. *Journal of Physiology and Pathophysiology*, *4*(4), 46–57. doi:10.5897/JPAP2013.0001

Pan, X. R., Yang, W. Y., Li, G. W., & Liu, J. (1997). Prevalence of diabetes and its risk factors in China, 1994. National Diabetes Prevention and Control Cooperative Group. *Diabetes Care*, *20*(11), 1664–1669. doi:10.2337/diacare.20.11.1664

Penckofer, S., Ferrans, C. E., Velsor-Friedrich, B., & Savoy, S. (2007). The psychological impact of living with diabetes: Women's day-to-day experiences. *The Diabetes Educator*, *33*(4), 680–690. doi:10.1177/0145721707304079

Pollack, C. E., Chideya, S., Cubbin, C., Williams, B., Dekker, M., & Braveman, P. (2007). Should health studies measure wealth? A systematic review. *American Journal of Preventive Medicine*, *33*(3), 250–264. doi:10.1016/j.amepre.2007.04.033

Polonsky, W. H., & Henry, R. R. (2016). Poor medication adherence in type 2 diabetes: Recognizing the scope of the problem and its key contributors. *Patient Preference and Adherence*, *10*, 1299–1307. doi:10.2147/PPA.S106821

Punthakee, Z., Goldenberg, R., & Katz, P. (2018). Definition, classification and diagnosis of diabetes, prediabetes and metabolic syndrome. *Canadian Journal of Diabetes*, *42*, S10–S15. doi:10.1016/j.jcjd.2017.10.003

Racicka, E., & Bryńska, A. (2015). Eating disorders in children and adolescents with Type 1 and Type 2 Diabetes: Prevalence, risk factors, warning signs. *Psychiatria Polska*, *49*(5), 1017–1024. doi:10.12740/PP/39536

Ramkisson, S., Pillay, B. J., & Sibanda, W. (2017). Social support and coping in adults with type 2 diabetes. *African Journal of Primary Health Care & Family Medicine*, *9*(1), e1–e8. doi:10.4102/phcfm.v9i1.1405

Rechenberg, K., Whittemore, R., & Grey, M. (2017). Anxiety in youth with type 1 diabetes. *Journal of Pediatric Nursing*, *32*, 64–71. doi:10.1016/j.pedn.2016.08.007

Rodin, G., Olmsted, M. P., Rydall, A. C., Maharaj, S. I., Colton, P. A., Jones, J. M., & Daneman, D. (2002). Eating disorders in young women with Type 1 diabetes mellitus. *Journal of Psychosomatic Research*, *53*(4), 943–949. doi:10.1016/S0022-3999(02)00305-7

Rodríguez Calvín, J. L., Zapatero Gaviria, A., & Martín Ríos, M. D. (2015). Prevalence of depression in type 2 diabetes mellitus. *Revista Clínica Española*, *215*(3), 156–164. doi:10.1016/j.rceng.2014.12.001

Roper, N. A., Bilous, R. W., Kelly, W. F., Unwin, N. C., & Connolly, V. M. (2001). Excess mortality in a population with diabetes and the impact of material deprivation: Longitudinal, population based study. *BMJ (Clinical Research Ed.)*, *322*(7299), 1389–1393. doi:10.1136/bmj.322.7299.1389

Sacco, W. P., & Yanover, T. (2006). Diabetes and depression: The role of social support and medical symptoms. *Journal of Behavioral Medicine*, *29*(6), 523–531. doi:10.100710865-006-9072-5

Salinero-Fort, M. A., Gómez-Campelo, P., San Andrés-Rebollo, F. J., Cárdenas-Valladolid, J., Abánades-Herranz, J. C., Carrillo de Santa Pau, E., ... De Burgos-Lunar, C. (2018). Prevalence of depression in patients with type 2 diabetes mellitus in Spain (the DIADEMA Study): Results from the MADIABETES cohort. *BMJ Open*, *8*(9), e020768. doi:10.1136/bmjopen-2017-020768

Sarwar, N., Gao, P., Seshasai, S. R., Gobin, R., Kaptoge, S., Di Angelantonio, E., ... Danesh, J. (2010). Diabetes mellitus, fasting blood glucose concentration, and risk of vascular disease: A collaborative meta-analysis of 102 prospective studies. Emerging Risk Factors Collaboration. *Lancet*, *375*(9733), 2215–2222. doi:10.1016/S0140-6736(10)60484-9

Scott, A., Chambers, D., Goyder, E., & O'Cathain, A. (2017). Socioeconomic inequalities in mortality, morbidity and diabetes management for adults with type 1 diabetes: A systematic review. *PLoS One*, *12*(5), e0177210. doi:10.1371/journal.pone.0177210

Secrest, A. M., Costacou, T., Gutelius, B., Miller, R. G., Songer, T. J., & Orchard, T. J. (2011). Associations between socioeconomic status and major complications in type 1 diabetes: The Pittsburgh epidemiology of diabetes complication (EDC) Study. *Annals of Epidemiology*, *21*(5), 374–381. doi:10.1016/j.annepidem.2011.02.007

Semenkovich, K., Brown, M. E., Svrakic, D. M., & Lustman, P. J. (2015). Depression in type 2 diabetes mellitus: Prevalence, impact, and treatment. *Drugs*, *75*(6), 577–587. doi:10.100740265-015-0347-4

Seshasai, S. R., Kaptoge, S., & Thompson, A.Emerging Risk Factors Collaboration. (2011). Diabetes mellitus, fasting glucose, and risk of cause-specific death. *The New England Journal of Medicine*, *364*(9), 829–841. doi:10.1056/NEJMoa1008862

Shrivastava, S. R., Shrivastava, P. S., & Ramasamy, J. (2013). Role of self-care in management of diabetes mellitus. *Journal of Diabetes and Metabolic Disorders*, *12*(1), 14. doi:10.1186/2251-6581-12-14

Singh, H., Raju, M. S., Dubey, V., Kurrey, R., Bansal, S., & Malik, M. (2014). A study of sociodemographic clinical and glycemic control factors associated with co-morbid depression in type 2 diabetes mellitus. *Industrial Psychiatry Journal, 23*(2), 134–142. doi:10.4103/0972-6748.151687

Smith, K. J., Béland, M., Clyde, M., Gariépy, G., Page, V., Badawi, G., ... Schmitz, N. (2013). Association of diabetes with anxiety: A systematic review and meta-analysis. *Journal of Psychosomatic Research, 74*(2), 89–99. doi:10.1016/j.jpsychores.2012.11.013

Snoek, F. J., Bremmer, M. A., & Hermanns, N. (2015). Constructs of depression and distress in diabetes: Time for an appraisal. *The Lancet. Diabetes & Endocrinology, 3*(6), 450–460. doi:10.1016/S2213-8587(15)00135-7

Stetson, B., Minges, K. E., & Richardson, C. R. (2017). New directions for diabetes prevention and management in behavioral medicine. *Journal of Behavioral Medicine, 40*(1), 127–144. doi:10.100710865-016-9802-2

Stoa, E. M., Meling, S., Nyhus, L. K., Stromstad, G., Mangerud, K. M., Helgerud, J., ... Storen, O. (2017). High-intensity aerobic interval training improves aerobic fitness and HbA1c among persons diagnosed with type 2 diabetes. *European Journal of Applied Physiology, 117*(3), 455–467. doi:10.100700421-017-3540-1

Stolar, M. W. (2010). Defining and achieving treatment success in patients with type 2 diabetes mellitus. *Mayo Clinic Proceedings, 85*(12 Suppl.), S50–S59. doi:10.4065/mcp.2010.0471

Strom, J. L., & Egede, L. E. (2012). The impact of social support on outcomes in adult patients with type 2 diabetes: A systematic review. *Current Diabetes Reports, 12*(6), 769–781. doi:10.100711892-012-0317-0

Tan, M. L., Manski-Nankervis, J. A., Thuraisingam, S., Jenkins, A., O'Neal, D., & Furler, J. (2018). Socioeconomic status and time in glucose target range in people with type 2 diabetes: A baseline analysis of the GP-OSMOTIC study. *BMC Endocrine Disorders, 18*(1), 47. doi:10.118612902-018-0279-6

Tang, T. S., Brown, M. B., Funnell, M. M., & Anderson, R. M. (2008). Social support, quality of life, and self-care behaviors among African Americans with type 2 diabetes. *The Diabetes Educator, 34*(2), 266–276. doi:10.1177/0145721708315680

Tiv, M., Viel, J. F., Mauny, F., Eschwège, E., Weill, A., Fournier, C., ... Penfornis, A. (2012). Medication adherence in type 2 diabetes: The ENTRED study 2007, a French Population-Based Study. *PLoS One, 7*(3), e32412. doi:10.1371/journal.pone.0032412

Trento, M., Passera, P., Tomalino, M., Bajardi, M., Pomero, F., Allione, A., ... Porta, M. (2001). Group visits improve metabolic control in type 2 diabetes: A 2-year follow-up. *Diabetes Care, 24*(6), 995–1000. doi:10.2337/diacare.24.6.995

Trief, P. M., Grant, W., Elbert, K., & Weinstock, R. S. (1998). Family environment, glycemic control, and the psychosocial adaptation of adults with diabetes. *Diabetes Care, 21*(2), 241–245. doi:10.2337/diacare.21.2.241

van der Heijden, M.M., van Dooren, F.E., Pop, V.J., &Pouwer, F. (2013). Effects of exercise training on quality of life, symptoms of depression, symptoms of anxiety and emotional well-being in type 2 diabetes mellitus: a systematic review. *Diabetologia, 56*(6), 1210-1225.

Van Dyck, D., De Greef, K., Deforche, B., Ruige, J., Tudor-Locke, C. E., Kaufman, J. M., ... Bourdeaudhuii, I. (2011). Mediators of physical activity change in a behavioral modification program for type 2 diabetes patients. *The International Journal of Behavioral Nutrition and Physical Activity, 8*(1), 105. doi:10.1186/1479-5868-8-105

Walker, R. J., Gebregziabher, M., Martin-Harris, B., & Egede, L. E. (2015). Quantifying direct effects of social determinants of health on glycemic control in adults with type 2 diabetes. *Diabetes Technology & Therapeutics, 17*(2), 80–87. doi:10.1089/dia.2014.0166

Westaway, M. S., Seager, J. R., Rheeder, P., & Van Zyl, D. G. (2005). The effects of social support on health, well-being and management of diabetes mellitus: A black South African perspective. *Ethnicity & Health, 10*(1), 73–89. doi:10.1080/1355785052000323047

Wisting, L., Reas, D. L., Bang, L., Skrivarhaug, T., Dahl-Jorgensen, K., & Ro, O. (2017). Eating patterns in adolescents with type 1 diabetes: Associations with metabolic control, insulin omission, and eating disorder pathology. *Appetite, 114*, 226–231. doi:10.1016/j.appet.2017.03.035

Wu, S. F., Young, L. S., Yeh, F. C., Jian, Y. M., Cheng, K. C., & Lee, M. C. (2013). Correlations among social support, depression, and anxiety in patients with type-2 diabetes. *The Journal of Nursing Research, 21*(2), 129–138. doi:10.1097/jnr.0b013e3182921fe1

Young, V., Eiser, C., Johnson, B., Brierley, S., Epton, T., Elliott, J., & Heller, S. (2013). Eating problems in adolescents with Type 1 diabetes: A systematic review with meta-analysis. *Diabetic Medicine, 30*(2), 189–198. doi:10.1111/j.1464-5491.2012.03771.x

Zagarins, S. E., Allen, N. A., Garb, J. L., & Welch, G. (2012). Improvement in glycemic control following a diabetes education intervention is associated with change in diabetes distress but not change in depressive symptoms. *Journal of Behavioral Medicine*, *35*(3), 299–304. doi:10.100710865-011-9359-z

Zanoveli, J. M., de Morais, H., Dias, I. C. da S., Schreiber, A. K., de Souza, C. P., & Cunha, J. M. (2016). Depression associated with diabetes: From pathophysiology to treatment. *Current Diabetes Reviews*, *12*(3), 165–178. doi:10.2174/157339981 1666150515125349

Zhang, W., Xu, H., Zhao, S., Yin, S., Wang, X., Guo, J., ... Tian, D. (2015). Prevalence and influencing factors of co-morbid depression in patients with type 2 diabetes mellitus: A General Hospital based study. *Diabetology & Metabolic Syndrome*, *7*(1), 60. doi:10.118613098-015-0053-0

Zhao, F. F., Suhonen, R., Katajisto, J., & Leino-Kilpi, H. (2018). The association of diabetes-related self-care activities with perceived stress, anxiety, and fatigue: A cross-sectional study. *Patient Preference and Adherence*, *12*, 1677–1686. doi:10.2147/ PPA.S169826

KEY TERMS AND DEFINITIONS

Anxiety: A feeling of worry, distress or unease caused by fear of danger, misfortune or an uncertain outcome.

Biopsychosocial: Relating or examining the interconnectedness of biological, physiological and social factors in health and illness.

Depression: An emotional state characterized by feelings of sadness, guilt, low self-worth or anger and decreased ability to enjoy life.

Diabetes mellitus: A chronic disorder of carbohydrate metabolism associated with unusually elevated levels of glucose in the blood due to insufficient insulin production or failure of the body to respond to insulin.

Psychological: Relates to things that involves the mental and emotional state of an individual.

Sociocultural: Relating or encompassing common social and cultural factors.

Socioeconomic: Refers to the interaction or combination of social and economic factors of a group of individuals.

Section 6
Stress

Chapter 8
Stress:
An Overview

Daniel Opotamutale Ashipala
University of Namibia, Namibia

Anna P. K. Shilunga
University of Namibia, Namibia

ABSTRACT

Stress has become part of life, and, as such, the best thing one can do to prevent a stress burden is to know the warning signs and symptoms. Since people handle stress differently, symptoms of stress may vary. The causes of stress depend partly on how a person perceives it and include a wide variety of negative and positive stressors. Therefore, stress can affect all aspects of life and no part of the body is immune to it. This chapter focuses on stress, defining the concept, outlining the causes, and identifying the warning signs and symptoms and the effects on health. The impact of stress in the workplace and strategies for managing stress are also discussed.

INTRODUCTION

Stress is very common and has become a universal human experience that affects almost everyone. Stress basically refers to the body's reaction to changes that create taxing demands (Middleton, Nicolson, & O'Neil, 2012). The word 'stress' is generally used to refer to unpleasant experiences that leave people feeling overwhelmed. As a result, many people believe that stress is always bad, hence all stress is bad. This is not true, as stress is not always a bad thing and may also be beneficial. Because stress has become pervasive in most of our lives, it is not always easy to avoid.

DOI: 10.4018/978-1-7998-2139-7.ch008

However, people can learn ways to deal with stress. It is therefore important to know the warning signs and symptoms of stress. In so doing, one is minimising the harmful effects of stress on one's physical and mental health. Life is not static; changes in people's lives such as moving away from home and getting promotion at work, to mention but a few, can be sources of stress.

Stressors can range from daily hassles to major traumatic experiences. However, a life event that may be experienced as stressful by one person may not necessarily lead to stress in another.

BACKGROUND

Stress has significant potential to be a major contributor to morbidity and mortality, if not taken care of which may lead to suicide, the incidence and adverse outcomes of medical illness, disruption in interpersonal relations and lost work time and productivity. Thus, an understanding about the meaning of the concept "stress" is necessary not only to the individual but, also by the public at large.

WHAT IS STRESS

There are several definitions of stress. Stress may be defined as a response to any demand or threat (Gardner, 2002; Kruger, Burke, & Harper, 2006); as well as a stimulus, wear and tear on the body, a body's reaction to a harmful situation (WebMD, 2019). Stress can be anything that causes physical and/or mental wear and tear on the body and mind, which can be negative or positive (Healtheirsf, 2019). The commonly accepted definition of stress is the negative emotional or physical responses that occur when someone perceives a demand or situation as exceeding their capabilities or resources.

Technically, however, stress is the body's reaction to any perceived threat. And, contrary to popular belief, this reaction is a functional one. Historically, when perceiving a threat, our bodies released hormones and other chemicals, increasing the heart rate and respiration, and tensing the muscles to enable us to run away or fight whatever it was that threatened us. Today, such reactions motivate us, help us to prepare for important events and even enhance our performance and productivity.

Many people believe that stress is always bad or only refers to negative events; however, certain experiences that are usually considered positive may stressful as well be. Positive (good) stress inspires a person to achieve a goal, become more confident or grow stronger physically. It gives a feeling of fulfilment and energy in our everyday lives. However, if the move is an exciting challenge, the same stressor is more likely to make a person excited and look forward to the change.

If stress leaves a person feeling depleted or anxious or overly excited, they may resort to poor practices for dealing with stress such as doing too much too fast or obsessing over possibilities that may never happen For example, if one is preparing for a move, thinking about the situation as overwhelming or scary or as too much to handle is likely to make you feel more anxious. Accordingly, the move becomes a source of negative (bad) stress.

As we do not typically have to run from or fight our stressors these days, the effects of the chemicals released in our bodies are not neutralised. Instead, they build up over time and, when excessive or prolonged, produce a range of physical and emotional health problems. No one is immune to stress and everyone is likely to have experienced stress in their lifetime, young or adult. Young people and/or students' stress is usually related to everyday experiences, worries and challenges at school, home, in the community and within their peer group.

CAUSES OF STRESS

The causes of stress depend partly on how a person perceives it. Stress can be caused by a wide variety of factors. What is regarded as stressful by one person may not necessarily be regarded as such by another. Deadlines, for example, which may motivate one person to perform to the best of their best ability may be a source of severe stress for another. In the workplace, people are subject to pressures (both personal and individual stress) and it can sometimes be a combination of these pressures that results in stress. Individual stress factors may include family and relationship problems, illness, financial worries, bereavement, and juggling the demands of work and life. Students and young people may experience stress resulting from bullying, name calling, social isolation, not getting what they want, body image, academic difficulties, and unsafe neighbourhoods. Occupational stress may include unreasonable workloads, poor working relationships, bullying or harassment, lack of training, role uncertainty, long working hours, and so on. Based on the above discussion, the causes of stress can be classified into negative and positive stressors (Kruger, Burke, & Harper, 2006). Examples of such stressors are listed in Table 1:

Table 1. Examples of negative and positive stressors

Negative stressors	Positive stressors
• The death of a loved one • Filing for divorce • Losing contact with loved ones • The death of a family member • Hospitalisation (oneself or a family member) • Injury or illness (oneself or a family member) • Being abused or neglected • Separation from a spouse or a committed relationship partner • Conflict in interpersonal relationships • Bankruptcy/money problems • Unemployment • Sleep problems • Children's problems at school • Legal problems	• Receiving a promotion or raise at work • Starting a new job • Marriage • Buying a home • Having a child • Moving • Taking a vacation • Holiday seasons • Retirement • Taking educational classes or learning a new hobby

The Holmes and Rahe Stress Scale list the top ten most stressful life events for adults that can contribute to illness:

1. Death of a spouse
2. Divorce
3. Marriage separation
4. Imprisonment
5. Death of a close family member
6. Injury or illness
7. Marriage
8. Job loss
9. Marriage reconciliation
10. Retirement

Immediate Stress Response in the Body

When you feel threatened, the nervous system responds by releasing a flood of stress hormones, and including adrenaline and cortisol, which rouse the body for emergency action. This stress response is also known as the fight-or-flight response because it evolved as a survival mechanism. This response causes the heart to beat faster, and muscles tighten, blood pressure rises, breath quickens, and sweating increases, the blood supply to the brain, muscles and limbs increases, more sugar for energy is released, and the senses become sharper. These physiological changes increase strength and stamina, speed up reaction time, and enhance focus – preparing to either fight or flee from the danger at hand.

SIGNS OF STRESS

It is not always easy to recognise the effects of stress. Stress may start to feel normal even if it is taking a heavy toll on a person. It is therefore important to be aware of the common warning signs and symptoms of stress are categorised into cognitive, behavioural, physical, psychological as well as social signs (Roncaglia, 2014; SSQ financial solution, 2013).

COGNITIVE SIGNS

- Memory loss
- Difficulty concentrating
- Poor judgement
- Imagine negative, worrisome, or terrifying scenes
- Nervous habits (e.g. nail biting, pacing)
- Feeling depressed or generally unhappy

BEHAVIOURAL SIGNS

The individual may be:

- Rushed
- Impatient,
- Demanding
- Demonstrate
- Aggression
- Miss work
- Seeing only the negative

PHYSICAL SIGNS

- Headaches
- Stomach aches including diarrhea or constipation
- Digestion problems
- Chronic fatigue
- Feel jumpy or exhausted all the time
- Aches and pains

- Nausea, dizziness
- Chest pain, rapid heart rate

PSYCHOLOGICAL SIGNS

- Anxiety
- Irritability
- Depression
- Loss of motivation

SOCIAL SIGNS

- Difficulty communicating
- Lack of interest
- Voluntary resentment
- Withdrawing from others
- Procrastinating or neglecting responsibilities (Roncaglia, 2014; SSQ financial solution, 2013).

EFFECTS OF STRESS

The effects of stress vary from person to person. Some of the most frightening findings include the over-production of the stress hormone, cortisol, which has the potential to shrink cells in a specific area of the brain (called the hippocampus) and inhibit the formation of new cells. The impact of ongoing and/or unresolved stress can lead to feelings of anxiety, depression, irritability, poor concentration, aggression, physical illness, fatigue, sleep disturbance and poor coping skills such as tobacco, drug and/or alcohol use.

A little stress every now and then is not something to be concerned about. However, ongoing stress can increase your risk of infectious diseases and may aggravate serious health problems. Not only are you more likely to catch whatever is going around but you will also probably have more severe symptoms after becoming ill than someone who is not chronically stressed.

Other negative physical effects include the following:

- **Cardiovascular Disease:** Stress can lead to high blood pressure, abnormal heartbeat, chest pains, and problems with blood clotting and hardening of the arteries. It is also associated with coronary artery disease, heart attack and heart failure.
- **Nervous System Responses:** Chronically stressed people often experience sleep deprivation, headaches, migraines, depression and chronic fatigue. Recent research even suspects a link between stress and Alzheimer's disease.
- **Muscle Tension and Pain:** People who are stressed often have neck, shoulder and lower back pain. This may be caused by constant tension in the muscles because of stress.
- **Stomach and Intestinal Problems:** Stress can cause diarrhea and constipation and may be a factor in gastro-esophageal reflux disease (GORD), peptic ulcer disease and irritable bowel syndrome.
- **Reproductive Organs:** Stress can cause painful menstrual periods, decreased fertility and sexual disorders (such as loss of libido, premature ejaculation or erection problems).
- **The Lungs:** Stress can make the symptoms of asthma and chronic obstructive pulmonary disease (COPD) worse.
- **Skin Problems:** Stress is a contributing factor in skin disorders such as hives, acne and psoriasis.
- Mental health problems may result such as depression, anxiety and personality disorders (National Institute for Health & Clinical Excellence, 2011).

Stress can affect all aspects of life. Apart from the physical symptoms, stress also affects one's thoughts, moods, behaviour and interactions with others. Therefore, no part of the body is immune to stress. Stressed individuals tend to be more irritable and moodier, and overreact easily, which leads to more confrontation, conflict, and in some instances even violence. In addition, stressed people are more anxious, have problems concentrating and remembering, and may be more prone to use drugs or drink excessively in an attempt to relax.

Stressed employees tend to be unhealthy, poorly motivated, and less productive at work. Their organisations tend to be less competitive in the market.

Moderate stress still has its place. The right level of stress motivates us, helps us to prepare for important events and even enhances our performance. But once we've reached that peak, stress turns into distress and we experience negative consequences.

IMPACT OF STRESS

For many years, stress was viewed as the unfortunate and inevitable consequence of having a job. Employers and managers equated it with performance and employees correlated it with just part of getting the job done.

Chronic, excessive stress is not only abnormal, but also detrimental to one's physical and mental health (Schneiderman, Ironson & Siegel, 2005; Mariotti, 2015). Furthermore, excessive stress in the workplace undermines an organisation's productivity and competitiveness in the marketplace.

Signs that your organisation may be negatively affected by employee stress include:

- Increased absenteeism
- Decreased commitment to work
- Increased staff turnover
- Impaired performance and productivity
- Increased unsafe working practices and accident rates
- Increased complaints from clients and customers
- Increasing liability to legal claims and actions by stressed workers.

The impact of unresolved stress can lead to feelings of anxiety, depression, irritability, poor concentration, aggression, physical illness, fatigue, sleep disturbance and poor coping skills such as tobacco, drug and/or alcohol use.

MANAGEMENT OF STRESS

There are many ways you can help or encourage colleagues to manage their stress. Some solutions blend relaxation techniques with nutrition and exercise. Others focus on specific issues such as time management, assertiveness training and improving social skills.

It is important to remember that not all stress management techniques are effective for everyone. Some people may find relaxation techniques very helpful, while others find they can only relax after vigorous exercise. The key is to find the healthy solution that works for you. According to the World Health Organisation, stress in an organisation can be reduced using the following methods:

Work Redesign

Strategies for work redesign usually focus on demands, knowledge and abilities, support and control (German Technical Cooperation, 2009; Wu, Hu & Zheng, 2019).

They include

- changing the demands of work (e.g. changing the way the job is done or the working environment, sharing the workload differently)
- ensuring that employees have or develop the appropriate knowledge and abilities to perform their jobs effectively (e.g. by selecting and training them properly and by reviewing their progress regularly)
- improving employees' control over the way they do their work (e.g. introduce flexi-time, job-sharing and more consultation about working practices)
- Increasing the amount and quality of the support they receive (e.g. introduce people management training schemes for supervisors, allow interaction among employees, encourage cooperation and teamwork) (Wu, Wu, Li, & Dan, 2018)

Ergonomics and Environmental Design

Improving the equipment used at work and the physical working conditions.

Stress Management Training

Asking employees to attend classes on relaxation, time management, assertiveness training or exercise.

Management Development

Improving managers' attitudes towards dealing with work stress, their knowledge and understanding of it and their skills to deal with the issue as effectively as possible.

Organisational Development

Implementing better work systems and management systems, as well as developing a more friendly and supportive culture.

Early Detection and Prevention of Work Stress-Related Problems

- Regularly monitoring staff satisfaction and health
- Making sure staff know whom to talk to about problems
- Knowing where to refer employees to for professional help when they appear to be experiencing real difficulties.

ACTIVITIES THAT ENHANCE RECOVERY FROM STRESS

Balanced Diet

Stressed people often crave foods that are high in fats and sugars. A high-fibre diet rich in fresh fruits, vegetables, nuts and whole grains provides greater appetite satisfaction over a longer period than processed, high-fat and high-sugar snacks. A balanced diet can reduce the impact of stress on the body. Stop or reduce the intake of alcohol, drugs and caffeine as they may worsen the level of stress.

Balance Between Rest and Work

Work-life balance involves adjusting one's day-to-day activities to achieve a sense of balance between work life and personal life. Get enough sleep, aim for at least six to eight hours every night.

Exercise

Physical activity helps to get rid of the physical and emotional effects that stress is having on the body. Exercise helps with the production of feel-good neurotransmitters which can relax the body. It also improves the mood by lowering the symptoms associated with mild depression and anxiety. Exercise can also improve your sleep, which is often disrupted by stress, depression and anxiety. Aim for at least 30 minutes of exercise every day.

Fun and Laughter

Laughter relaxes the whole body. A good, hearty laugh relieves physical tension and stress. Laughter makes a person feel good, increases energy, enabling a person to stay focused and accomplish more. Hence, a regular dose of fun and laughter is essential.

Creative and Relaxing Activities

Creative activities help the mind to recover from work stress (Scott, 2019). People who focus on such activities are completely consumed by what they are doing which counters stress. The following creative activities can greatly reduce stress:

- Stress Reduction Activities for Students Introduction
- Deep Breathing Exercise (Belly Breathing)
- Progressive Relaxation (Deep Muscle Relaxation) Simple Meditation
- Visual Imagery
- Peer Sharing (Co-listening)
- Animal Charades (Physical Activity)
- Silent Ball (Physical Activity)
- Dancing
- Writing a poem
- Playing with a pet

Additional strategies German Technical Cooperation (2009) which may be helpful especially for young people and/or students can be:

- State feelings in a clear way (for example: "I feel angry when you yell at me.")
- Decrease negative self-talk (for example: transform "My grades will never get any better." to "I may not be doing too well now, but my grades can improve if I get extra help and I do all my homework.")
- Be with friends who help you cope in a positive way
- Learn relaxation techniques (such as: deep breathing, muscle relaxation, meditation)
- Talk to a caring adult for some advices.

STRATEGIES THAT CAN SERVE AS BUFFERS AGAINST STRESS

Open and Effective Communication

Share your problems with trusted others; try out peer support groups. Seek help from others and remember you are not alone. Be caring to colleagues and accept support from them, accept that it is okay to be seen to be vulnerable.

Healthy Relationships

It is important to be part of a group of people that support and understand you. Develop support systems among co-students, friends, colleagues and family to bolster resources. Do not isolate yourself. Develop an honest relationship with yourself.

Through reflection you can learn to live consciously and be aware of what you are experiencing and how you are coping with it. Make your friendships meaningful and cherish them.

Time Management

Do not allow little things to take your time, making you put off doing important things. Remember, procrastination is said to be the art of keeping up with yesterday. Manage your time to increase your sense of control and organisation. Set priorities and stick to them. Plan and organise ahead to allow enough time to get tasks done. Do not waste time feeling guilty about what you haven't done. Make use "to do" lists and set priorities to help you achieve your goals.

Problem Solving and Goal Setting

Effective problem solving reduces stress greatly. It is important to analyse your problems and develop a strategy to tackle them. Make use of your support group to help you. Set small, manageable and achievable goals. Try to worry less about things you can't control, and make plans for dealing with the things that can be controlled.

Attitudes and Belief

Develop a hopeful and positive attitude. Face your disappointments and try again. Accept your weaknesses but be aware of your strengths and use them. Remember that it is not whether people fail that determines their success but how they cope with failure.

Be aware that going the extra mile in everything you do generates excitement, fulfilment and a sense of purpose.

COPING STYLES

There are two fundamental types of coping: problem-focused coping and emotion-focused coping.

Problem-Focused Coping

This type of coping involves identifying the problem, considering possible solutions, weighing the costs and benefits of these solutions, and then selecting an alternative (Uys & Middleton, 2014). Efforts are directed at changing or acting on the source of the problem by exploring solutions and planning actions and by getting assistance or information from others. It can also involve a deliberate effort to control the meaning of the problem by recognising only the creative and growth potential it offers. A problem-focused approach to managing stress means people actively try to do things to address the problem at hand (Roncaglia, 2014). Problem-focused coping is more likely to occur when encountering stressors that are perceived as controllable (Uys & Middleton, 2014).

Emotion-Focused Coping

In this coping style, efforts are directed at changing or reducing the negative emotions associated with stress (Uys & Middleton, 2014). These efforts may include denying, avoiding, minimising, or distancing oneself from the problem or positive comparisons with others (e.g. "I'm not as badly off as he is") or seeking something positive in a negative event (e.g. "Now that I've failed my grade, I can sleep in for a few days"). The focus here is on changing how the person feels about the problem.

In some instances, coping efforts can be destructive such as blaming or direct frustration and aggression towards others or objects (Roncaglia, 2014). Some people can withhold their emotions by inhibiting feelings and refusing to acknowledge how they feel. They may be unwilling either to seek or accept assistance from others and unwilling to express feelings of vulnerability or dependency. They criticise themselves for failing to cope, and may adopt self-destructive behaviours such drinking, troublemaking and suicide.

In some cases, emotion-focused coping strategies involve reappraisal, where the stressor is interpreted differently without changing its objective level of threat. Emotion-focused coping is more likely to predominate when people are faced with stressors they believe they are powerless to change (Uys & Middleton, 2014).

FUTURE RESEARCH DIRECTIONS

Future studies should focus their efforts to explore other types of early-life stress that may set in motion similar neuroimmune processes such as war, natural disasters, bullying, familial dysfunction, discrimination n). There is emerging evidence implicating inflammation in the etiology of numerous emotional and physical disorders. In addition, it strongly suggested that future explore future directions should focus on theory, research, and interventions with children and adolescents.

CONCLUSION

Stress is a part of life. Recognising the warning signs and symptoms of stress is the best thing one can do to alleviate the stress burden. In this way, people will be better placed to help not only themselves but their families, friends and communities at large. While stress cannot be entirely avoided, what matters most is how you handle it.

REFERENCES

Gardner, R. M. (2002). *Psychology Applied to everyday life*. Belmont: C Thomson/ Wadsworth.

German Technical Cooperation. (2009). Health and wellness: Peer educator handbook. Windhoek.

Kruger, G., Burke, A., & Harper, M. (2006). *Psychology for nurses*. Pretoria: Van Schaik.

Mariotti, A. (2015). The effects of chronic stress on health: New insights into the molecular mechanisms of brain-body communication. *Future Science OA*, *1*(3), FSO23. doi:10.4155/fso.15.21

Middleton, L., Nicolson, G., & O'Neil, V. (2012). *Juta's nursing psychology: Applying psychological concepts to nursing practice*. Johannesburg: Juta.

National Institute for Health & Clinical Excellence. (2011). COMMON MENTAL HEALTH DISORDERS: The nice guideline on identification and pathways to care. The British Psychological Society & The Royal College of Psychiatrists. Leicester. United Kingdom. Retrieved from: https://www.ncbi.nlm.nih.gov/books/NBK92266/pdf/Bookshelf_NBK92266.pdf

Roncaglia, I. (2014). Coping Styles: A Better Understanding of Stress and Anxiety in Individuals With Autism Spectrum Conditions Through Sport and Exercise Models. *Psychological Thought*, *7*(2), 134–143. doi:10.5964/psyct.v7i2.115

Schneiderman, N., Ironson, G., & Siegel, S. D. (2005). Stress and health: Psychological, behavioral, and biological determinants. *Annual Review of Clinical Psychology*, *1*(1), 607–628. doi:10.1146/annurev.clinpsy.1.102803.144141

Scott, E. (2019). 17 Highly Effective Stress Relievers. Very Well Mind. Retrieved from https://www.verywellmind.com/tips-to-reduce-stress-3145195#citation-5

SSQ financial solution. (2013). Reference document: Stress management. Paris. France. Retrieved from https://ssq.ca/sites/default/files/archives/ac/Chroniques_sante/Stress_management_-reference_document-.pdf

Uys, L., & Middleton, L. (2014). *Mental health nursing: A South African perspective* (6th ed.). Johannesburg: Juta.

Wu, G., Hu, Z., & Zheng, J. (2019). Role Stress, Job Burnout, and Job Performance in Construction Project Managers: The Moderating Role of Career Calling. *International Journal of Environmental Research and Public Health*, *16*(13), 2394. doi:10.3390/ijerph16132394

Wu, G., Wu, Y., Li, H., & Dan, C. (2018). Job Burnout, Work-Family Conflict and Project Performance for Construction Professionals: The Moderating Role of Organizational Support. *International Journal of Environmental Research and Public Health*, *15*(12), 2869. doi:10.3390/ijerph15122869

ADDITIONAL READING

Avison, W. R., & Gotlib, I. H. (1994). Future Prospects for Stress Research. In W. R. Avison & I. H. Gotlib (Eds.), *Stress and Mental Health. The Springer Series on Stress and Coping*. Boston, MA: Springer. doi:10.1007/978-1-4899-1106-3_12

Demerouti, E., & Bakker, A. B. (2011). The Job Demands–Resources model: Challenges for future research. *SA Journal of Industrial Psychology*, *37*, 2.

Hostinar, C. E., Nusslock, R., & Miller, G. E. (2018). Future Directions in the Study of Early-Life Stress and Physical and Emotional Health: Implications of the Neuroimmune Network Hypothesis. *Journal of clinical child and adolescent psychology*, *47*(1), 142–156. doi:10.1080/15374416.2016.1266647

Koivu, A., Saarinen, P. I., & Hyrkas, K. (2012). Does clinical supervision promote medical–surgical nurses' well-being at work? A quasi-experimental 4-year follow-up study. *Journal of Nursing Management*, *20*(3), 401–413.

May, R. W., Seibert, G. S., Sanchez-Gonzalez, M. A., & Fincham, F. D. (2018). School burnout and heart rate variability: Risk of cardiovascular disease and hypertension in young adult females, *Stress*. Kocaekşi, S. (2016). The evaluation of burnout levels of sports sciences faculty students. *Educational Research Review*, *11*, 4.

Ross, W., May, R. W., Bauer, K. N., & Fincham, F. D. (2015). School burnout: Diminished academic and cognitive performance. *Learning and Individual Differences*, *42*, 126.

Wortman, C. B., Sheedy, C., Gluhoski, V., & Kessler, R. C. (1992). Stress, coping, and health: Conceptual issues and directions for future research. In H. S. Friedman (Ed.), *Hostility, coping, & health* (pp. 227–256). Washington, DC, US: American Psychological Association; doi:10.1037/10105-016

Chapter 9
Stress and Trauma:
Negative Outcomes

Dana C. Branson
Southeast Missouri State University, USA

ABSTRACT

Toxic stress and trauma are common occurrences that can create physiological and psychological changes with negative short- and long-term effects. Research has clearly established a correlation between adversity and negative outcomes. However, there are a number of factors involved in the development, intensity, and severity of outcomes, specifically the type of stress or trauma experiences, temperament, personality type, repertoire of coping skills, and level of resiliency. This chapter reviews the definitions of different types of stress, the neurological changes that can occur as a result of adversity, common and paradoxical reactions to trauma, and the ability of coping skills and resilience to change the trajectory from negative outcomes to opportunities for positive growth.

INTRODUCTION

Stress is an unavoidable physical occurrence that creates a palatable presence of adversity and anxiety (Segal, Gerdes, & Steiner, 2019), straining one's coping abilities (Weiten, 2017). However, not all stressors are the same. Identified types of stress are positive stress, tolerable stress, toxic stress, and chronic stress. Additionally, trauma is a phenomenon that can be a significant influence on a person's physical development, health, childhood and adult behaviors, and worldview (Branson, Radu, & Loving, in press; Francis, DePriest, Wilson, & Gross, 2018). These terms have different definitions; however, it is common for toxic stress, chronic stress, and

DOI: 10.4018/978-1-7998-2139-7.ch009

trauma to co-occur, creating increased potential for physical and emotional damage through complicated biological, psychological, and social channels (Corbin et al., 2013; Nurius, Green, Logan-Greene, Longhi, & Song, 2016; O'Connor, Finkbiner, & Watson, 2012; Reinert, Campbell, Bandeen-Roche, Lee, & Szanton, 2016; Shern, Blanch, & Steverman, 2016).

A significant research study clearly demonstrates the dangers of childhood toxic stress and trauma. The Adverse Childhood Experiences (ACE) study was innovative research conducted by Drs. Felitti and Anda that found a formidable positive correlation between childhood trauma and negative health outcomes and social problems in adolescents and adults. Elevated ACE scores corelated to an increased prevalence of numerous negative medical issues, lifestyle behaviors, and mental health (Anda et al., 1999; Dube et al., 2001; Felitti et al., 1998).

Research further indicates that children exposed to toxic stress and trauma may incur physiological changes to their brain development, putting them at risk for lifetime negative outcomes (Nurius et al., 2016). Exposure to trauma and toxic stress has been shown to have strong correlations to negative outcomes, yet it is the coping techniques that one engages in that serve as the conduit for the negative medical and mental health issues experienced later in life. Coping techniques borne from traumatic events are often survivalist, serving a purpose at the time of crisis. However, as time progresses and the crisis subsides, the coping skills remain, turning into a negative set of activities that begets additional negative consequences (Herman, 1997). It is here that interruption and change can occur to alter the trajectory of poor lifestyle choices and habits. Learning and using positive coping skills is a significant component of resiliency training (Dias & Cadime, 2017). With the use of the biopsychosocial lens, the intersection of toxic stress, trauma, and trajectory of one's healthy and behavioral outcomes can be better understood, while also promoting helpful interventions for purposeful and action-oriented change through the adoption of positive coping skills and resiliency techniques. The chapter will discussed the following objectives: (a) the presence and commonality of toxic stress, with a specific focus on findings from the Adverse Childhood Experiences (ACE) study, (b) the complexity of traumatic aftermath: biologically, psychologically, and socially; long-term medical and mental health trajectory, and (c) high-risk negative coping techniques, protective positive coping techniques, resilience, and related future outcomes.

BACKGROUND

Adverse Childhood Experiences (ACE)

In 1998, Drs. Felitti and Anda conducted the original Adverse Childhood Experiences (ACE) survey with mostly college-educated, middle-class, and gainfully employed adults. The results indicated a strong positive correlation between negative childhood events and negative health outcomes in adulthood. Research has consistently found a strong correlation between childhood abuse, trauma, and adversity with negative behavioral outcomes in adolescence and adulthood (Asok, Benard, Roth, Rosen, & Dozier, 2013; Francis et al., 2018; Hillis, Mercy, & Saul, 2017; Power, et al., 2013; Shern et al., 2016). However, Felitti et al. (1998) were pioneering in their findings that showed a correlation between childhood adversity and physical illness. Along with medical history and assessment of a comprehensive medical exam by a physician, study participants were asked 10: yes/no questions to calculate a simple score ranging from 0 – 10 to represent their experience of adversity. An endorsement of "yes" equaled one (1) point, while an endorsement of "no" equaled zero (0) points in the following categories:

- Emotional abuse
- Physical abuse
- Sexual abuse
- Emotional neglect
- Physical neglect
- Parental separation/divorce/death
- Domestic abuse—specifically of mother-figure
- Living with someone struggling with mental health issues
- Living with someone struggling with substance use disorders
- Incarceration of a household member

According to the results of the study, 67 people out of 100 would have at least one (1) ACE score. Furthermore, the correlations between childhood adversity and negative health outcomes were significant. Results indicated that as ACE scores increased, so did the occurrence of physical problems in adulthood. The prevalence of obesity, diabetes, ischemic heart disease, stroke, cancer, and emphysema all increased with the number of ACE scores (Danese & McEwen, 2012; Felitti et al., 1998). Additionally, increased ACE scores also correlated with high-risk behaviors, such as smoking, recreational drug use, sedentary lifestyle, poor eating habits, sexual permissiveness, and poor safer sex practices (Anda et al., 1999; Dube et al., 2001; Reinert et al., 2016). Furthermore, the presence of mental health issues also increased, as did the occurrence of poorly regulated clinical depression, self-harm ideation, and suicide attempts (Felitti et al., 1998; Zare et al., 2018). Childhood adversity can shape lifelong issues and behaviors so much that those with an ACE score of 6 or more have been found to have an average decreased life expectancy of 20 years (Redford, 2015).

ACE scores occur across all demographic categories, income levels, and cultures. However, vulnerable populations, persons of color, members of traditionally oppressed groups, and those living in poverty have the highest concentrations of ACE scores (Blosnich & Anderson, 2015). Disparities of ACE scores across categories of privilege add an additional layer of vulnerability for some people who are already living logistically, socially, and politically difficult lives due to social constructs of difference (Sher et al., 2016). Therefore, inequality in health care and the increased ACE scores add to the compounding negative outcomes childhood adversity and trauma can create (Miller-Cribbs et al., 2016). This generates important implications for social services, health providers, educators, and the judicial system, as well as the need to account for the presence of ACE scores and the corresponding substantial influence adversity might have on people, especially their behaviors (Branson et al., in press).

STRESS AND TRAUMA

Stress is a word commonly used to describe difficulty of some sort; however, there are different types of stress and it is important to understand the differences. Positive stress occurs due to changes to one's homeostasis. Usually short-lived, positive stress is generally viewed as acceptable, as it is part of a desired change or goal (Segal et al., 2019). An example of positive stress would be nervous feelings before a test, performance, or a first date. Although uncomfortable, this level of stress has been shown to increase positive performance. Positive stress helps put the mind in a state of heightened alert, allowing students to readily remember the information they studied, athletes to run faster and jump higher, and for a couple on a first date to put their best foot forward and remember proper table manners and socially acceptable talking points. Like all categories of stress, it exists on a continuum. A little positive stress is good for performance; not enough can cause a less than optimal performance, and too much can cause debilitation and negative performance. Professional athletes and sports trainers work to cultivate the right amount of positive stress to put athletes in the best place for peak performance (Gandhe, 2014).

Tolerable stress, however, is different. This type of stress is aversive, as it is unwanted, but logical due to the commonality of such events (Segal et al., 2019).

Examples of tolerable stress are events such as being laid-off from a job, the ending of a romantic relationship, moving to a new town, or the death of a loved one. These events are often viewed as a part of life, and in time, the feelings of adversity will subside. Those struggling with tolerable stress understand that they are not going to feel like this forever and things will get better eventually. However, if tolerable stress is extreme or continues too long, it has the potential to become toxic stress. This level of stress is characterized as damaging stress due to the persistent physiological and psychological distress and response of the body (De Jong, 2016; Francis et al., 2018; Shern et al., 2016). Examples of toxic stress include working 40 hours a week at a job that one finds appalling, but having no realistic means to find something better; growing up in a home with a parent struggling with active substance use dependence; or living with an abusive partner and feeling as if there is no way out. A closely related stress that often occurs with toxic stress is chronic stress. Chronic stress is an additional type of stress that is endured over a long period of time and can influence one's worldview, such as being a member of an oppressed population and/or living in poverty (Segal et al., 2019). For the purposes of this chapter, the terms toxic stress and chronic stress will be combined into one term—toxic stress. An additional term to appreciate is trauma, which results from an event(s) that is perceived as a real threat to survival and can create adverse effects to a person physically, psychologically, socially, and spiritually (Substance Abuse and Mental Health Services Administration [SAMSAH], 2014). Traumatic events suffered by children can produce toxic stress, resulting in neurological changes that can set into motion a sequela of negative coping skills, activities, and behaviors that can result in lifelong challenges. However, this is not a prescriptive relationship, as positive coping and life-long trajectory can also occur. There are numerous elements involved in how the aftermath of trauma unfolds; however, key determining factors are temperament, personality, coping skills and resiliency.

Stress and Trauma-Induced Neurological Changes

Trauma is a highly individual and fickle phenomenon. Twins growing up in the same household with the same parenting, teachers, and support system can experience the same trauma at the same time and have completely opposite outcomes. One child may come through the event seemingly unaffected, while the other child's life is forever defined by the experience. Several factors influence a person's response to trauma and aftermath: the intensity and frequency of the event(s), the meaning of the event for the traumatized person, individual characteristics, temperament, personality type, biological make-up, availability of quality supports, prior experiences with trauma, presence of positive and/or negative coping skills, individual reaction to the trauma, ability to accurately reflect on the event, willingness to share about the event, the cultural response of one's community, and a myriad of other factors (Enlow, Blood, & Egeland, 2013; Milburn et al., 2019; Regehr, 2018; Shern et al., 2016).

To understand behavioral issues that accompany trauma, it is important to understand the neurological events that occur in the brain of a child exposed to toxic stress and trauma. Children's brains are especially vulnerable to the damages of toxic stress due to the rapid rate of physical and neurological development of childhood (van der Kolk, 2014). Humans are uniquely created for survival through a network of biological and instinctual processes. The brain and the hypothalamic-pituitary-adrenal center work together when threatened to create a response to danger (Cross, Fani, Powers, & Bradley, 2017). This is a process that allows humans to deal with danger and crisis in an optimal manner. However, what happens when this system is engaged too often for too long of a period of time? What was good for survival now becomes destructive and hurtful. This is an example of too much of a good thing. Much like Thanksgiving dinner, some is delicious and makes for a wonderful memory, while too much makes for a miserable afternoon and a trip to the medicine cabinet.

The brain is a highly complex organ. Reactions to trauma start in the brain. When looking at different parts of the brain, it is important to appreciate the function of certain areas. The neocortex is a large portion of the brain, and among other things, is partly responsible for thinking and rational decision making. The neocortex sits on top of the limbic section of the brain, which is a primary source of emotions and displayed feelings. Deeper still, under the neocortex and limbic sections of the brain is the reptilian brain or the instinctual part of the brain. This is the automatic part of one's brain that is responsible for basic body functions, such as breathing, heartbeat, and blood circulation. Two other important parts of the brain involved in trauma reactions are the amygdala and the hippocampus. These two areas are nestled in the limbic system, but also close to the autonomic portion of the brain (Hines, 2018). When a person is threatened and/or senses danger, the amygdala sends out the alarm signal to the rest of the brain. The hippocampus, which normally is concerned with filing and storing of memories, decreases its regular memory functions and begins to pump out cortisol, a stress hormone that decreases pain and provides extra strength to deal with the trauma at hand (Burke-Harris, 2018). When this occurs, the body switches from the auto-pilot of the parasympathetic nervous system to the sympathetic nervous system. The telltale signs of this system are dilated pupils to increase accuracy of vision, decrease of saliva and stomach activity resulting in a lack of appetite, accelerated heartbeat, dilated bronchi for increased oxygen flow, glycogen converted to glucose for quick energy, and adrenaline secreted for increased reaction time (Weiten, 2017). Although all of these changes serve a survivalist function in the crisis response, it is physically uncomfortable to the system and the host usually desires to return to the norm of the parasympathetic nervous system.

Additionally, the hypothalamus-pituitary-adrenal access center is also activated, which diverts blood and oxygen to muscles and safety measures kick in: fight, flight, or freeze (Duros & Crowley, 2014). Depending on the trauma that one is facing, all three of these responses might be appropriate. For example, as a 10-year-old child is watching his mother be abused by her partner, he might attack (fight) the abuser to interrupt the event, giving his mother an opportunity to get into her own fighting stance and overpower the abuser. For the 7-year-old child in same household, it might be appropriate for the child to run away (flight) to a grandparents' house to escape possible violence, witnessed or experienced. Furthermore, the 14-year-old in the house might crouch behind a sofa and try not to make any noise (freeze), hoping that the abusive event will be over quickly, and she will not be on the receiving end of any abuse herself. Because the body's trauma response cycle, involving these different areas of the brain and the hypothalamus-pituitary-adrenal access center is instinctual and happens much faster than the rational part of one's brain, which takes time to deliberate and make a decision, one does not choose the trauma reaction—the behavior simply occurs. However, when the person begins to reflect on the event, often in isolation of one's own thoughts, thinking errors begin to develop. The fighter believes he should have fought harder—he did not give his all. If he had just been stronger and tried harder, he could have stopped the violence. Therefore, he is a failure. The child that took flight may believe that he should have stayed and helped. Therefore, any damage that was done is partially his fault. The girl who froze and hid behind the couch may believe that she is truly a terrible person who allowed someone she loved to be harmed and did nothing about it. Not only did she allow her mother to suffer, but she also did nothing to help her younger brother who tried to fight off the abuser. She is the oldest, she should have done something, but she froze and did nothing. Therefore, she is just as bad as the abuser for her lack of action. All three children negatively judge themselves for reactions to a crisis that occurred before they had time to think about it. Therefore, they run the risk of holding themselves accountable to mistaken thinking errors of what they should/should not have done and the compounding negative aftermath of guilt and shame. If this cascade of events can result after a single crisis event, imagine the totality of a childhood filled with ongoing events creating the physiological trauma response, followed by the cognitive and emotional aftermath.

Research indicates that on-going exposure to toxic stress can be especially damaging to a child's brain; physically, functionally, cognitively, emotionally, and the overall size and quality function of the brain (Cross et al., 2017; Tomoda et al., 2009). Severe toxic stress and trauma have been correlated with decreased development of the corpus callosum, the largest part of the brain and the site of neurological nerve connections. Other parts of the brain to show decreased volume are the prefrontal cortices, hippocampus, temporal lobes, and the amygdala, which are central to decision making, regulating social behavior, memory formation, and emotional regulation (De Bellis & Keshavan, 2006; Teicher, Samson, Polcari, & McGreenery, 2006). Additionally, toxic stress can become physically corrosive due to the overexposure to the separate components of the sympathetic nervous system. For example, if the system overly stimulates the system to convert glycogen to glucose, an increased risk for diabetes can result (Reinert et al., 2016).

Stress, Trauma, and Behavior

Because trauma and toxic stress have the potential to change neurological development of the brain, both in functionality and physical composition, additional domains might also be affected, such as memory, emotions, mental health, and resulting behaviors (Cross et al., 2017; Nurius et al., 2016; Sperry & Widom, 2013). Negative sequela from traumatic aftermath can compound and complicate the physical and emotional healing process; contribute to self-blame pathological guilt, shame, and stigmatization; increase risk factors of mental health issues; and promote repressed or false memories (van der Kolk, 2014; Zare et al., 2018). As these dynamics manifest in dysfunctional behaviors, acting out, and coping skills, survivors of trauma are quickly labeled as liar, troublemaker, attention seeking, poor historian, criminal, unreliable sources of information, sexually permissive, lazy, obstinate, disrespectful, and a host of other negative personal characteristics (Milburn et al., 2019; Nurius et al., 2016).

The implications of trauma creating negative behaviors that can correlate to lifelong physical and emotional problems need to be appreciated, especially by those who work with people, such as teachers, social service workers, medical professionals, and those involved with corrections. Children and adolescents struggling with trauma may display several problematic behaviors that setup a snowball effect. Specific examples might include exaggerated mood changes, which causes a child to be unpredictable and labeled as a "drama queen/king" or "diva." This results in the child not being taken seriously, and complaints and protests being pushed aside, which can lead a child to act out in a more severe fashion to get his/her needs met. If this sequela of behavior occurs in an educational setting, it does not take long for the child to have a negative reputation that proceeds him/her in additional classes, with other teachers, students, and school administration. Other times, a child might appear to be emotionally numb, uncaring, having no conscious, or uninterested in others. Children struggling with emotional numbness often experience difficulty in forming friendships, are social isolated, struggle with trust issues, and have trouble forming healthy romantic and platonic bonds in their relationships. Additionally, as a means of combating emotional numbness, these children are at a greater risk for substance use disorders and involvement in nonsuicidal self-injury (formally known as self-mutilation; Andover & Morris, 2014).

Another common behavioral challenge is a cluster of issues resulting from poor emotional regulation, specifically explosive anger, incongruent affect, exaggerated sensitivity to non-verbal communication, and/or overreaction to events (SAMHSA, 2014). Even more confusing are opposite reactions or paradoxical reactions to trauma. The term paradoxical reaction is a common term used in medical science to describe contradictory reaction to medications or treatment regimens (Farkas, 2015). Reactions and aftermath of trauma can also appear to be paradoxical in that the behaviors displayed are incongruent with how one typically acts after experiencing a traumatic event or exposure to toxic stress. Examples of paradoxical behaviors are sexually assaulted women becoming sexually permissive with strangers in an attempt to seek control over their sexuality, or war-ravaged soldiers struggling with post-traumatic stress disorder signing up for the most dangerous missions with a high probability of human atrocity. Additional examples of paradoxical behaviors that sometimes create the most troublesome consequences are when children who are sexually abused become the perpetrator of sexual trauma on others (Parkhill & Pickett, 2016). Therefore, although one child survivor of trauma may struggle with poor emotional regulation and be easily angered and hypervigilant to non-verbal cues, another child may exhibit issues of poorly developed social skills and miss non-verbal cues completely. This is often mistaken as intentional misbehavior, selective listening, or diagnostic symptoms of mild Autism (formally known as Asperger's; Freeman, 2015). Furthermore, research indicates that children and adolescents who struggle with emotional regulation issues are also at a higher risk for suicidal ideation in later life (Glenn et al., 2017; Milburn et al., 2019).

Stress, Trauma, and Cognitions

Toxic stress and trauma can also negatively affect cognitive domains, specifically decision-making processes, impulsivity, and difficulties with attention, focus, and follow-through (Burke-Harris, 2018). Specific trauma related to physical abuse, severe physical or emotional neglect, or extreme poverty can result in decreased intelligence and overall cognitive ability (De Jong, 2016; Francis et al., 2018). When children are struggling with chaotic environments common to toxic stress, they may simply be unable to be completely present in school settings. The concerns of what happened in the past and what might continue to happen is cognitively distracting, keeping a child from being able to focus on educational tasks. Research indicates the earlier one is exposed to toxic stress and/or trauma the greater the risk of negative outcomes (Glenn et al., 2017). Therefore, cognitive deficits experienced early in a child's life can set into play a negative and compounding trajectory of educational problems and lack of learning. These same patterns occur in adulthood, as those struggling with unresolved trauma find that their minds are often flooded with racing thoughts, causing distraction. This can lead to social problems, as one might appear disinterested in topics of conversation. Additionally, life partners may feel that they are not being listened to or validated due to the emotional unavailability of their partner. Employment can also be threatened, as one might make costly mistakes due to not listening to directives or poorly retaining training materials due to general inattentiveness (Hillis et al., 2017). Furthermore, negative cognitive consequences could create misinterpretations of one's overall attitude, creating negative evaluations of one's work ethic, ability to work well with colleagues, and potential as a team player (Felitti et al, 1998; Shern et al., 2016).

Additionally, emotional consequences noted in research are undeveloped skills in perspective taking, poor or inflated self-esteem, and erroneous locus of control. All these issues can create significant problems with relationships as adults including life partners, loved ones, co-workers, and peers (Hyu, Sun-Young, Jeong, & Jeong-Ho, 2014). Additionally, those struggling with toxic stress are at an increased risk for anxiety disorder, depression issues, and other mood-regulation disorders (Zare et al., 2018). This places those who have already struggled with injustice and maltreatment in a position to be oppressed by stigmatizing labels associated with mental health issues, increased medical costs, and complications common to logistically obtaining needed services due to lack of transportation, inability to pay, and/or lack of resources.

Toxic stress and trauma can also be physically internalized, placing one at an increased vulnerability for high-risk health behaviors, like smoking, substance use, eating disorders—both restrictive and overindulgent, stress-induced disease processes, and somatic complaints (Anda et al., 1999; D'Andrea, Stolbach, Ford, Spinazzola, & van der Kolk, 2012; Felitti et al., 1998). Research has long indicated that prolonged stress signaling is correlated with development of physical illness, to include coronary heart disease, high blood pressure, inflammation, periodontal disease and other dental problems, decreased immunity, increased respiratory problems, reproductive health issues, obesity, diabetes, kidney disease, and some cancers (Francis et al., 2018; Reinert et al., 2016; Shern et al., 2016). Additionally, there is an increased risk in disease processes through exposure to high-risk coping techniques, behaviors, and related violence resulting in personal injuries, traumatic brain injury, sexually transmitted infections (STI, formally known as sexually transmitted diseases [STD]), and other contagious diseases (Gurel et al., 2019; Hillis et al., 2017; Reinert et al., 2016; Weiten, 2017), all of which can result in lifelong disabilities. Each of these elements can create significant problems during any developmental life phase and across all life domains. However, rarely do negative sequela from trauma or toxic stress occur in silos. As life domains (physical, emotional, mental, social, cognitive, and spiritual) bleed into one another, so does negative aftermath of trauma and toxic stress. Below is a list of immediate and delayed traumatic symptoms from SAMHSA (2014).

Table 1. Reactions to trauma

Immediate Emotional Reactions: • Numbness and detachment • Anxiety or severe fear • Guilt (including survivor guilt) • Exhilaration as a result of surviving • Anger • Sadness • Helplessness • Feeling unreal; depersonalization (e.g., feeling as if you are watching yourself) • Disorientation • Feeling out of control • Denial • Constriction of feelings • Feeling overwhelmed	**Delayed Emotional Reactions** • Irritability and/or hostility • Depression • Mood swings, instability • Anxiety (e.g., phobia, generalized anxiety) • Fear of trauma recurrence • Grief reactions • Shame • Feelings of fragility and/or vulnerability • Emotional detachment from anything that requires emotional reactions (e.g., significant and/or family relationships, conversations about self, discussion of traumatic events or reactions to them)
Immediate Physical Reactions: • Nausea and/or gastrointestinal distress • Sweating or shivering • Faintness • Muscle tremors or uncontrollable shaking • Elevated heartbeat, respiration, and blood pressure • Extreme fatigue or exhaustion • Greater startle responses Depersonalization	**Delayed Physical Reactions** • Sleep disturbances, nightmares Somatization (e.g., increased focus on and worry about body aches and pains) Appetite and digestive changes • Lowered resistance to colds and infection Persistent fatigue • Elevated cortisol levels • Hyperarousal • Long-term health effects including heart, liver, autoimmune, and chronic obstructive pulmonary disease
Immediate Cognitive Reactions • Difficulty concentrating • Rumination or racing thoughts (e.g., replaying the traumatic event over and over again) • Distortion of time and space (e.g., traumatic event may be perceived as if it was happening in slow motion, or a few seconds can be perceived as minutes) Memory problems (e.g., not being able to recall important aspects of the trauma) Strong identification with victims	**Delayed Cognitive Reactions** • Intrusive memories or flashbacks Reactivation of previous traumatic events Self-blame • Preoccupation with event • Difficulty making decisions • Magical thinking: belief that certain behaviors, including avoidant behavior, will protect against future trauma • Belief that feelings or memories are dangerous • Generalization of triggers (e.g., a person who experiences a home invasion during the daytime may avoid being alone during the day) • Suicidal thinking

continued on following page

Table 1 continued

Immediate Behavioral Reactions • Startled reaction • Restlessness • Sleep and appetite disturbances • Difficulty expressing oneself Argumentative behavior • Increased use of alcohol, drugs, and tobacco • Withdrawal and apathy • Avoidant behaviors	**Delayed Behavioral Reactions** • Avoidance of event reminders • Social relationship disturbances Decreased activity level • Engagement in high-risk behaviors Increased use of alcohol and drugs Withdrawal
Immediate Existential Reactions • Intense use of prayer • Restoration of faith in the goodness of others (e.g., receiving help from others) Loss of self-efficacy • Despair about humanity, particularly if the event was intentional • Immediate disruption of life assumptions (e.g., fairness, safety, goodness, predictability of life)	• **Delayed Existential Reactions** Questioning (e.g., "Why me?") • Increased cynicism, disillusionment Increased self-confidence (e.g., "If I can survive this, I can survive anything") • Loss of purpose • Renewed faith • Hopelessness • Reestablishing priorities • Redefining meaning and importance of life Reworking life's assumptions to accommodate the trauma (e.g., taking a self-defense class to reestablish a sense of safety)

Adapted from SAMHSA, 2014, p. 62-63

Temperament and Personality

Research has clearly demonstrated a positive correlation between toxic stress, trauma, and negative life events. However, exposure to adversity is not prescriptive. Although some people struggle with the aftermath of trauma, others prosper and experience life-changing growth and development. The difference between those who struggle and those who prosper is a complex formula, often consisting of personality, temperament, supportive resources, coping skills, and resilience. Personality and temperament are personal characteristics one is born with and has little control over to change. Infants come equipped with temperaments at birth, commonly described as easy or difficult. Those babies described as having easy temperaments are usually good sleepers, cry less, and seem to be naturally laid-back. Difficult temperament babies are often the opposite: poor sleepers, fussy with excessive crying, and sensitive to slight changes to schedules (Zastrow & Kirst-Ashman, 2015). Adding to the presence of temperament is the interaction this characteristic has with caregivers and environment. Easy temperament babies create less stress for parents, and therefore may receive different interactions and bounding opportunities. However, difficult temperament babies may increase the stress of parenting, evoking negative experiences and be placed at a higher risk for abuse and neglect (Voorthuis et al., 2014). Therefore, there are those who seem to come equipped to deal more effectively with life's adversities and perhaps avoid them altogether, while there are those that are naturally more vulnerable to trauma and toxic stress, as well as being more likely to experience it.

Personality is the predictable actions and reactions a person demonstrates over the course of a lifetime (Weiten, 2017). Because personality is such a static dynamic, if a person's personality (i.e. behaviors, actions, and reactions) suddenly changes, it is an indicator that something significant has occurred, such as a significant medical problem, emotional crisis, and/or change in lifestyle (Hanson, Venturelli, & Fleckenstein, 2018). McCrae and Costa (2008) identified five specific personality types. Most people are conglomerates of each of these five different personality types, some more prevalent than others. The identified traits are: (a) openness (those amenable to new experiences, intellectually curious, and tolerant of difference), (b) conscientiousness (those who are self-disciplined, dependable, and purposeful in their behaviors), (c) extraversion (those who are outgoing, friendly, and enjoy social attention), (d) agreeableness (those who are naturally empathetic, humble, and help others), (e) neuroticism (those who struggle with emotional instability, personal insecurity, impulsivity, and can be demanding). Research implies that those who score high on extraversion and/or openness are more likely to have positive aftermath from traumatic events, whereas those who score high on neuroticism are more likely to struggle with traumatic aftermath, to be diagnosed with post-traumatic stress disorder, and negative lifelong consequences (Aldemi, Dalbudak, & Topcu, 2015; Weinberg & Gil, 2016). Therefore, a difficult temperament child who scores high on neuroticism personality trait is likely to struggle with an aversive childhood more than a child born with an easy temperament and an extraversion personality. Consequently, there are certain people that seem to simply be set up to deal with trauma better than others. Additionally, there are those who are more vulnerable to the negative effects of trauma and toxic stress.

Trajectory of Coping Skills and Resilience Training

Temperament and personality traits are dynamics that resist change; however, understanding about one's personal make-up allows one to cater a plan that works for them for positive change. Additional dynamics that one has significant control over and can augment for purposeful change are coping skills. Coping skills are those efforts used to conquer, decrease, extinguish, or endure adversity (Weiten, 2017). These skills emerge from different circumstances, events, and experiences, and can sometimes be as complicated as the adversity that set them into place. Sometimes one finds comfort in an arbitrary activity that is paired with stress relief and it becomes a conditioned response, and other times coping activities are modeled by others of influence (Powell, Honey, & Symbaluk, 2016). Coping skills can be positive, negative, or both. When working with those struggling with trauma and toxic stress, coping skills can be seen as a means to deal with the crisis situation and survival (Levine, Proulx, & Schwartz, 2018). Additionally, what was once a productive and positive coping skill for a child can become negative as one develops and becomes an adult. For example, if a child is raised in a home with a parent with persistent mental illness, she might learn to not talk back to her mother who is making verbal comments that do not make sense due to an episode of psychosis. The child learns not to defend herself when being accused of being an FBI agent planted in the home to spy on her mother and to obediently take a shower with all her clothes on to ensure the listening devises are destroyed by water. This is a much easier and more effective way to deal with her mother who struggles with schizophrenia. However, as the child grows, this coping technique of not standing up for herself and obedience to avoid conflict can create significant problems in a toxic relationship with an abusive partner. Coping skills are dynamic, fluid, and need to be modified as life and personal development evolves.

Resiliency is the ability to adapt and cope with negative events (Tassie, 2015). Although some people are born with temperaments, personality traits, and/or privilege that simply make them more resilient, this dynamic can also be artificially enhanced with purposeful attention and conscious behavior (Gul & Karanci, 2017; Moore & Woodcock, 2017). Resiliency is a natural counterweight to adversity, and increased resilience is correlated with increased positive coping and aftermath from negative situations. Even though resiliency is a personal trait that individuals possess in varying amounts, it is also a skill that can be taught, learned, and practiced. Additionally, not all adversity is bad. Dooley, Slavich, Moreno, and Bower (2017) found that some adversity in a person's life can be helpful in developing positive resiliency that can be adapted and applied to other difficult life experiences. Therefore, when looking for a way to decrease the negative consequences of trauma and toxic stress for children, adolescents, and adults, the answer may lie in the need to increase resilience and teach skills that reinforce the use and expansion of resiliency skills in daily life. Furthermore, the use of positive techniques begets modeling of positive behaviors, cognitive approaches, and attitudes for others, especially younger generations to emulate. Humans are one of the most resilient creatures on the planet due to opportunities, networks, evolving medical care, and ability to evolve, adapt, and welcome change (Scheffer et al., 2018). Therefore, assisting those struggling with toxic stress and trauma with practical and purposeful ways to increase their level of resiliency is a viable means of tipping the direction of future outcomes.

SOLUTIONS AND RECOMMENDATIONS

Practical factors for increasing resiliency are having reliable resources and supports, including access to basic daily needs, financial capital, transportation, health care, education, and employment. Often this means making new connections and opportunities to help fill in the gaps. Cognitive resiliency skills involve purposefully approaching adversity as an opportunity to grow, working to be less crisis-oriented and more goal-oriented with recovery efforts, focusing more on the future and less on the past, remaining flexible, and consciously adopting an attitude of gratitude. Furthermore, adversity needs to be processed outside of one's own mind and worldview (Lam, 2015). This can be accomplished through journaling, guided artistry, sharing with others, being part of a group with others who have experienced similar adverse events, drama-related storytelling, learning more about the complexity of trauma reactions and recovery, and creating a realistic plan to create desired change (Palidofsky & Stolbach, 2012; Zerrudo, 2016). Additional sources of support are spirituality, which is loosely and independently defined by those seeking this arena for assistance (Reinert et al., 2016). Finally, one of the most importantly factors of resiliency, especially for children, is at least one dependable and emotionally stable person who is actively involved in the child's life and supporting of his/her holistic growth (Redford, 2015). Research indicates that with calculated deliberation, one can decide to grow from adversity, but this often requires support, coaching from others, purposeful steps to make change happen, and time (Ben-Porat, 2015). It is possible that one might experience post traumatic growth spontaneously and in isolation; however, it is far more likely if the change one desires is carefully planned out and executed.

FUTURE RESEACH AND DIRECTION

The best way to deal with negative traumatic aftermath is to prevent adversity from occurring. Unfortunately, trauma and toxic stress are common occurrences that likely will continue. Social service and social sciences have been actively involved in research and education of trauma care as a means of ensuring social service workers provide more holistic and effective care. Due to the complex and intricate nature of trauma and toxic stress and the potential effects to a person's physical, emotional, mental, cognitive, social, and spiritual life, research is still needed. Exploring the relationship between trauma and toxic stress with a variety of variables, including temperament, personality traits, parenting styles, cognitive processes, purposeful recovery approaches, and resiliency factors, would yield further interventions for positive outcomes. Although trauma and toxic stress can create a host of short- and long-term negative consequences, with the right approach, it can also be a springboard for growth and positive outcomes.

CONCLUSION

Understanding the components of toxic stress, trauma, and negative medical and mental health outcomes is important in creating proactive and purposeful interventions to reverse damage and improve outcomes. Due to biological changes in the chronically stressed brain, the on-going presence of increased cortisol levels, and other areas of the central nervous system, the body remains at high alert and has a reduced capacity to rest and repair. Psychological issues of hypervigilance, mental arousal, and anxiety develop, causing one to desire physical and emotional relief. Coping skills exist on a continuum, with a varying degree of what is healthy and unhealthy. Additionally, the comprehensive wellness aspects of coping skills change as one moves into different periods of human development. Related social aspects can also occur due to the concentration of toxic stress and trauma in certain communities. This creates social networks of people engaging and modeling negative coping skills to each other, resulting in habit-forming activities and behaviors that potentially breed negative medical and mental health issues later in life. By using a biopsychosocial perspective, we can assess the development of problematic issues, understand the individual, environmental, and communal aspects of the issues, and find meaningful methods to interrupt and reverse negative outcomes. Through purposeful intervention, planning, and cognitive approaches, negative life experiences can become opportunities for personal growth and intentional behaviors can produce positive physical and emotional health outcomes.

REFERENCES

Aldemi, S., Dalbudak, E., & Topcu, M. (2015). Relationship of posttraumatic stress symptoms with depression, anxiety, childhood trauma and personality characteristics. *Klinik Psikofarmakoloji Bülteni*, *25*, S98.

Anda, R. F., Croft, J. B., Felitti, V. J., Norenberg, D., Giles, W. H., Williamson, D. R., & Giovino, G. A. (1999). Adverse childhood events and smoking during adolescence and adulthood. *American Medical Association, 282*(17), 1652-1658.

Andover, M. S., & Morris, B. W. (2014). Expanding and clarifying the role of emotional regulation in nonsuicidal self-injury. *Canadian Journal of Psychiatry*, *59*(11), 569–575. doi:10.1177/070674371405901102

Asok, A., Bernard, K., Roth, T. L., Rosen, J. B., & Dozier, M. (2013). Parental responsiveness moderates the association between early-life stress and reduced telomere length. *Development and Psychopathology*, *25*(3), 577–585. doi:10.1017/S0954579413000011

Ben-Porat, A. (2015). Vicarious post-traumatic growth: Domestic violence therapists versus social service department therapists in Israel. *Journal of Family Violence*, *30*(7), 923–933. doi:10.100710896-015-9714-x

Blosnich, J. R., & Anderson, J. P. (2015). Thursday's child: The role of adverse childhood experiences in explaining mental health disparities among lesbian, gay, and bisexual U.S. adults. *Social Psychiatry and Psychiatric Epidemiology*, *50*(2), 335–338. doi:10.100700127-014-0955-4

Branson, D. C., Radu, M. B., & Loving, J. D. (in press). Adverse Childhood Experiences (ACE) scores: When social work students and trauma mix. *The Journal of Baccalaureate Social Work*.

Burke-Harris, N. (2018). *The deepest well: Healing the long-term effects of childhood adversity*. London, England: Bluebird.

Corbin, T. J., Purtle, J., Rich, L. J., Rich, J. A., Adams, E. J., Yee, G., & Bloom, S. L. (2013). The prevalence of trauma and childhood adversity in an urban, hospital-based violence intervention program. *Journal of Health Care for the Poor and Underserved*, *24*(3), 1021–1030. doi:10.1353/hpu.2013.0120

Cross, D., Fani, N., Powers, A., & Bradley, B. (2017). Neurobiological development in the context of childhood trauma. *Clinical Psychology: Science and Practice*, *24*(2), 111–124. doi:10.1111/cpsp.12198

D'Andrea, W., Ford, J., Stolbach, B., Spinazzola, J., & van der Kolk, B. A. (2012). Understanding interpersonal trauma in children: Why we need a developmentally appropriate trauma diagnosis. *The American Journal of Orthopsychiatry*, *82*(2), 187–200. doi:10.1111/j.1939-0025.2012.01154.x

Danese, A., & McEwen, B. S. (2012). Adverse childhood experiences, allostasis, allostatic load, and age-related disease. *Physiology & Behavior*, *106*(1), 29–39. doi:10.1016/j.physbeh.2011.08.019

De Bellis, M. D., Keshavan, M. S., Shifflett, H., Iyengar, S., Beers, S. R., Hall, J., & Moritz, G. (2006). Cerebellar volumes in pediatric maltreatment-related posttraumatic stress disorder: A sociodemographically matched study. *Biological Psychiatry*, *52*(11), 1066–1078. doi:10.1016/S0006-3223(02)01459-2

De Jong, A. R. (2016). Domestic violence, children, and toxic stress. *Widener Law Review*, *22*(2), 201–213.

Dias, P. C., & Cadime, I. (2017). Protective factors and resilience in adolescents: The mediating role of self-regulation. *Psicologia dell'Educazione*, *23*(1), 37–43. doi:10.1016/j.pse.2016.09.003

Dooley, L. N., Slavich, G. M., Moreno, P. I., & Bower, J. E. (2017). Strength through adversity: Moderate lifetime stress exposure is associated with psychological resilience in breast cancer survivors. *Stress and Health*, *33*(5), 549–557. doi:10.1002mi.2739

Dube, S. R., Anda, R. F., Felitti, V. J., Chapman, D. P., Williamson, D. F., & Giles, W. H. (2001). Childhood abuse, household dysfunction, and the risk of attempted suicide throughout the life span: Findings from the Adverse Childhood Experiences study. *American Medical Association, 286*(24), 3089-3095.

Duros, P., & Crowley, D. (2014). The body comes to therapy too. *Clinical Social Work Journal*, *42*(3), 237–246. doi:10.100710615-014-0486-1

Enlow, M. B., Blood, E., & Egeland, B. (2013). Sociodemographic risk, developmental competence, and PTSD symptoms in young children exposed to interpersonal trauma in early life. *Journal of Traumatic Stress*, *26*(6), 686–694. doi:10.1002/jts.21866

Farkas, J. (2015, September). *Recognizing and managing paradoxical reactions from benzodiazepines and propofol*. Retrieved from https://emcrit.org/pulmcrit/recognizing-and-managing-paradoxical-reactions-from-benzodiazepines-propofol/

Felitti, V. J., Anda, R. F., Nordenberg, D., Williamson, D. F., Spitz, A. M., Edwards, V., ... Marks, J. S. (1998). Relationship of childhood abuse and household dysfunction to many of the leading causes of death in adults: The Adverse Childhood Experience (ACE) study. *American Journal of Preventive Medicine*, *14*(4), 245–258. doi:10.1016/S0749-3797(98)00017-8

Francis, L., DePriest, K., Wilson, M., & Gross, D. (2018). Child poverty, toxic stress, and social determinants of health: Screening and care coordination. *Online Journal of Issues in Nursing*, *23*(3), 2. doi:10.3912/OJIN.Vol23No03Man02

Freeman, J. (2015). Developing social skills and relationships. *Reclaiming Children and Youth*, *23*(4), 48–51.

Gandhe, R. J. (2014). Positive stress: Review of relevant theories and an alternative conceptualization. *Indian Journal of Positive Psychology*, *5*(3), 260–266.

Glenn, C. R., Lanzillo, E. C., Esposito, E. C., Santee, A. C., Nock, M. K., & Auerbach, R. P. (2017). Examining the course of suicidal and nonsuicidal self-injurious thoughts and behaviors in outpatient and inpatient adolescents. *Journal of Abnormal Child Psychology*, *45*(5), 971–983. doi:10.100710802-016-0214-0

Gul, E., & Karanci, A. N. (2017). What determines posttraumatic stress and growth following various traumatic events? A study in a Turkish community sample. *Journal of Traumatic Stress*, *30*(1), 54–62. doi:10.1002/jts.22161

Gurel, N. Z., Carek, A. M., Inan, O. T., Levantsevych, O., Abdelhadi, N., Hammadah, M., ... Shah, A. J. (2019). Comparison of autonomic stress reactivity in young healthy versus aging subjects with heart disease. *PLoS One*, *14*(5), 1–16. doi:10.1371/journal.pone.0216278

Hanson, G. R., Venturelli, P. J., & Fleckenstein, A. E. (2018). *Drugs and society* (13th ed.). Burlington, MA: Jones & Bartlett Learning.

Herman, J. (1997). *Trauma and recovery: The aftermath of violence-from domestic abuse to political terror*. New York, NY: Basic Books.

Hillis, S. D., Mercy, J. A., & Saul, J. R. (2017). The enduring impact of violence against children. *Psychology Health and Medicine*, *22*(4), 393–405. doi:10.1080/13548506.2016.1153679

Hines, T. (April 2018). *Anatomy of the brain*. Mayfield Brain and Spine. Retrieved from https://mayfieldclinic.com/pe-anatbrain.htm

Hyu, J. H., Sun-Young, K., Jeong, J. Y., & Jeong-Ho, C. (2014). Childhood trauma and adult interpersonal relationship problems in patients with depression and anxiety disorders. *Annals of General Psychiatry*, *13*(1), 1–23. doi:10.118612991-014-0026-y

Lam, K. Y. (2015). Disclosure and psychological well-being of sexually abused adolescents in Hong Kong. *Journal of Child Sexual Abuse*, *24*(7), 731–752. doi:10.1080/10538712.2015.1077364

Levine, K. A., Proulx, J., & Schwartz, K. (2018). Disconnected lives: Women with intellectual disabilities in conflict with the law. *Journal of Applied Research in Intellectual Disabilities*, *31*(2), 249–258. doi:10.1111/jar.12387

McCrae, R. R., & Costa, P. T. (2008). The five-factor theory of personality. In O. P. John, R. W. Robins, & L. A. Pervin (Eds.), *Handbook of personality: Theory and research* (Vol. 3, pp. 159–181). New York, NY: Guilford Press.

Milburn, N. G., Stein, J. A., Lopez, S. A., Hilberg, A. M., Veprinsky, A., Arnold, E. M., ... Comulada, W. S. (2019). Trauma, family factors and the mental health of homeless adolescents. *Journal of Child & Adolescent Trauma, 12*(1), 37–47. doi:10.100740653-017-0157-9

Miller-Cribbs, J. E., Wen, F., Coon, K. A., Jelley, M. J., Foulks-Rodriguez, K., & Stearns, J. (2016). Adverse childhood experiences and inequalities in adult health care access. *International Public Health Journal, 8*(2), 257–270.

Moore, B., & Woodcock, S. (2017). Resilience, bullying, and mental health: Factors associated with improved outcomes. *Psychology in the Schools, 54*(7), 689–702. doi:10.1002/pits.22028

Nurius, P. S., Green, S., Logan-Greene, P., Longhi, D., & Song, C. (2016). Stress pathways to health inequalities: Embedding ACEs within social and behavioral contexts. *International Public Health Journal, 8*(2), 241–256.

O'Connor, C., Finkbiner, C., & Watson, L. (2012). *Adverse childhood experiences in Wisconsin: Findings from the 2010 behavioral risk factor survey*. Madison, WI: Wisconsin Children's Trust Fund and Child Abuse Prevention Fund of Children's Hospital and Health System.

Palidofsky, M., & Stolbach, B. C. (2012). Dramatic healing: The evolution of a trauma-informed musical theatre program for incarcerated girls. *Journal of Child & Adolescent Trauma, 5*(3), 239–256. doi:10.1080/19361521.2012.697102

Parkhill, M. R., & Pickett, S. M. (2016). Difficulties in emotion regulation as a mediator of the relationship between child sexual abuse victimization and sexual aggression perpetration in male college students. *Journal of Child Sexual Abuse, 25*(6), 674–685. doi:10.1080/10538712.2016.1205161

Powell, R. A., Honey, P. L., & Symbaluk, D. G. (2016). *Introduction to learning and behavior* (5th ed.). Belmont, CA: Wadsworth Publishing Company.

Power, R. A., Lecky-Thompson, L., Fisher, H. L., Cohen-Woods, S., Hosang, G. M., Uher, R., ... McGuffin, P. (2013). The interaction between child maltreatment, adult stressful life events and the 5-HTTLPR in major depression. *Journal of Psychiatric Research, 47*(8), 1032–1035. doi:10.1016/j.jpsychires.2013.03.017

Redford, J. (Producer). (2015, September 21). *ACES primer* [Video file]. Retrieved from https://vimeo.com/139998006

Regehr, C. (2018). *Stress, trauma, and decision-making for social workers*. New York, NY: Columbia University Press. doi:10.7312/rege18012

Reinert, K., Campbell, J., Bandeen-Roche, K., Lee, J., & Szanton, S. (2016). The role of religious involvement in the relationship between early trauma and health outcomes among adult survivors. *Journal of Child & Adolescent Trauma, 9*(3), 231–241. doi:10.100740653-015-0067-7

Scheffer, M., van de Leemput, I. A., van Nes, E. H., Gijzel, S. M. W., Romero, L. M., & Bolhuis, J. E., … Martin, C. M. (2018). Quantifying resilience of humans and other animals. In *Proceedings of the National Academy of Sciences of the United States of America* (pp. 11883–11890). Academic Press. 10.1073/pnas.1810630115

Segal, E. A., Gerdes, K. E., & Steiner, S. (2019). *An introduction to the profession of social work* (6th ed.). Boston, MA: Cengage Learning.

Shern, D. L., Blanch, A. K., & Steverman, S. M. (2016). Toxic stress, behavioral health, and the next major era in public health. *The American Journal of Orthopsychiatry, 86*(2), 109–123. doi:10.1037/ort0000120

Sperry, D. M., & Widom, C. S. (2013). Child abuse and neglect, social support, and psychopathology in adulthood: A prospective investigation. *Child Abuse & Neglect, 37*(6), 415–425. doi:10.1016/j.chiabu.2013.02.006

Substance Abuse and Mental Health Services Administration. (2014). Trauma-Informed Care in Behavioral Health Services. Treatment Improvement Protocol (TIP) Series 57. Rockville, MD: Author.

Tassie, A. K. (2015). Vicarious resilience from attachment trauma: Reflections of long-term therapy with marginalized young people. *Journal of Social Work Practice, 29*(2), 191–204. doi:10.1080/02650533.2014.933406

Teicher, M. H., Samson, J. A., Polcari, A., & McGreenery, C. E. (2006). Sticks, stones, and hurtful words: Relative effects of various forms of childhood maltreatment. *The American Journal of Psychiatry, 163*(6), 993–1000. doi:10.1176/ajp.2006.163.6.993

Tomoda, A., Suzuki, H., Rabi, K., Sheu, Y. S., Polcari, A., & Teicher, M. H. (2009). Reduced prefrontal cortical gray matter volume in young adults exposed to harsh corporal punishment. *NeuroImage, 47*, T66–T71. doi:10.1016/j.neuroimage.2009.03.005

van der Kolk, B. (2014). *The body keeps the score: Brain, mind, and body in the healing of trauma*. New York, NY: Penguin Books.

Voorthuis, A., Bhandari, R., Out, D., Veen, R., Bakermans-Kranenburg, M., & IJzendoorn, M. (2014). Childhood maltreatment experiences and child abuse potential: Temperamental sensitivity as moderator? *Journal of Family Violence*, *29*(7), 749–756. doi:10.100710896-014-9624-3

Weinberg, M., & Gil, S. (2016). Trauma as an objective or subjective experience: The association between types of traumatic events, personality traits, subjective experience of the event, and posttraumatic symptoms. *Journal of Loss and Trauma*, *21*(2), 137–146. doi:10.1080/15325024.2015.1011986

Weiten, W. (2017). *Psychology: Themes and variations* (10th ed.). Boston, MA: Cengage Learning.

Zare, M., Narayan, M., Lasway, A., Kitsantas, P., Wojtusiak, J., & Oetjen, C. A. (2018). Influence of Adverse Childhood Experiences on anxiety and depression in children aged 6 to 11 years. *Pediatric Nursing*, *44*(6), 267–274.

Zastrow, C., & Kirst-Ashman, K. K. (2015). *Empowerment series: Understanding human behavior and the social environment* (10th ed.). Boston, MA: Cengage Learning.

Zerrudo, M. R. (2016). Theater of disaster, folk stories as vehicles for healing and survival. *Teaching Artist Journal*, *14*(3), 161–170. doi:10.1080/15411796.2016.1209073

ADDITIONAL READING

Building Resiliency Toolkit. (n.d.). Koru Development. Retrieved from https://www.korudevelopment.co.uk/building-resilience/

Center on the Developing Child at. https://developingchild.harvard.edu/resources/aces-and-toxic-stress-frequently-asked-questions/

Centers for Disease Control and Prevention. (n.d.). Retrieved from https://www.cdc.gov/violenceprevention/acestudy/index.html

Cori, J. L. (2007). *Healing from trauma: A survivor's guide to understanding your symptoms and reclaiming your life*. Boston, MA: Da Capo Lifelong Books.

Edwards, K. M., Murphy, S., Palmer, K. M., Haynes, E. E., Chapo, S., Ekdahl, B. A., & Buel, S. (2017). Co-occurrence of and recovery from substance abuse and lifespan victimization: A qualitative study of female residents in trauma-informed sober living homes. *Journal of Psychoactive Drugs*, *49*(1), 74–82. doi:10.1080/02791072.2016.1273566

Leppin, A. L., Bora, P. R., Tilburt, J. C., Gionfriddo, M. R., Zeballos-Palacios, C., Dulohery, M. M., ... Montori, V. M. (2014). The efficacy of resiliency training programs: A systematic review and meta-analysis of randomized trials. *PLoS One*, *9*(10), 1–15. doi:10.1371/journal.pone.0111420

Phifer, L., Crowder, A., Elsenraat, T., & Hull, R. (2017). *CBT toolbox for children and adolescents: Over 200 worksheets & exercises for trauma, ADHD, autism, anxiety, depression & conduct disorders*. Eau Claire, WI: PESI Publishing and Media.

Scaer, R. (2005). *The trauma spectrum: Hidden wounds and human resiliency*. New York, NY: W. W. Norton and Company.

Sciaraffa, M. A., Zeanah, P. D., & Zeanah, C. H. (2018). Understanding and promoting resilience in the context of adverse childhood experiences. *Early Childhood Education Journal*, *46*(3), 343–353. doi:10.100710643-017-0869-3

Substance Abuse and Mental Health Services Administration (SAMHSA). (n.d.). Retrieved from https://www.samhsa.gov/capt/practicing-effective-prevention/prevention-behavioral-health/adverse-childhood-experiences

Toxic Stress Toolkit. (n.d.). Early Childhood Colorado Partnership. Retrieved from http://eccp.civiccanopy.org/resources/toolkits/toxic-stress-toolkit/#1474411393133-9f4e52ad-0fb9

Trauma-informed Toolkit Part 1. (n.d.). Government of Manitoba, Department of Health Living and Health. Retrieved from https://trauma-informed.ca/wp-content/uploads/2013/10/Trauma-informed_Toolkit.pdf

van der Kolk, B. (2015). *The body keeps the score: Brain, mind, and body in the healing of trauma*. London, United Kingdom: Penguin Books.

Yoon, S. (2018). Fostering resilient development: Protective factors underlying externalizing trajectories of maltreated children. *Journal of Child and Family Studies*, *27*(2), 443–452. doi:10.100710826-017-0904-4

Chapter 10
IOT Applications to Cure TTH Using Different Biofeedback:
A Statistical Approach in Healthcare

Rohit Rastogi
https://orcid.org/0000-0002-6402-7638
Dayalbagh Educational Institute, India & ABES Engineering College, India

Devendra Kumar Chaturvedi
https://orcid.org/0000-0002-4837-2570
Dayalbagh Educational Institute, Agra, India

ABSTRACT

The most common type of primitive headache is the tension type headache (TTH). The focus of complete research work was to compare the impression of EMG, GSR and EEG integrated biofeedback on stress due to headache and quality-of-life of the subjects under consideration. EMG biofeedback (BF) and galvanic skin resistance (GSR) are considered effective therapy for headaches. There are no such comparative effects of visual and auditory EMG biofeedback for headaches. Twenty subjects were subjected to EEG therapy. The variables for stress (pain) and SF-36(Quality of life) scores were recorded at starting point, 30 days and 90 days after the starting of GSR and EMG-BF therapy.

DOI: 10.4018/978-1-7998-2139-7.ch010

INTRODUCTION

More than half of the world experiences TTH in one form or the other. It has been called by different names over the years for example tension headache, muscle contraction, etc. (Cassel, 1997).

It is not accompanied by nausea or vomiting and is also not affected by physical factors. Thus, one will continue to do his daily task without even knowing if he is suffering from such headache or not. It also does not have any visual disturbances.

TTH (Tension Type Headache)

TTH stands for tension-type headache. It is a condition of the body in which one experiences ache/ pain like a physical weight or a tight band around your head. It can generally last for some days or can even continue long. TTH is different from migraine as it can be affected due to everyday activities, which is not in the case of TTH.

Tension-type headache arises due to

- Constant stress
- Incomplete sleep
- Anxiety
- Depression
- Emotional Disturbance

The pain in TTH spreads all over the head, unlike migraine which pains only on a particular side of your head. Symptoms of TTH include:

- The feeling of pressure across the forehead
- Aching head all over the area
- Tenderness of head and neck muscles, etc. (Cassel, 1997).

TTH can be divided into two main types: Chronic and Episodic

Episodic Tension Headaches

They can last from 30 minutes to about a week. It can also vary from 15 days in a month to about 3 months. It can also become chronic. One can have migraines if episodic headaches occur frequently.

Chronic Tension Headaches

If the headache lasts for 15-20 days out of a month continuing for about 3 months it becomes chronic. It occurs early in the morning and its symptoms include poor appetite, restlessness, lack of concentration and depression.

TTH varies in intensity, duration, and location. Use of alcohol, stress, caffeine, cold, dental problem, eye strain, excessive smoking, tiredness, etc. are the triggers of tension headaches. However one must remember they are not a brain disease. An individual may suffer from this TTH in any age group however they are normal in adult age and older teens. It generally runs in families and is common in women. Earlier reports which show the occurrence of tension-type headaches are given below:

Figure 1. Stats of occurrence of TTH as per different countries (Episodic vs. Chronic) (Boureau et al., 2001)

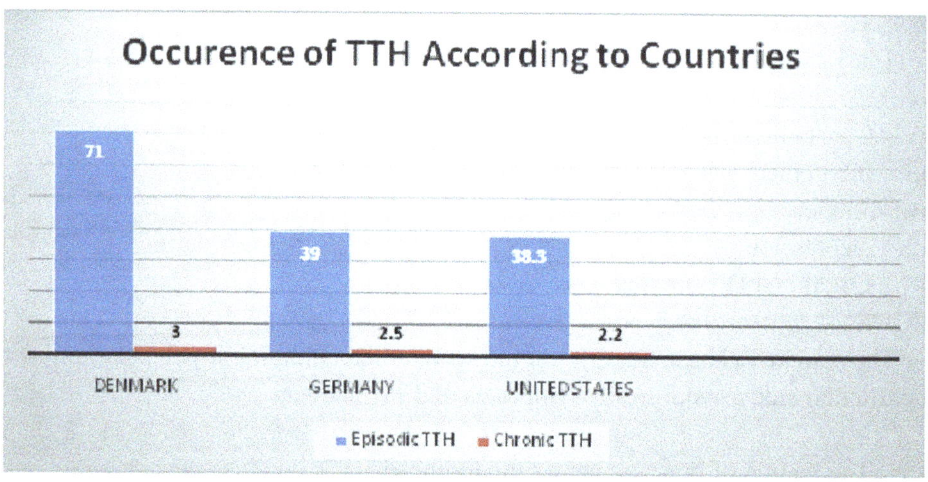

This graph shows various countries in which Episodic TTH and Chronic TTH is experienced by the people whether it is man or women. Around 71% and 3% people in Denmark are suffering, 39% & 2.5% in Germany and around 38.3% & 2.2% all are suffering by this disease.

Treatment

Massaging scalp, temples or bottom of your neck can help to relieve pain in a headache.

Over the countries, painkillers such as ibuprofen, aspirin, paracetamol, and naproxen are mostly used by patients suffering from TTH. These painkillers are used when the condition of headache becomes uncontrollable and interferes with your physical activities. However, the treatment of TTH can vary according to the symptoms and triggers causing it.

Taking painkillers more than thrice a weak can be harmful and thus avoided by the patient. An individual is suggested to be in relaxation stage and tension free to avoid TTH. It is also suggested by experts to have a full sleep of 7-8 hours a day in order to be away from headaches. Another way is the use of tricycle antidepressants. If your headache is caused due to psychological factors it may be hard to tackle. It is then advised to see a counselor or psychotherapist. If home remedies do not work, then medical assistance may be needed by the doctor. Consumption of a high quantity of acetaminophen can damage the liver. The heavy dose of analgesics like ibuprofen or aspirin can disturb one's stomach or damage the kidneys too.

It is a non-pharmacologic, majorly used to treat the stress and headache and tension-type headache. The key factors of efficiency, specificity and treatment moderators are measured by the meta-analysis of biofeedback for TTH (Rastogi et al., 2018f).

It is suggested that biofeedback is a good exercise for overcoming headache mainly tension-type headache. Many studies have been carried out for Biofeedback for the treatment of TTH and migraine. It was revealed that out of the last three months at least four patients were harmed by this technique to cure headache (Chaturvedi et al., 2017b).

When to Seek Medical Emergency?

One must seek a medical emergency if

- Loss of balance, vision, speech, etc. occurs
- The headache starts suddenly and becomes uncontrollable
- Headache accompanied by high fever
- Headache pattern changes
- Medicines fail
- One has side effects from medicines such as pale skin, rashes, depression, nausea, vomiting, cramps, dry mouth, etc.
- One is pregnant

One needs to learn to keep balance among alternative therapy with no-drug consumption, using right and necessary medications only and nurturing healthy habits. It is not necessary that one is having TTH only whenever headache happens. There may be sufficient chances of brain tumor or rupture of a weakened blood vessel also known as an aneurysm in heavy TTH cases. One might also face headaches after a severe head injury. Protecting your head from such injuries is very important. Tension headaches are very common and it marks the QoL and efficiency and productivity in the job along with life satisfaction. Such kind of aches checks an individual from active participation in different activities. One may need to take a break from the job and be at home or even if one goes to work it may make your work impaired (Satya et al., 2019a and Wenk-Sormaz, 2005).

Preventions of Tension Type Headache

Biofeedback Training

It is used to check some predefined body responses in a constrained environment to decrease the pain. Some important body indications are used as parameters like muscle tension, heart rate, and blood pressure.

Cognitive Behavioral Therapy

The method supports individual to learn how to handle stress and helps to shorten the frequency and severity of one's headaches.

Other Relaxation Techniques

Includes effective alternative therapies like deep breathing, yoga, meditation, and progressive muscle relaxation, etc.

As per different studies and reports, it has been found and established that TTH is directly correlated with demographical conditions, social culture across the region as per age, the gender of individual and stats analysis of data assessment. Large range of risk factors, new researches in genetic and neurobiological research have given a clear insight and in-depth know-how for TTH.

A majority of people with TTH do not seek medical attention thus it has been proven to be difficult to completely diagnose the exact effects, causes, and preventions of TTH. Even adults with new bodily changes are likely to go through TTH. This report thus proves that further research is very necessary on this particular topic and must be done by the medical associations (Carlson, 2013).

Biofeedback Therapy

History of Biofeedback Therapy

The concept of homeostasis, i.e. the tendency of the body to stay hold in the inner environment, was introduced by Claude Bernard in the year 1865. It was shown by J.R. Tarchan off in the year 1885 that the voluntary control of the heart rate could be precisely direct without changing the breathing rate. The voluntary control of the responsible muscle which wriggles the ear was studied by J.H. Blair in the year 1901. He discovered that this skill was learned by the subjects by inhibiting interfering muscles and by the demonstration of the self-regulation of the skeletal muscles. Conscious efforts were made by Alexander Graham Bell used 2 devices, the phonautograph invented by Edouard-Leon Scott's and a manometric flame, where he tried best to enable a deaf to speak. A theory was developed by mathematician, Norbert Wiener, proposing that control of systems is possible by monitoring their results. The popular word 'biofeedback' was given feedback of Wiener in the conference in Santa Monica in 1969. As a result, the Bio-Feedback Research Society was founded that allowed isolated researchers to collaborate with each other and it popularised the term 'biofeedback' as well (Chauhan et al., 2018d).

Biofeedback and TTH

Many techniques were used to survey this problem one of the techniques is electromyography feedback (EMG-FB). Many factors are been observed for making the survey like Temperature feedback, galvanic skin response feedback, and electroencephalography feedback. Many teenagers in this world are facing this problem a lot and they all are unaware of this technique. Biofeedback techniques are simply cured of TTH and other headache problems.

Biofeedback Application in Headache

Biofeedback is a technique where our body is been carried out by an electrical sensor to monitors. It monitors the activities that are not able to recognize by our physical body.

Biofeedback takes many measurements, like the important human body parameters heart rate, blood pressure, brain waves, skin temperature, anxiety, breathing rate, etc. This helps us recognized that what inner problem our body is facing and we are not able to cure that in time (Chauhan et al., 2018d).

By this treatment, we are able to cure our headache and other problem like anxiety, high blood pressure, etc. But in today world TTH i.e. tension-type headache is the main problem that every single person in the present generation is facing day by day. So it is a simple technique to cure headache. By doing many physical activities instead of eating medicines that can affect our body biofeedback technique in which a person is not being affected by another problem.

Social Impact of TTH

TTH though is not very harmful as it is present in the majority of the population. But to be true there are various social impacts of TTH. They can be described as below:

- It can result in a lack of concentration at work.
- One may not be able to go to work due to this and constantly stay unhappy.
- It can also lead to anger and disturbed state of mind leading to unhealthy relationships with others.
- One may not be able to spend quality time with friends and family.
- The person suffering TTH may stay in depression and anxiousness for a prolonged period of time.
- The person will find it difficult to stay socially active.

Social Records of TTH According to Gender and Age

Figure 2. Representation of Impact of TTH on Age between Male and Female (Haynes et al., 2005)

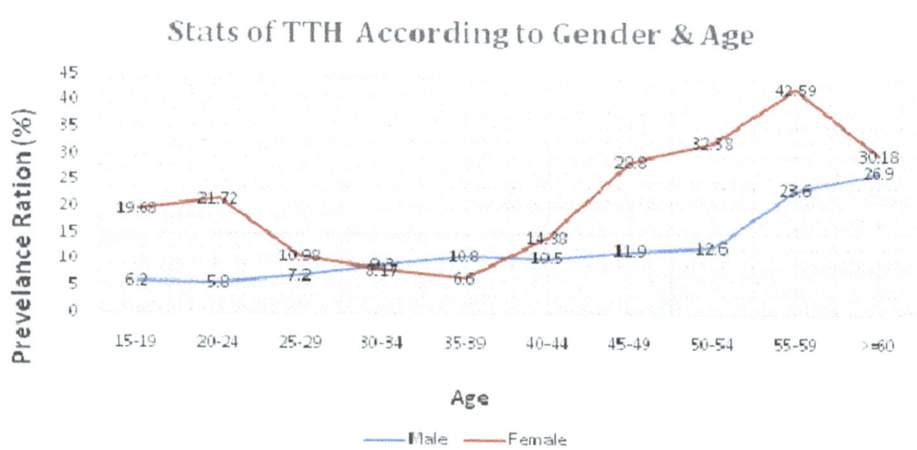

Type of TTH

Figure 3. Prevalence of different types of TTH (Journal of Neurology & Neuroscience, 2007)

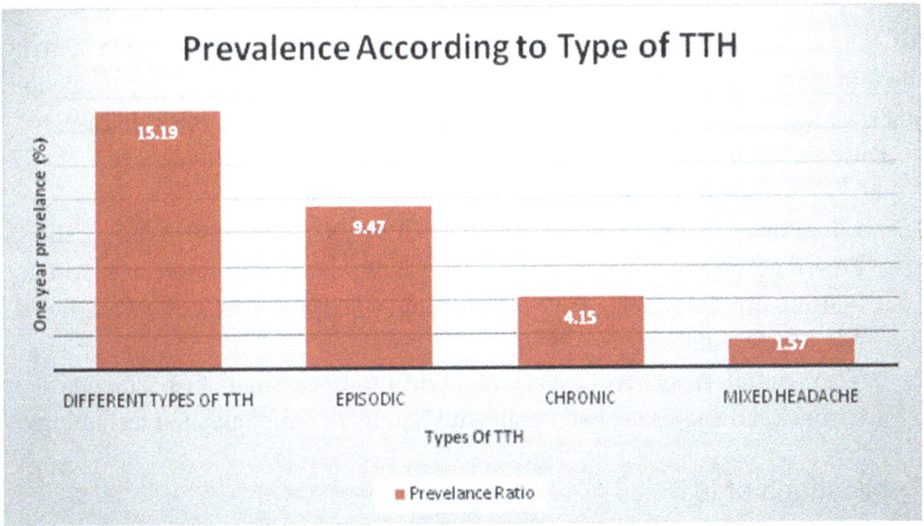

Internet of Things (IoT)

Relation between IoT and Big Data

The quantity of gadgets inter joined to the internet is growing day by day at a rapid rate. These devices will obviously generate a huge amount of data which will increase in quantity with the number of devices. This data will need to be stored, organized and processed and hence, big data comes into the picture.

History of IoT

IoT has evolved and has been a famous term now such as machine language, commodity analysis, etc. IoT has brought automation, control system, wireless sensor networks that are connected to the internet and helps us to make us easier to do work.

Kevin Ashton in 1999 was first who coined the term IoT i.e. "Internet of Things". But in earlier the concept of IoT was purposed in Carnegie Mellon University in 1982 that work on the concept of network smart devices (Rubin, 1999).

Nowadays technology is increasing day by day like CISCO is introducing new technology and in the future, the technology will replace every human work with this technology (Rubin, 1999).

Remarks for IoT

IoT is a very useful technology in every field because it plays a crucial role in every filed. In the field of medical, it is very important and by this, we can help the people and save them even they are suffering from TTH, stress, or any other disease.

Different kind of networks used here are as below,

1. **Low-Power Wide-Area Networking (LPWAN):** Wireless networks, allows Low data rate communication in long-rang, decreases power and cost for transmission. Available LPWAN technologies and protocols: LoRaWan, Sigfox, NB-IoT, Weightless.
2. **Very Small Aperture Terminal (VSAT):** Uses small dish antennas for narrowband and broad band-data with Satellite communication technology.

Applications of IoT

The application of IoT is usually bifurcated among infrastructure, industry, commercial and consumer spaces. Many technologies have been evolved in this field to describe it. IoT can also be used to manage mental health.

Mental Health

Importance of Mental Health, Stress and Emotional Needs and Significance of Study

From ages, human has always been in search of peace. From 5000 B.C. to till date in the first quarter of the 21st century, from a long time, man has developed many methods for recreation, entertainment, and synergy. As much as the lifestyle went on hectic, the population was increasing; limited resources of earth were not enough for all. To grab more and more resources, the natural lifestyle vanished and the human race was collectively gripped into a materialistic culture and accumulating tendency with the consumerist lifestyle.

It generated a mass of stress and consequently clashes, disharmony, anxiety, depression and in extreme situation, the suicidal tendency. To meet these issues, the psychiatrist, psychologist, social analysts did in-depth studies in their own ways and they found many alternative methods and treatments for the same. In recent studies of this century, it has been well established that most of the human body diseases and abnormality are psychosomatically generated. In this research, the scholar has tried best the recent method(s) of alternative therapy like biofeedback which is getting popular due to their ease of applicability and no side effects on human brain and body (Satya, 2018e).

The Biofeedback therapies have been popular for long for the treatment of various mental challenges, stress and chronic headache like TTH type headache. Stress due to TTH headache is a very frequent occurrence in all our lives. A TTH symptom experienced for long by an individual with no relief or with increased frequency, it is termed as "distress". Weakened cognitive and physiological control is due to TTH originated stress and results in performance reduction. It can lead to symptoms like headache, gastrointestinal disturbances, elevated blood pressure, chest pain, insomnia, peptic ulcers, sexual dysfunction, skin ailments, etc.(Satya, 2018e).

In this crucial time, mostly the teenagers lose their mental balance, get violent and are unable to handle the pressure from peer, friends, parents, and society. In opposition to this, those parents who rightly care about their youngsters and treat them friendly behave sympathetically, less suffer from these issues in their families.

Major emotions of an individual are fear, anger, love, jealousy, guilt, and worries. Wise people handle them carefully and stop the cycle within them instead of spreading them. They enjoy their family relations, office work, and social relations and treat them as their duty. So in this research work, the author team tried to find the impact of positive ideas on mood states of personality for mental health (Anxiety, Stress, Depression, Aggression, Fatigue, Guilt, Extraversion and Arousal on the students and technocrats of our institutes (DSVV and ABES Engineering College, Ghaziabad and Mayur et al., 2018f and Scott et al., 2004).

Mental Health Introduction

Mental Health has been always the prime concern of intellectuals, behavioral scientists and social study makers. Nowadays, it's of a prime concern and happiness index has been considered as an integral part of the progress of any country. Less work has experimented in the South Asian region regarding mental health correlated with social parameters of age, gender defined by Kornhauser (1965)"connotates those behaviors, perceptions, and feelings that determines a person's overall level of personal effectiveness, success, happiness, and excellence of functioning as a person" (Sharma et al., 2018g).

It depends on the development and retention of goals that are neither too high nor too low to permit realistic successful maintenance of belief in one's self as a worthy, effective human being (Lakshminarayan & Prabhakaran, 1993). So, a mentally healthy person is firm in his intentions and is least distributed by strains and stresses of day to day life (Haddock et al., 1997).

As per the Med lexicon's medical dictionary, "A state of emotional and psychological wellbeing in which an individual is able to use his or her cognitive and emotional capabilities, function in society, and meet the ordinary demands of everyday life."

The WHO has also accepted the fact and reframe its definition of complete health as individual mental, physical, social and spiritual well-being is termed complete health.

Therefore has found a balance in his or her social, emotional and psychological areas of life.

In 2007, WHO has stated, mental health is about: the feeling for ourselves, others, and our demands from life. It has also stated the difference between mental ill-health and illness. It states that mental unfitness vanishes the chance of potentials and causes serious problems.

In the case of mental issues, recovery/management may be ensured in the form of counseling or psychotherapy, drug treatment, and lifestyle changes. Stats says that approximately 25% of the people in the UK have mental health problems during their lives whereas the USA is said to have the highest incidence of people diagnosed with mental health (Arora et al., 2019b and Vyas et al., 2018h).

Factors Affecting Mental Health

According to Joel L. Young M.D, there are 9 main symptoms or components that challenge to individual's mental health- Daily exercise and social activity Level, Smoking, Diet pattern, Physical activity in form of bodily work, abuse or misbehave, social and community activities in residence, relationships with peer and office mates, practice of meditation and other relaxation techniques, use of alternative therapies and priority to healthy sleep (Rastogi et al., 2018i and McCror et al., 2001).

Problems and Needs of Adolescents

On the basis of age, group adolescence is categorized into 20-26 years of age or according to early principles 13-18 years that mainly depends on physical growth and development. Physical, Emotional, Social and Intellectual Development are 4 major types. Following needs and life goals appear to be a source of many emotional problems of adolescents. Need for social status, acceptance and security, independence, adventure, self-support, belongingness. Adjustment to personal appearance, physical and psychological changes, use of alcohol and drugs, need of heterosexual relations and a theory of life (Saini et al., 2018j; Turk et al., 2008).

IoT helps in the medical field to make our future bright such as, major technology has been evolved in this field such as a pace-maker. With the help of IoT, we can create digitalized health care facilities; we can connect to medical resources easily and can get medical facilities easier.

Devices enabled with IoT services are applicable for remote health monitoring and especially in emergency notification facilities. They may help us in from blood pressure and heart rate monitors and latest gadgets like pacemakers to monitor specialized implants.

Nowadays "smart beds" can be seen in the medical facilities that are another feature of IoT. A doctor can interrogate their patient with the help of video call from far away from the place, even the nurses can be appointed through internet facilities. A 2015 Goldman Sachs reported that by increasing revenue and decreasing cost, gadgets being used for health care devices in the USA are helping to save nearly $300 billion in annual expenditures in the health sector.

Moreover, a special monitoring sensor is being setup in the parks, shop, medical shops, hospitals, etc. To ensure the medical health care of the people. These sensors are being connected to a database system that is been collected server and information is being gathered out. These ways scientists are researching their on the human being that how they are developing day by day.

Machines are being built on the bases of application on IoT that help the doctor to study properly to their patients and collect and store data in the form of big data that is a subclass of IoT. Many types of research are being done by collecting the data from the sensor. Chronic Disease control and prevention of them is being wisely cared for by IoT in health sector plays a fundamentally. Mighty wireless connections have proved remote monitoring a reality; this fast connectivity has made easy the application of recording of subject data and analysis of complex algorithms on it (Rubin, 1999).

Big Data

Characteristics

There are major four characteristics of big data, namely volume, variety, velocity, and veracity. Volume is the quantity of the data which is to be stored and which determines whether a data set is large enough to be considered big data or not. The nature and type of generated data are known as variety whereas the processing speed of data and its generation to handle a specific need is called velocity. Veracity characterizes the quality and value of the available data (Fumal, Scohnen, 2008).

Applications of Big Data

Healthcare

Big data finds a major application in the healthcare industry. Nowadays, in major hospitals and large healthcare centers, there is a huge influx of patients suffering from a wide variety of ailments. Thus, the doctors rely more on the patient's clinical health record which means gathering a huge amount of data and that too for different patients. This is not possible with the help of traditional data processing and storing software. Hence, big data comes into the picture.

Predictive analysis is an important result of big data which ensures the patient's quality care and safety. It helps the doctors to give the right prescriptions to their patients keeping their medical histories in mind. Analytics can also be used by the medical researchers to observe the recovery rates of various cancer patients which may help them to find the treatments that have the highest rates of success. As the number of patients' increases, the volume of medical records also increases which stems the need of adopting a new approach called Electronic Health Records (EHRs) that organizes this data and makes it easier to have access to such data. Various real-time monitoring systems and tools are offered by many healthcare centers to their patients like new wearable sensors which keep track of the patient's health trends right at their home, which will reduce the patient's visits to the clinics (Chaturvedi et al., 2018b).

Media and Entertainment

The media and entertainment sector is rapidly developing day by day. The development brings about the creation of new content and an improvement in marketing and distribution. Many actionable points of action are provided by big data about thousands of individuals which are collected through various different data mining activities. Big data helps this sector by:

- Considering the needs and requirements of the audience
- Being open to optimization
- Consumer targeting for advertisement and marketing purposes
- New content development and content monetization (Boureau, Luu, and Doubrere, 2001).

Government

In government processes, the same sets of data are used again and again across multiple platforms. Big data allows this and also offers cost innovation and productivity, thus allowing different departments to work together in association. As the government works in almost all the important sectors, the role of big data increases. Some major areas include:

- **Crime Prevention and Prediction:** Real-time analytics systems can be used by the police and intelligence departments to observe and track crime patterns and criminal behavior.
- **Weather Forecasting:** Large amount of data at every instance of each day by using high-end sensors and then use this information to predict the forecast for coming instances of time as used by NOAA.
- **Tax Fraud Identification:** Tax organizations can use big data to identify suspicious behavior and multiple or duplicate identities.
- **Drug Evaluation:** Big data can be used to access large amounts of data and help in the evaluation of treatment and drugs and thus save millions of dollars for pharmaceutical companies.
- **Traffic Optimization:** The real-time traffic data collected from sensors, GPS navigators, CCTV cameras, etc. can be used to solve the traffic problems in dense or congested areas by adjusting transportation routes accordingly (Chaturvedi et al., 2018b and Boureau et al., 2001).

Role of Big Data in IoT

In a big data system, a heavy quantity of unorganized data is generated by IoT devices and stored. Then this data can be processed or organized accordingly. Analysis of this data can be done using tools like Spark or Hadoop, Map-Reduce. This data needs the light fastening speed of analysis as it is collected through the internet.

Interdependency Between Big Data and IoT

Big Data and IoT are not only mutually dependent but also hugely impact each other. As the number of IoT devices will increase, the demand for Big Data services will also increase gradually. This is because as the quantity of the generated data increases, traditional storage technology will be pushed to its limits and the demand for Big Data, which is a more advanced and developed data storage technology, will increase drastically. Therefore, more and more organizations will update, develop and work on their Big Data storage systems (Arora et al., 2017a).

Big Data Tools

For storage and analysis of the big data, there are few intelligent applications which are advance tools, very easy to use and getting popular in today's scenario. Some of the main tools are described as below (Fumal, Scohnen, 2008).

Apache Hadoop

Java-based free software framework to store a heavy amount of data effectively in the form of a cluster, Runs in parallel on a cluster to enable the user to process data across all the nodes.

Microsoft HD Insight

Big Data solution by Microsoft, using Azure Blob storage as the default file system, provides high availability with low cost.

Big Data in Excel

MS Excel can be used to access Big Data. MS Excel 2013 has a feature which allows the user to access the stored data in a Hadoop platform.

Presto

Open source Query engine, developed by Face book, used to handle large amounts of data, not works on Map-Reduce data and can quickly retrieve data.

PolyBase

Works on SQL Server 2012 Parallel Data Warehouse (PDW), accesses the data stored in PDW, an appliance for data warehousing to process any related data and provide connectivity with Hadoop as well (Haynes et al., 2005).

Big Data Security

It is a term used for all measures and techniques to secure the data and all the data analysis processes. The threats to data can include information thefts which can endanger critical and confidential information stored online. There are several ways to implement data security. One simple way is encryption. Encrypted data is useless to any third party as long as it does not have the key to access it. Data stays protected during both input and output processes. Another way of securing the data is by building a strong firewall, which acts as strong data filters and avoids any external sources or third parties (Rastogi et al. 2018c).

Fog Computing

Carla Mouradian, Diala Naboulsi, Sami Yangui, Roch H. Glitho, Monique J. Morrow, Paul A. Polakos experimented in their research that Fog computing is introduced to tackle problems like connectivity between end devices and cloud storage, high-latency, to situate components of application over multiple clouds separately, overhead of latency induced by inter-cloud communications and many more. Fog computing provide benefits such as low latency, allowing instruction processing to take place at the edge of the network etc. Fog system consists of three level architecture. It has three levels: The cloud level, the fog level, and the IoT/end-users level. Fog layer is formed by single or more fog domains which in turn are formed by fog nodes. IoT layer is formed by two domains, end-user devices and IoT devices (Carla et al., 2017).

Biofeedback with EEG Instrument (Earlier Experiments)

Biofeedback is a method of Neurotherapy, a forward-moving regression, and self-controlled relaxation technique to handle the stress and TTH (Wenk, 2005). It helps subject to know the current stress level and to handle them.

The Biofeedback is an alternative popular therapy used for QoL and strengthens adjustment skills (Baum, Herberman, & Cohen, 1995). Mcdowelll (2015) found that silent meditation, yoga, and Indian spiritual exercises have a very deep effect on the subconscious of the patient and refines their ill personality factors. Chambers et al.(2008) in their research, recruited 20 mediation practitioners for 10 days meditative therapy process and established the high reported concentration, confidence and peace of mind. They also reported the decrement in the negative emotions and ill effects as compared to the non-experimental control group. They also witnessed fewer demotivating components and reduced rumination (Fig. 7).

Sensor Modalities

Popularly 3 standard organizations responsible for controlling and marking the biofeedback process, therapy, symptoms, and effects are AAPB, BCIA, and ISNR, they unanimously reached the common definition of biofeedback in 2008: "Biofeedback is a process to make capable an individual to learn to alter physiological activity to strengthen the purposes rectifying the health and performance.

Figure 4. Experiment using biofeedback machines

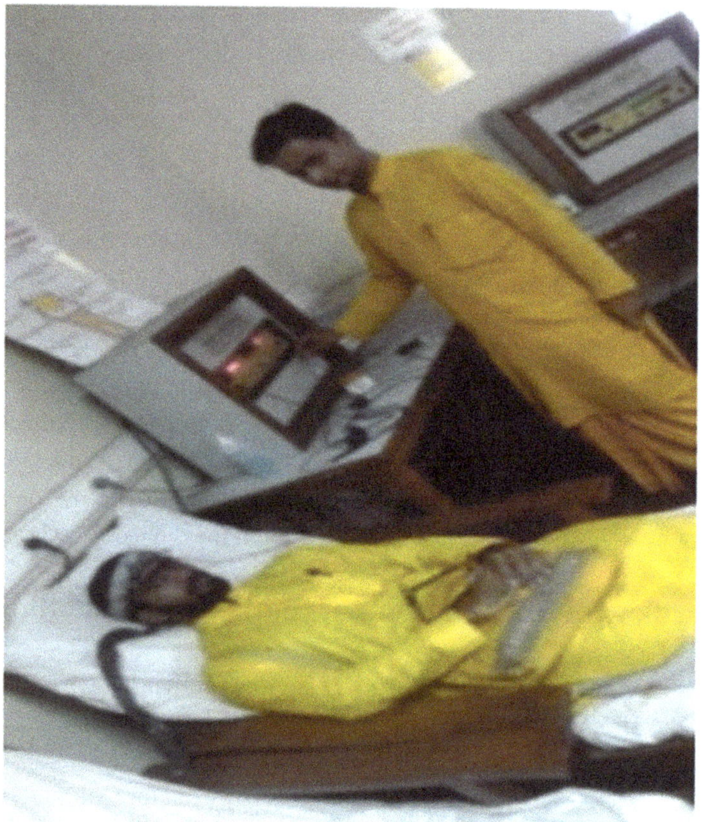

Types of Biofeedback

Electroencephalography (EEG)

It is an electrophysiological monitoring technique which is used to track the brain's electrical activity. EEG is generally non-invasive, electrodes are placed along the scalp, although sometimes invasive electrodes may be used too. Brain neurons have an ionic current which is measured by voltage fluctuations. It is generally used to diagnose epilepsy. It can also be used to diagnose coma, brain death, sleep disorders, encephalopathy, depth of anaesthesia, stroke, tumours and other brain disorders (Rastogi et al., 2018f).

Figure 5. Recording of biofeedback data

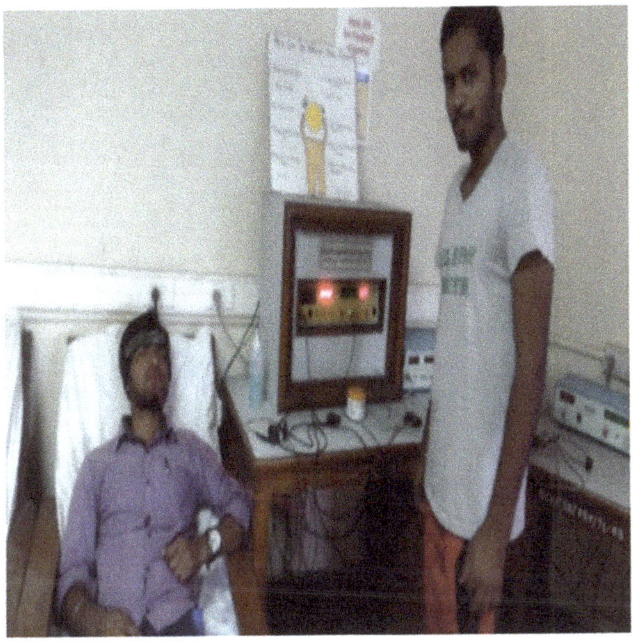

Figure 6. Eight factors of mood state (Arora, 2019b)

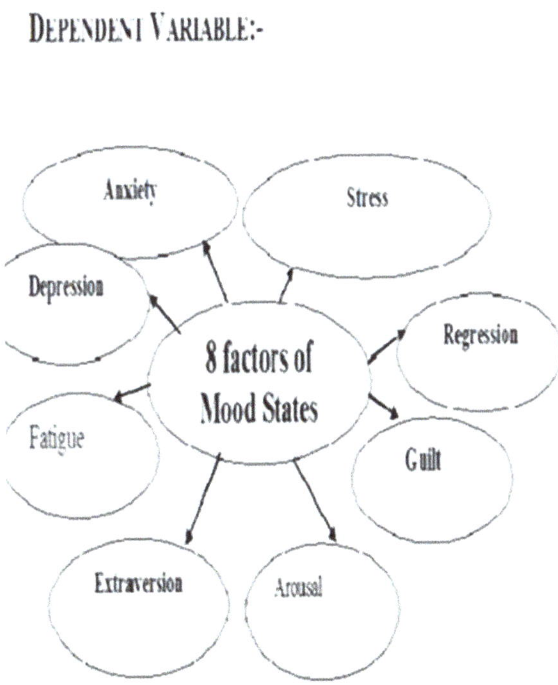

Figure 7. Process of mind (Arora, 2019b)

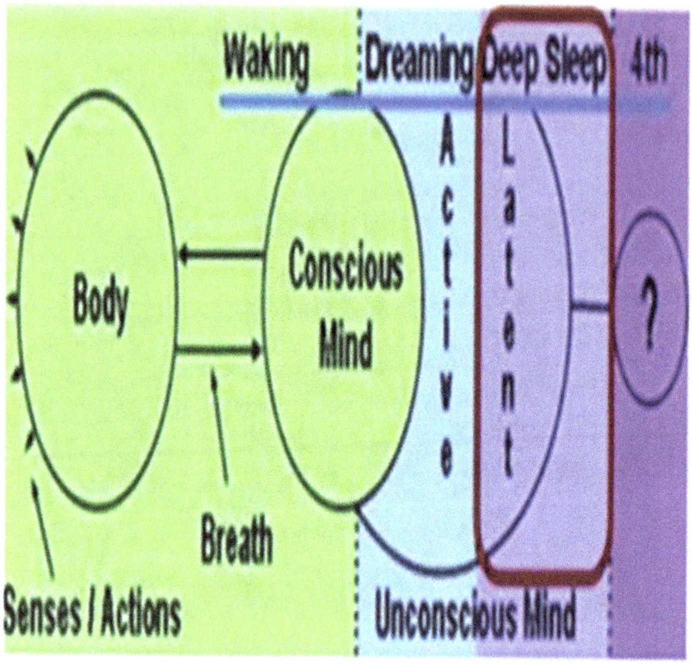

Figure 8. Stress and syndromes (Arora, 2019b)

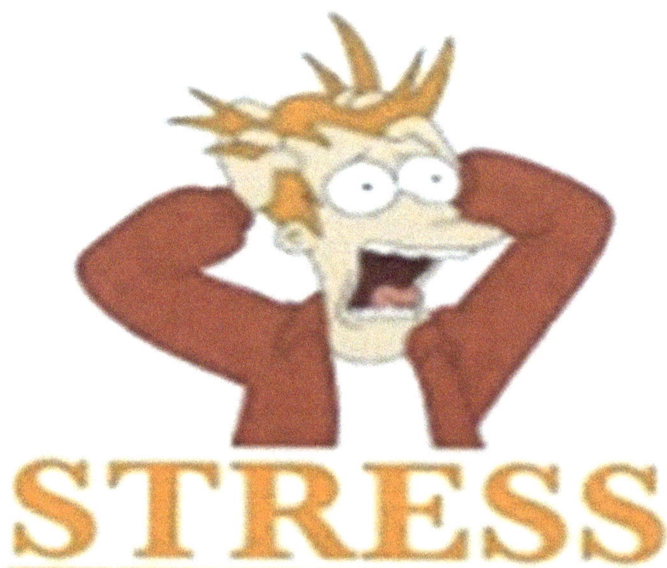

Table 1. Primary and secondary variables of EMG-GSR biofeedback process (Hayness et al., 2005)

Variables	EMG	GSR	Control
Average Frequency of Headache per Week	56	55.9	25.8
Average Intensity of Headache per Week	58.2	56.3	46.5
Average Duration of Headache per Week	75.7	63.6	49
SF-36 Physical Scores	25	26	21
SF-36 Mental Scores	25.1	19.5	21.7
SF-36 Total Scores	28.5	30.5	21.7

Electrocardiography (ECG)

The process of generating an electrocardiogram, electrodes are placed on the skin, is called electrocardiography (ECG). Small electrical changes produced as a result of the cardiac muscle polarisation and depolarisation during each heartbeat is detected by these electrodes. Inadequate artery blood flow, electrolyte disturbances, and numerous cardiac abnormalities can result in changes in the normal ECG pattern (Scott and Lundeen, 2004).

Electromyography (EMG)

The electro diagnostic technique used to track and evaluate the electrical activity of the skeletal muscles is known as electromyography (EMG). It is carried out by using an instrument known as electromyography, which generates a record called electromyogram. The electric potential produced by the electrically or neurologically activated muscle cells are detected by the electromyography. Upon evaluation and analysis, to analyze the biomechanics of human and animal movement, these signals can be used to detect recruitment order, medical abnormalities or activation level (Sharma et al., 2018g).

Galvanic Skin Response (GSR)

The features and characteristic of our body where rapid variations on the electrical characteristic of skin are measured I very important biofeedback indicator. The gadget to record this feature is called Galvanic Skin Response (GSR). The resistance of the skin changes as per nature of the sweat glands in the individual's skin. Skin conductance indicates physiological or psychological arousal. If the sympathetic nervous system gets aroused, then sweat gland activity increases, which results in the increase of skin conductance. Skin conductance measures sympathetic and emotional responses. Recent studies show that there is much more about GSR than meets the eye, and further research and study is going on this field. It is also known as Electrodermal activity (EDA), Electrodermal response (EDR), skin conductance, psycho galvanic reflex (PGR), etc (Haddock et al., 1997).

Electrical characteristic of the skin of the human body is measured under electrodermal activity (EDA)(Fig.8) EDA has also been known as Skin Conductance, Galvanic Skin Response (GSR), Electro Dermal Response (EDR), Psycho Galvanic Reflex (PGR), Skin Conductance Response (SCR), Sympathetic Skin Response (SSR) and Skin Conductance Level (SCL) (Rastogi, et al., 2018i).

At Subconscious state, the cognitive and emotional level of human behaviour is modulated by an autonomous way for the sympathetic activity of skin conductance. So it helps to get the right evaluation of autonomous emotional regulation. Fingers, palms, and soles of feet and other human extremities exhbi- various bio-electrical phenomena (McCrory et al., 2001).

Stress

Models of Stress (Headache)

3 Models are in practice to medically define the stress which is described as below.

- General Adaptation Syndrome (Fig.9 and Fig.10) Stages-Alarm, Resistance
- Exhaustion: Selye Eustress and Distress (Fig.11)
- Lazarus: Cognitive appraisal Model

Types of Stress

Stress management can be very much worrying and disturbing, with three types of stress Acute stress containing Emotional Problem, Muscular Pressure, episodic acute stress and chronic stress each with its own characteristics, symptoms, duration, and treatment approaches (Fig. 12 and Fig. 13).

Figure 9. Phases of stress (Arora et al., 2019b)

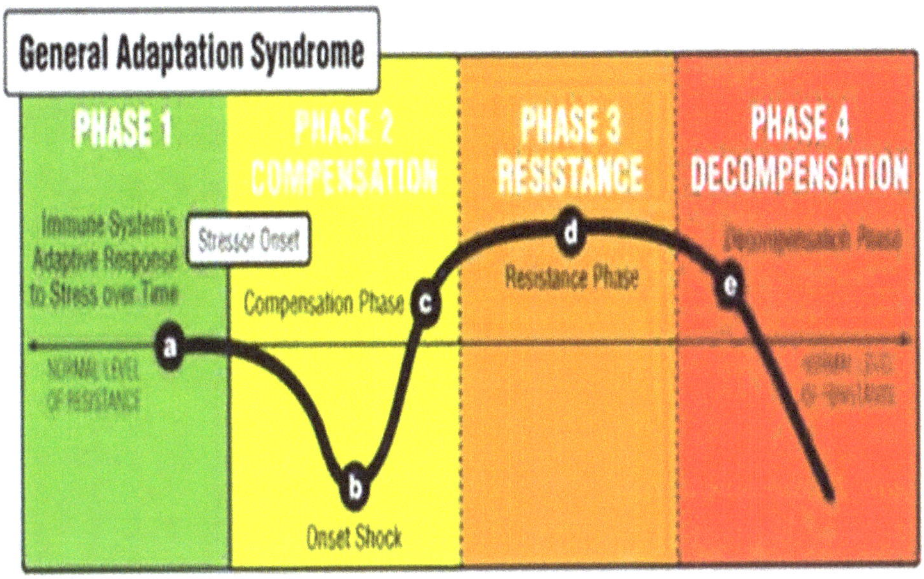

Figure 10. Graphical updates for stress (Arora et al., 2019b)

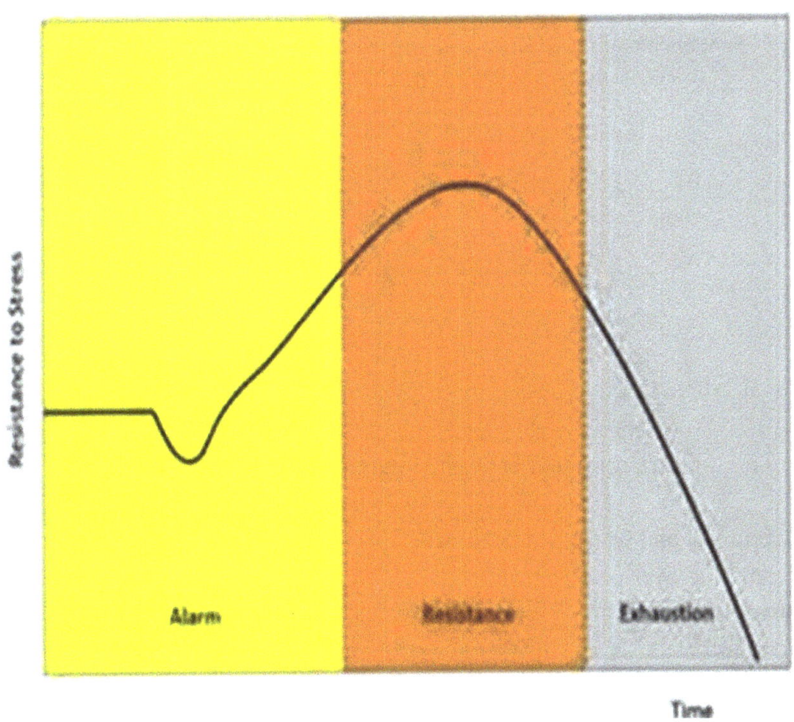

Figure 11. Different body / mood states (Arora et al., 2019b)

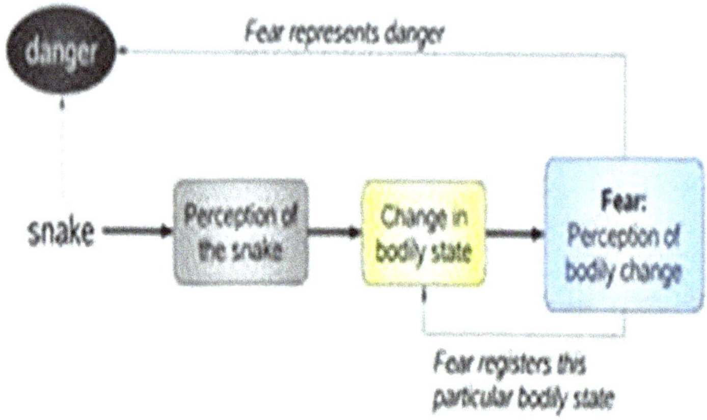

Figure 12. Stress vs. distress (Arora et al., 2019b)

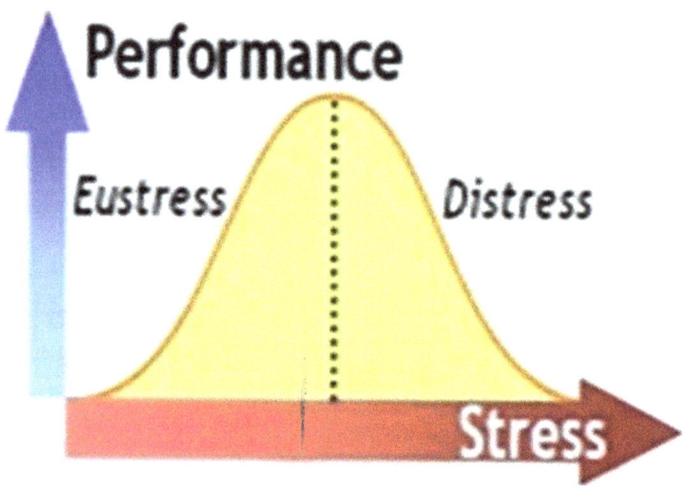

Causes of Stress

In 1965, Korchin differentiated categories panic situations as below:

- Uncertainty and under-stimulation
- Informative overload
- Danger
- Ego control failure
- Ego-mastery failure

Figure 13. Levels of stress (Arora et al., 2019b)

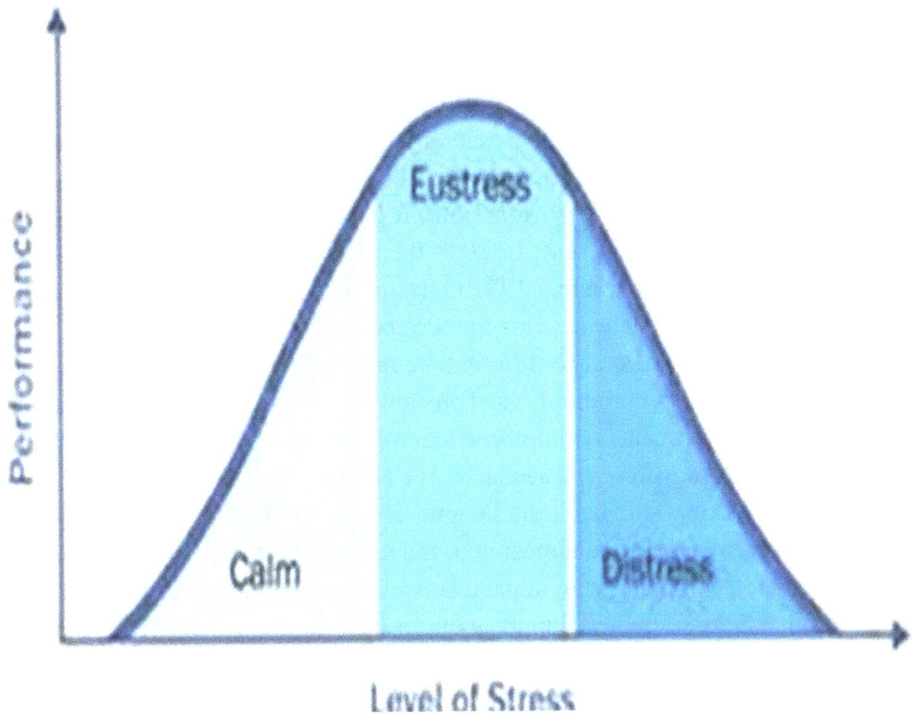

- Self-esteem danger
- Other esteem danger.

Symptoms of Stress

Stress Warning indicators and Symptoms are as below:

Cognitive symptoms consist of memory problem, inability to concentrate, poor judgment, seeing only the negative, anxious or reaching thoughts, constant worrying, the emotional symptoms deals with moodiness, irritability or short temper, agitation, inability to relax, feeling overwhelmed, sense of loneliness and isolation, depression or general unhappiness and physical symptoms covers aches and pains, diarrhea or constipation, nausea, dizziness, chest pain, rapid heartbeat, low of sex drive, frequent colds, there is last variety of behavioural symptoms which deals with procrastinating or neglecting responsibilities, isolating oneself from others, sleeping too much or too little, eating more or less, nervous habits (e.g. nail biting, pacing), using alcohol, cigarettes, or drugs to relax (Costa, 2014; Yadav et al., 2018j).

BACKGROUND

There are various researches are carried out on stress and illness. Design of EMG model for biofeedback is efficient and it decides some protocol that would be for TTH. The main mode to treat people who are affected by TTH is Pharmacotherapy; it is very effective in decreasing the extent and duration of TTH. But it also has a drawback as it is all overused as antidepressant medicine and those have the risk of having an adverse effect. Other than that, it has a potential risk for analgesic medication because of the overuse. In 2008 there was an article which states the efficiency of biofeedback in treating TTH. Galvanic skin resistance (GSR) therapies are used to treat these headaches and are found very effective. At times, it can be very severe that it becomes difficult to differentiate among tension-type headache and migraine attack. The most commonly used preventive measures include medications such as allopathic treatments and non-medication treatments such as biofeedback therapies. The term "tension-type headache" (TTH) has been declared through the International Classification Headache Diagnosis I (ICHD I). The terms "tension" and "type" represents its different meanings and reflect that there is a sort of mental or physical tension could cause an impact. However, studies at a large extent at this topic shows that there somehow a doubt about its neurobiological nature (McCrory, 2001).

TTH is the most basic form of headache occurring in about three-quarters of the world. Tension-type headache can usually last from 31 minutes to 8 days. The pain is generally mild and moderate in most of the times and sometimes it is worst. There are no diagnostic tests to confirm to tension-type headache. Galvanic skin resistance (GSR) therapies are used to treat these headaches and are found very effective. At times, it can be very severe that it becomes difficult to distinguish between tension-type headache and migraine attack. The most commonly used preventive measures include medications such as allopathic treatments and non-medication treatments such as biofeedback therapies. The term tension-type headache has been declared by the International Classification Headache Diagnosis I (ICHD I). The terms "tension" and "type" represents its different meanings and reflect that some sort of mental or muscular tension could cause an impact. However, studies at a large extent at this topic shows that there somehow a doubt about its neurobiological nature (Rubin, 1999). It is one of the common forms for headache and in normal cases, people took it lightly and they don't consult to the doctor and they treat themselves with various drugs in most cases people got cured but sometimes the drugs have a chronic impact on the health which could be severe. To our knowledge, no study has been done so far to find out the effectiveness of auditory, visual or integrated (audiovisual) EMG feedback in TTH patients (Bansal et al., 2018k; Kropotov, 2009; Millea, 2002).

In a study, auditory EMG BF was used in TTH patients and it was found that the subjects were not only able to maintain low frontalis EMG levels but also managed to remain headache-free during follow-up11. Similar studies utilizing only auditory BF have been performed in both TTH and migraine patients (Arora et al., 2017a and Carlson (2013)). Visual EMG BF has been used less compared to auditory feedback15. In another study, TTH patients received both visual and audio EMG feedback and found a significant decrease in headache (Mullaly et al., 2009 and Crystal et al., 2010).

Though there is evidence pointing out the efficacy of BF in tension headache patients, it is not advocated very frequently in India which could due to the cost of the equipment involved and hence the added cost to the patient as well. Most BF equipment provides both visual and audio feedback, hence if the equipment could be designed to provide only the form of feedback which is the most effective, it could automatically reduce the equipment cost as well as the cost to the patient making it more economical for both practitioner as well as the patient.

No controlled trials have been done so far to compare the efficacy of visual EMG feedback or auditory EMG BF separately in tension-type headache. This study, therefore, was conducted to find out relative efficacy of visual and auditory BF in isolation or combination in TTH subjects (Zanella et al., 2004 and Lee et al., 2017).

Emotional Fulfillment

Basic human needs for emotional fulfillment are universal and include:

Love, Acceptance, Affection, and Feeling valued, Appreciated, Secure, Companionship, Admiration, Trust, Respect, Understanding, Conversation, and Communication.

In the theory of Self Actualization, Maslow in 1954 has given a hierarchy of human needs which are Psychological, safety, belonging, love, esteem needs and need of self-actualization.

Murray in his studies proposed 12 physical needs and 28 psychological needs. Among them 20 important needs are as follows: Dominance, Sentience, Deference, Exhibition, Autonomy, Play, Aggression, Affiliation, Abasement, Rejection, Achievement, Succorance, Sex, Nurturance, avoidance, Ham avoidance, Dependence, Order, Counteraction, Understanding.

10 Steps to Emotional Fulfillment in Psychology Today

We all want to feel happy, and each one of us has different ways of getting there. Here are ten steps that help us to bring more happiness in our life.

- Be with others who make you smile.
- Hold on to your values.
- Accept the good.
- Imagine the best.
- Do things you love.
- Find purpose.
- Listen to your heart.
- Push yourself and not others.
- Be open to change.
- Bask in the simple pleasure (Binder and Blettner, 2015).

STUDY PLOTAND EXPERIMENTAL SETUP OF BIOFEEDBACK

Study Duration and Approval from Candidates

The candidates were taken from Middle of January 2017 till May 2018 and up to July 2018. Candidates were taken in the experiment only after when we got a consent approval signed from them. Another information-Consent Form was signed by the ethical committee was got completed by the subjects and clinical verification for the experiment was recorded and clearance was given by the ethical committee formed by the University. All the experiments are done in a randomized, single-blinded and protected environment so that the results wouldn't deviate much. Subjects are taken from various neurology clinics and subjects referred by neurologists to the OPD of Hardwar Physiotherapy University.

Intervention on Experimental Study Conducted

When all the candidates are divided into three groups, all the candidates are informed about the treatment that is going to be tested upon them. They were given biofeedback training in a separated room of, Hardwar research laboratory, which had very low lighting and negligible external noise so that they could remain in a relaxation state. All candidates underwent respective (EMG/GSR) BF training for 20 minutes per session for 07 sessions (Turk et al., 2008; Kropotov, 2009).

METHODOLOGY and COLLECTION OF DATA

Study Design

This study was a randomized, single-blinded, prospective controlled trial.

Source of Data

Data will be obtained from the subjects recruited from various neurology clinics and subjects referred by neurologists to the outpatient department of psychology, DevSanskriti Vishwavidyalaya, Hardwar, Uttarakhand and ABESEC, Ghaziabad for biofeedback therapy.

Study Duration

Subjects will be recruited from June-2019 up to June-2020 and followed up till October-2020.

Informed Consent

Subjects will be recruited in the trial only after obtaining informed consent from them. (Informed Consent Form approved by the ethical committee attached).

Sampling Design

Simple random sampling will be used with the lottery method for allocation of subjects to seven groups. Subjects with stress and TTH (Tension-Type Headache) will be enrolled in the study. Subjects who will not give consent and who will not meet the eligibility criteria will be excluded from the study. The rest of the subjects will be randomized using the lottery method for allocation. They will also be scrutinized after 30 days, 60 days.

Allocation Procedure

Chits numbered one to seven will be placed in a bowl and the subjects will be asked to pick the chits. Subjects with the following chit numbers will be allocated to the corresponding groups:

- EMG auditory biofeedback (EMGa) group
- EMG visual biofeedback (EMGv) group

- EMG auditory +visual (EMGav) group
- GSR auditory (GSRa) group
- GSR visual (GSRv) group
- GSR auditory +visual (GSRav) group
- Control group

Sample Size: Sample size will be calculated using the following formula:

Probability of Type I error will be set at 0.05 Power of the study is expected to set at 80% (0.8).

Let p1= 1.0 and p2=0.75 are the mean differences of pre and post (baseline to one year) average frequency of headache per month in the EMG biofeedback training group and pain management group respectively from a study by (Mullay et al., 2009).

Let p = 0.875 was calculated as (p1+p2)/2 and q = 0.125 was calculated as 1-p. The sample size thus calculated was 26.6 per group. To accommodate for dropouts the sample size was chosen as 30 per group.

Universe and Sample

This study will be a randomized single-blinded controlled prospective study. We will select a no. of recruited subjects n, h (f and m males) will be randomly assigned to seven groups receiving electromyography feedback auditory (EMGa) (let n = 27), visual (EMGv) (let n = 28), combined audio-visual (EMGav) (let n=27), galvanic skin resistance biofeedback auditory (GSRa) (let n =26), visual (GSRv) (let n=29) and combined audio-visual (GSRav) (let n=28) and a control group (let n = 27). Each subject (except the control group) will receive 10 sessions of respective biofeedback for 15 minutes each in an isolated room. The control group will receive only the medication prescribed by their treating doctor. Each patient will be kept blinded to the type of biofeedback (EMG or GSR) being given. Pain variables (average frequency, duration, and intensity of headache per week), SF-36 quality of life scores will also be measured from survey to all n subjects.

The entire psycho challenged cases living in Uttarakhand and NCR region (Delhi, Meerut, Ghaziabad, Faridabad, Gurugram, Modinagar, and Muradnagar) will be the universe of study. The college-going students and Technocrats of different giant MNCs will be understudy.

A control group of around 100 to 150 persons will be chosen and for carrying out this work the methodology employed shall be as follows:

- Literature survey.
- Identification of the location (Cluster near the region of NCR-national capital region Zone) and perform the study of different given parameters of

the psychosomatic disorders due to life deregulation which disturbs one's complete health.

- Development of a model of Biofeedback based experiments which will be performed at Research Labs and Scientific Spirituality Centers of DevSanskriti VishwaVidyalaya, Hardwar and Patanjali Research Foundations, Uttarakhand.
- Experimental investigation of Mental and spiritual health will be on various medical parameters.
- We will Apply some spiritual techniques as per the symptoms observed, suitable to the patient as per his/her age, diet, culture and habits.
- Data Analysis of the Comparative study of both EMG and GSR machines with various spiritual techniques (Guided meditations) will be applied over the patients and their performance.
- Analysis of the results obtained and verification of the efficiency of the technique and suggesting appropriate one will be done in a repeated process in case the method doesn't work.
- Impact of the result obtained on the society, the employee, company/ college and environment.
- 25% area (approximately 25 wards) out of 103 wards will be selected as samples purposively.

In the present study, samples of 95 adolescents are selected from ABESEC, Ghaziabad and DSVV Hardwar of graduation. Among this sample 55 are from urban area i.e. Lalquan and 50 are from rural area i.e. near to Pilkhua township in Ghaziabad.

SOLUTIONS BY EXPERIMENTS AND RESULTS

Hypothesis

There is a significant effect of Bio-Feedback based self guided meditation on mental health, stress management (headache). There is a significant increase in the level of stress management (TTH) and emotional needs by meditation practices. The hypothesis which proved true by this experiment are as below

- There is no significant difference in the mental health of adolescents due to meditation and therapy by EEG, GSR, and EMG integrated audio-visual biofeedback.
- There is no significant relationship between mental health and stress relief practices.

Variables in the Study

Independent Variables- EEG inputs, Audio-visual EMG and GSR Biofeedback therapy, Mindful Meditation, Spiritual Attitude.

Dependent Variables- Stress Management, Tension-Type Headache, Mental Health of Adolescents.

Experiment with Audio-Visual EMG and GSR

Graphs were plotted in Anaconda framework with the help of python programming.

Figure 14. The graph shows the SF-36 scores of 27 patients over the period of starting point, 30 days, 90 days, 180 days and 365 days with EMGav therapy

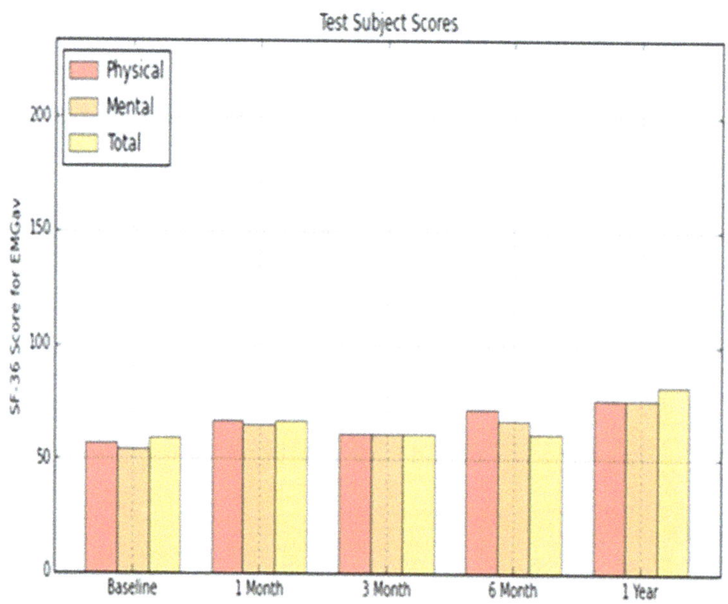

The analysis in Figure 14 shows the SF-36 test applied on different subjects who experienced the audio-visual EMG therapy and graph shows the SF-36 scores of 27 patients over the period 30 days, 90 days, 180 days, and 365 days. From the bar graph it is observed that the relative scores of all the patients have been increased. The x axis shows the time duration in months.

Figure 15. The graph shows the SF-36 scores of 28 patients which were given audio-visual GSR therapy for 10 sessions each 15 minutes

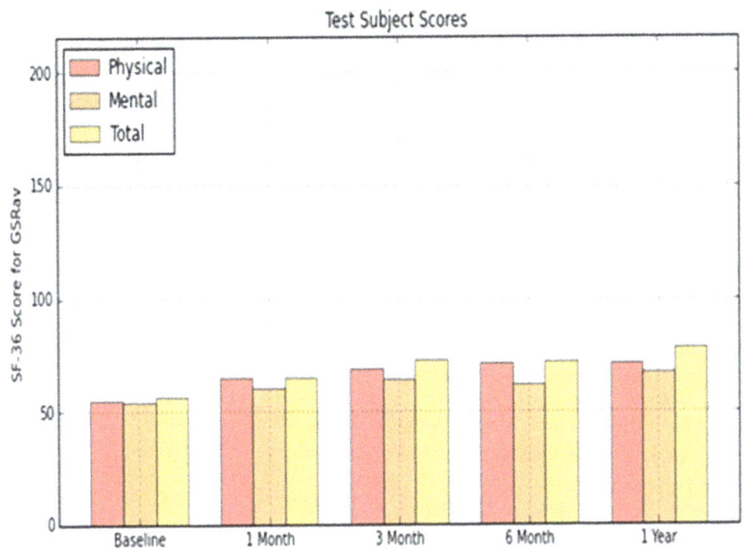

Figure 16. SF-36 scores of 27 subjects chosen for non-experiment (control) group were recorded over a period

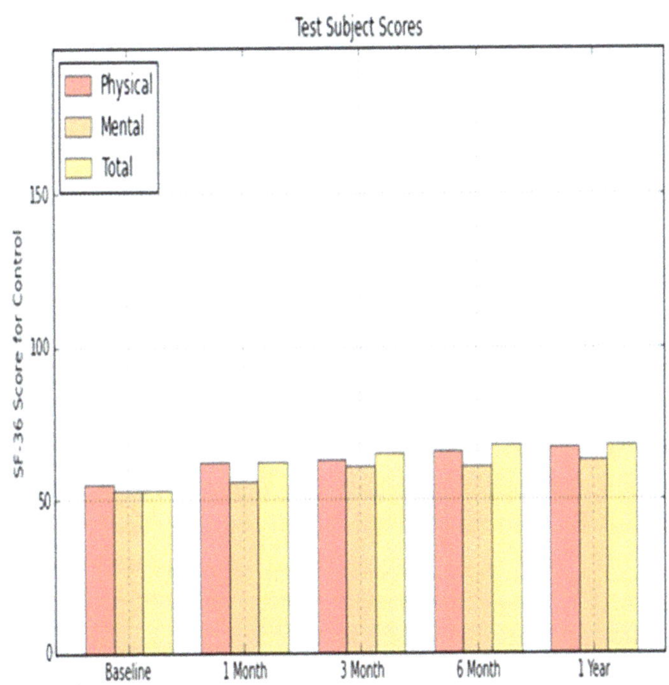

The analysis in Figure 15 shows the SF-36 scores of 28 patients which gave audio-visual GSR therapy for 10 sessions each 15 minutes. Records were taken over the period of 30 days, 90 days, 180 days, and 365 days. From the graph we may conclude that the relative scores of all the patients have been increased, so it validates the utility of the therapy. The x axis shows the time duration in months.

The analysis shown in Figure 16 shows 27 other subjects chosen for non-experiment group and their SF-36 scores were recorded but it has been observed that over the period of baseline, 1 month, 3 month, 6 month, and 1 year. From the graph, it is observed that the above scores increased. X Axis shows the time duration in months.

From all 3 bar graphs, simultaneous observations may be made that relatively EMG and GSR group has experienced more growth than the control group in their physical, mental and total scores than the control group. BFB therapy application has shown a significant reduction in stress (TTH).

In EMG, physical scores were constant for 6 months and gradually increased in the next half. In GSR, physical scores kept on varying to increment continuously. In EMG, mental scores were continuously increasing. In GSR, physical scores kept on increasing continuously. Total scores in both were under fluctuation and varying but increasing timely.

The analysis, Figure 17, shows the relation between physical scores of audio-visual EMG, GSR, and control categories over the period of a starting point, 30 days, 90 days, 180 days, and 365 days. From the graphs, it is clear that the physical scores of EMG and GSR were better than have increased over the period of time. Initially, the GSR superseded the EMG therapy up to around 6 months but in the next half, EMG therapy showed significant increment over GSR and control groups.

The analysis in Figure 18 shows the relation between mental scores of audio-visual EMG, GSR, control categories over the time period of baseline, 1 month, 3 month, 6 month, and 1 year. From the very starting point, the EMG therapy showed the drastic increment continuously over GSR and control groups in the overall experiment period.

The analysis shown in Figure 19 shows an overall score of EMG, GSR, and control categories, we found that initially GSR and EMG were competing but in the latter half, EMG showed a clear win over GSR technique in dealing with the stress issue of subjects.

The analysis in Figure 20 shows the relation between average frequency of headaches for audio-visual EMG category over the period of 30 days, 90 days, 180 days, and 365 days. From the graphs, it is clear that the frequency of EMG and GSR were decreased over the period of time. The y-axis is episodes per week.

The analysis in Figure 21 shows the relation between average frequency of headaches for audio-visual GSR categories over the period of 30 days, 90 days, 180

Figure 17. The line graph shows the relationship between physical scores of audio-visual EMG, GSR, control categories over the period of the starting point, 30 days, 90 days, 180 days and 365 DAYS

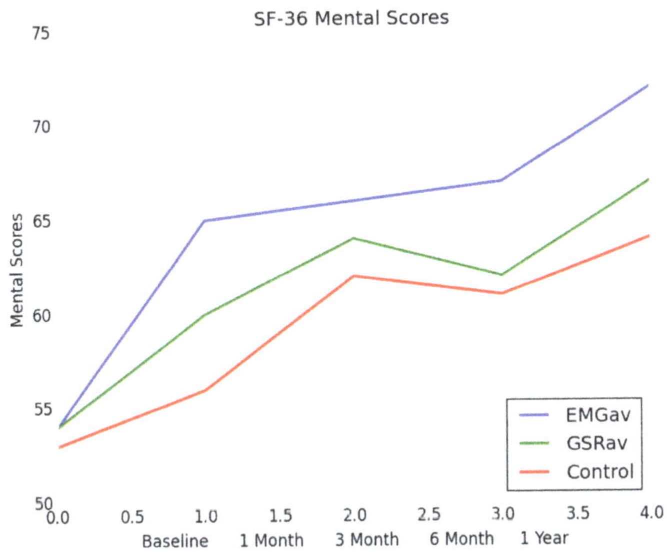

Figure 18. Graph showing the relation between mental scores of audio-visual EMG, GSR, control categories over the time period of baseline, 1 month, 3 months, 6 months, 1 year

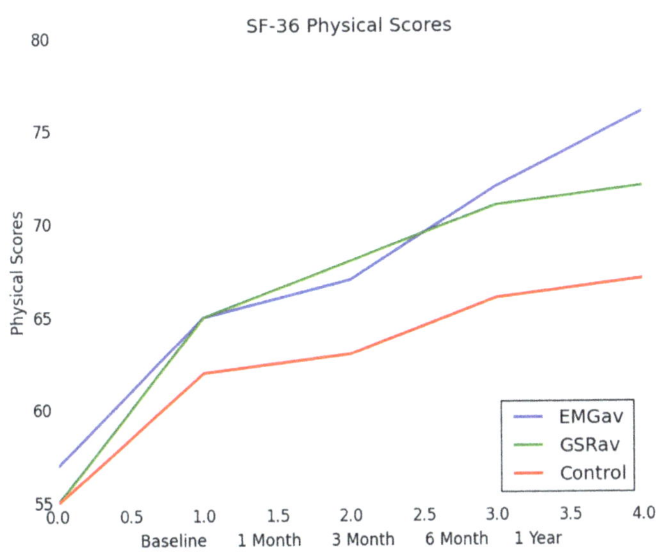

Figure 19. Shows the overall score of EMG, GSR and control categories

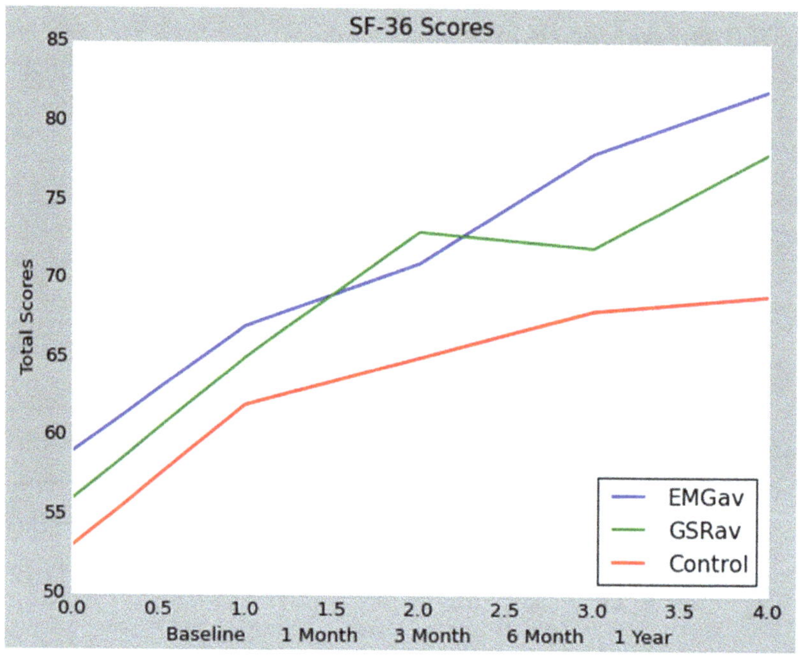

Figure 20. Above the line, the graph shows the relation between the average frequency of headache for audio-visual EMG category over the period of starting point, 30 days, 90 days, 180 days and 365 days

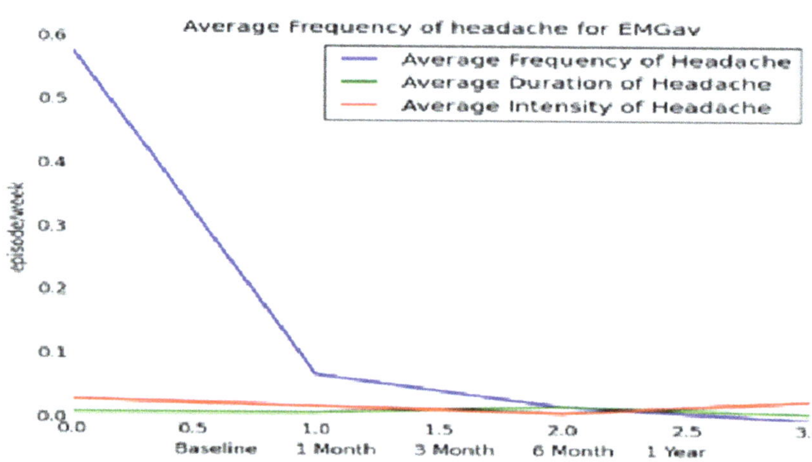

Figure 21. The line graph shows the relation between the average frequency of headache for audio-visual GSR category over the period of starting point, 30 days, 90 days, 180 days and 365 days

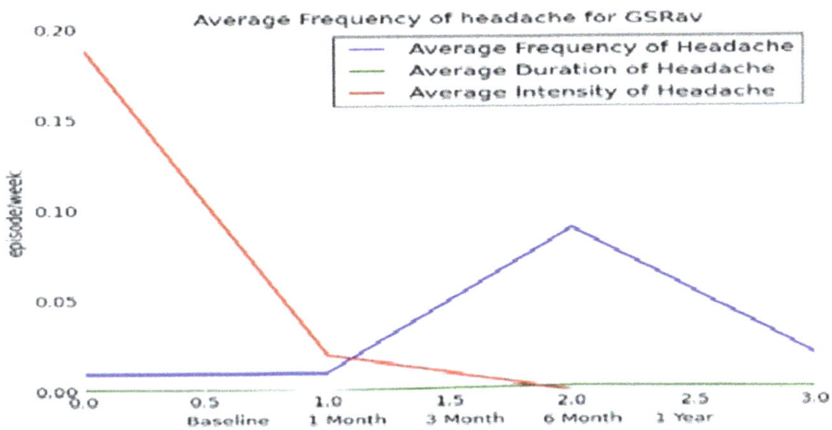

days, and 365 days, From the graphs, it is clear that the frequency of EMG and GSR were decreased over the period of time. The y-axis is episodes per week.

The analysis shown in Figure 22 shows the relation between average frequency of headaches for the control category over the period 30 days, 90 days, 180 days, and 365 days, From the graphs, it is clear that the frequency of EMG and GSR were decreased over the period of time. On the other hand, their control groups do show such results. The y axis is episodes per week.

Figure 22. The line graph shows the relation between the average frequency of headache for control category over the period of starting point, 30 days, 90 days, 180 days and 365 days

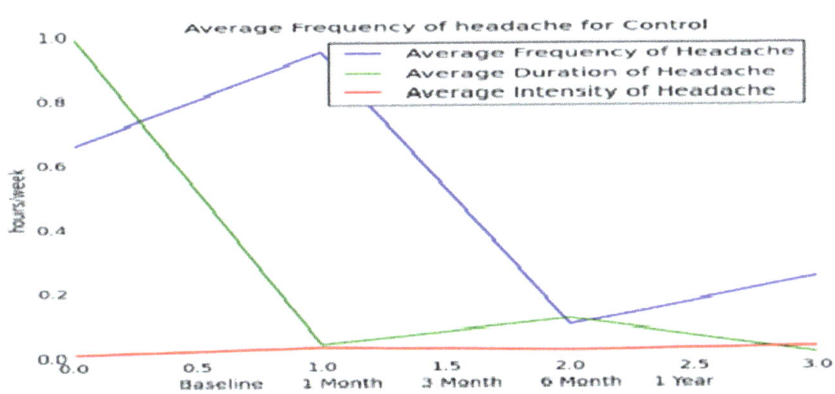

Figure 23. The graph shows the score of REMG & VAS of 51 patients

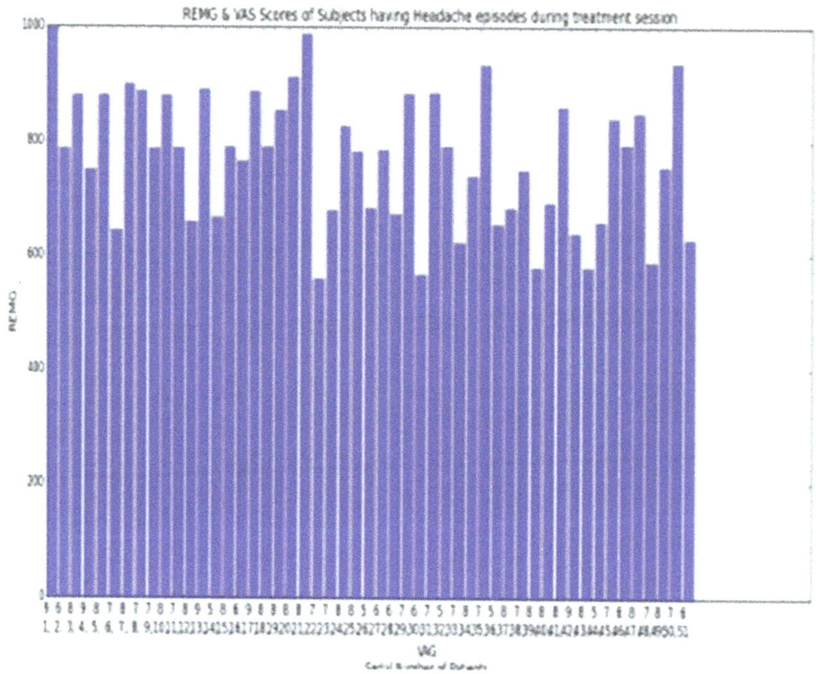

The analysis in Figure 23 shows the score of REMG & VAS of 51 patients. The x axis shows the score of VAG and REMG score is shown on y axis. The x axis also shows the serial number of patients. The graph shows the fluctuating records of different patients with respect to their relative EMG scores and visual analog score of headache intensity on a scale of 10. The x axis is the visual analogue score (VAS).

Experiments and Discussion With EEG

Analysis (Fig. 25): The waves are categorized majorly into four types i.e. alpha,beta,gamma, and theta. Alpha waves are considered to be the best while the tatobe the worst as per the literature available. The super most form of waves is the alpha waves for human being which are considered to be released during the meditation process (as per Table 2 and Table 3). This is the meditative state.

Our experiment focuses don to measure the alpha waves before and after meditation and also considering the use of EEG for the same. The EEG machine we haved one the experimentis32-channels andthe64-channels could not be used because it was costly. Observations were recorded with and without EEG machine and for pre and post-meditation.

Figure 24. The graph shows the alpha waves for some subjects recorded within a particular interval of time

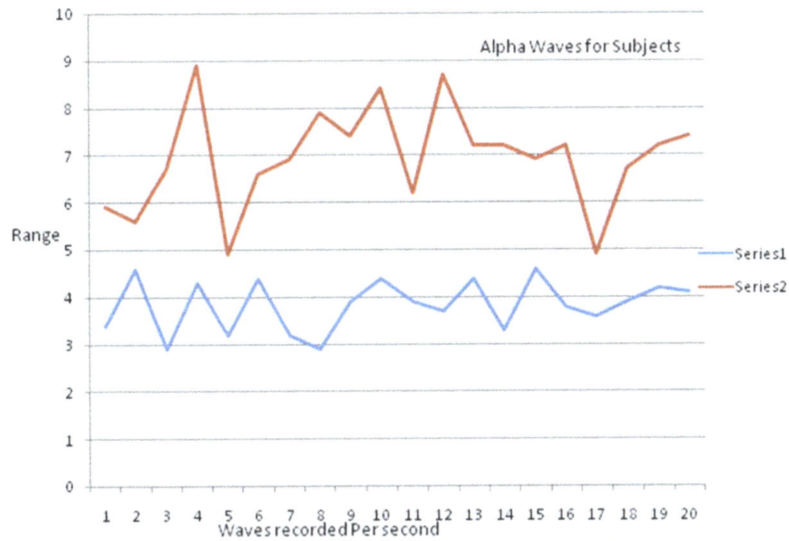

Table 2. EEG recordings data in the first experiment

M1	3.84
M2	6.94
R	0.18
SDx	0.53
S	1.06
SED	0.25
t-value	12.6

The initial experiment was for a group of 13 subjects of different genders. There readings for alpha-waves without using guided meditation through EEG were 3.4, 4.6, 2.9, 4.3 and soon while for after using guided meditation through EEG were 5.9, 5.6 and so on respectively. We then calculated the standard derivative and the rank relation coefficient for the two values and concluded that they are very less correlated (0.18). The value of SD1 and SD2 were 0.53 and 1.06 respectively. Also, the test conducted result in at-value of 12.6.

Figure 25. The graph shows the alpha waves of subjects recorded after meditation

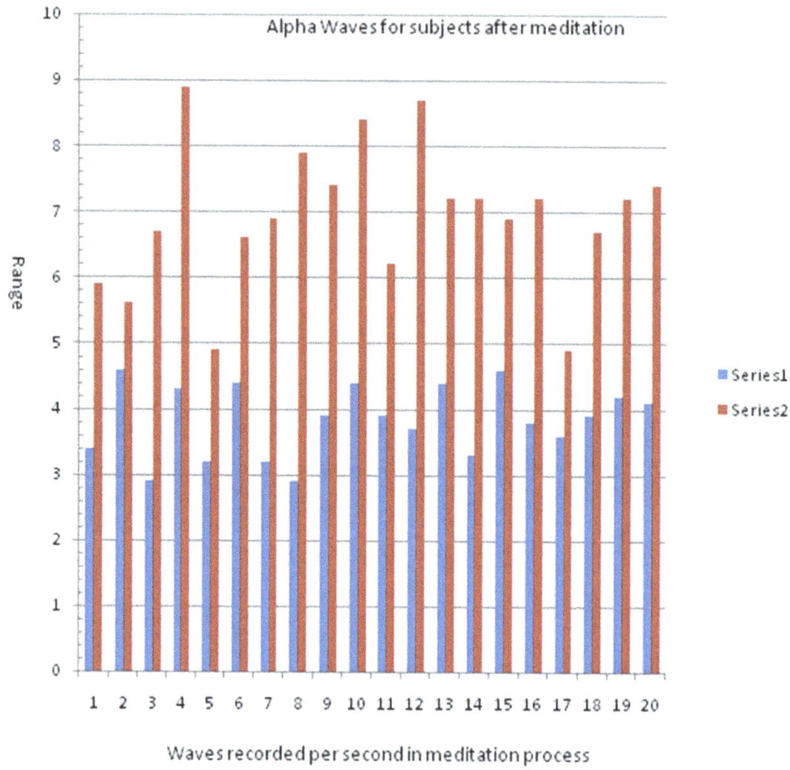

Experiment 2 Graphs

The same experiment was repeated for another 18 subjects for pre and post- stress relief exercises. The observations were recorded as they were previously done. The alpha waves measured for before experiment was recorded to be 5.17, 4.13, 6, 7.37 and so on. The observations were, however, this time divided based on gender and also a combined observation was recorded. The readings were different for some subjects while the same for some subjects and differed for each subject. The value of SD1 and SD2 for combined data was recorded to be 1.02 and 1.62 respectively. The rank correlation coefficient was 0.52. However, a very low value of T was recorded i.e. 0.01. The study could be better experimented using 64 channels EEG but due to some limitations, we were unable to do so. The 64 channel EEG machine is costly and can be used for a large sample of data (as per Table 4 and Table 5).

Table 3. EEG recordings data in the first experiment

Before experiment reading						After experiment reading					
Name	**Pre**	**Post**	**Alpha Waves/ sec..X**	**x=X-M1**	**x^2**	**Pre**	**Post**	**Alpha Waves/ sec..Y**	**y=Y-M2**	**y2**	**X*Y**
Raj	10	34	3.4	-0.44	0.189225	10	59	5.9	-1.04	1.0816	0.452
Radha	10	46	4.6	0.77	0.585225	10	56	5.6	-1.34	1.7956	-1.03
Monika	10	29	2.9	-0.94	0.874225	10	67	6.7	-0.24	0.0576	0.224
Harish	10	43	4.3	0.47	0.216225	10	89	8.9	1.96	3.8416	0.911
Ganga	10	32	3.2	-0.64	0.403225	10	49	4.9	-2.04	4.1616	1.295
Mradul	10	44	4.4	0.57	0.319225	10	66	6.6	-0.34	0.1156	-0.19
Mukesh	10	32	3.2	-0.64	0.403225	10	69	6.9	-0.04	0.0016	0.025
Savitri	10	29	2.9	-0.94	0.874225	10	79	7.9	0.96	0.9216	-0.9
Jaya	10	39	3.9	0.06	0.004225	10	74	7.4	0.46	0.2116	0.03
Rekha	10	44	4.4	0.57	0.319225	10	84	8.4	1.46	2.1316	0.825
Poornima	10	39	3.9	0.06	0.004225	10	62	6.2	-0.74	0.5476	-0.05
Manoj	10	37	3.7	-0.14	0.018225	10	87	8.7	1.76	3.0976	-0.24
Mukul	10	44	4.4	0.57	0.319225	10	72	7.2	0.26	0.0676	0.147
Suresh	10	33	3.3	-0.54	0.286225	10	72	7.2	0.26	0.0676	-0.14
Savita	10	46	4.6	0.77	0.585225	10	69	6.9	-0.04	0.0016	-0.03
Anmol	10	38	3.8	-0.04	0.001225	10	72	7.2	0.26	0.0676	-0.01
Mradul	10	36	3.6	-0.24	0.055225	10	49	4.9	-2.04	4.1616	0.479
Veerendra	10	39	3.9	0.06	0.004225	10	67	6.7	-0.24	0.0576	-0.02
Akhilesh	10	42	4.2	0.37	0.133225	10	72	7.2	0.26	0.0676	0.095
Nupur	10	41	4.1	0.27	0.070225	10	74	7.4	0.46	0.2116	0.122
Sum			76.7	Ex	5.6655			138.8	Ey	22.668	2.012
M1			3.835		0.283275		M2	6.94		1.1334	
SD1					0.532236		SD2			1.0646	

The Discussion on Quality of Life

Since in the duration of1year, only 22 subjects participated fully so we are considering only them. Likewise, BF too is a learning process which therefore can be assumed to be facilitated by providing audio and visual cues to the patients. In our study, there was a significant improvement of stress variables and SF-36 sum and sub-scores in audio-visual EMG group indicating that integrated feedback is effective than that of GSR.

Increasing stress levels in people nowadays are creating higher tension levels ultimately results in chronic headaches. One of the most prominent headaches is Tension-Type Headache (TTH) creating unendurable mental disorders. Main life events such as divorce, surgery, and loss of close relatives, family members inculcate

Table 4. Second experiment readings data on EEG

Alpha EEG for combined subjects Before Experiment Reading								Alpha EEG for combined subjects After Experiment Reading					
Name	**Age**	**Sex**	**Pre**	**Post**	**Alpha Waves/ sec..X**	**x=X-M1**	**x^2**	**Pre**	**Post**	**Alpha Waves/ sec..Y**	**y=Y-M2**	**y2**	**X*Y**
Rakhi	23	F	10	51.7	5.17	0.04	1.600E-03	10	92.7	9.27	2.25	5.0625	0.09
Anamika	24	F	10	41.3	4.13	-1	1.000E+00	10	72.3	7.23	0.21	0.0441	-0.21
Sanjeev	23	M	10	60	6	0.87	7.569E-01	10	100.3	10.03	3.01	9.0601	2.6187
Sudha	25	F	10	73.7	7.37	2.24	5.018E+00	10	97	9.7	2.68	7.1824	6.0032
Ankita	26	F	10	46.7	4.67	-0.46	2.116E-01	10	63	6.3	-0.72	0.5184	0.3312
Satyendra	24	M	10	63	6.3	1.17	1.369E+00	10	78	7.8	0.78	0.6084	0.9126
Sumit	21	M	10	29.7	2.97	-2.16	4.666E+00	10	64	6.4	-0.62	0.3844	1.3392
Jitendra	22	M	10	56	5.6	0.47	2.209E-01	10	68.7	6.87	-0.15	0.0225	-0.0705
Chhaya	22	F	10	44.7	4.47	-0.66	4.356E-01	10	102.3	10.23	3.21	10.3041	-2.1186
Aneeta	24	F	10	41.3	4.13	-1	1.000E+00	10	70.7	7.07	0.05	0.0025	-0.05
Shobheet	32	M	10	44	4.4	-0.73	5.329E-01	10	63.3	6.33	-0.69	0.4761	0.5037
Ajeet	25	M	10	47.3	4.73	-0.4	1.600E-01	10	60.7	6.07	-0.95	0.9025	0.38
Swati	24	F	10	43	4.3	-0.83	6.889E-01	10	67.7	6.77	-0.25	0.0625	0.2075
Naveen	24	M	10	53.3	5.33	0.2	4.000E-02	10	59	5.9	-1.12	1.2544	-0.224
Meenakshi	23	F	10	47.7	4.77	-0.36	1.296E-01	10	43.3	4.33	-2.69	7.2361	0.9684
Anshu	21	M	10	67.7	6.77	1.64	2.690E+00	10	52	5.2	-1.82	3.3124	-2.9848
Surakhsha	21	M	10	40.7	4.07	-1.06	1.124E+00	10	64.3	6.43	-0.59	0.3481	0.6254
Sheela	24	M	10	52.3	5.23	0.1	1.000E-02	10	52	5.2	-1.82	3.3124	-0.182
Asif	24	M	10	60.3	6.03	0.9	8.100E-01	10	52.7	5.27	-1.75	3.0625	-1.575
Sameer	26	M	10	64.3	6.43	1.3	1.690E+00	10	63.5	6.35	-0.67	0.4489	-0.871
Sum					102.87	Ex				138.75	Ey		5.694
M1					5.134		M2			7.02			0.2847
SD1				1.02				SD2			1.62		

major negative effects. Such events in the previous year have been considered related to the persistence of headache.

The main aim of our research is to study the effects of tension-type headache using biofeedback therapies on various modes such as audio modes, visual modes, and audiovisual modes. The experiment was conducted on 90 people out of whom 78 people remain till the end of medical treatment. In 78 people, 46 were females and 32 were males and it was recorded that females had higher levels of headaches in younger ages. The groups were randomly allocated for GSR therapies and the other one was a control group (the group which was not under any type of allopathic or

Table 5. Second experiment gender-based readings on EEG

Alpha EEG-Combine		Alpha EEG-For Male		Alpha EEG-For Female	
M1	5.134	M1	4.98	M1	5.28
M2	7.02	M2	5.94	M2	4.73
N	20	N	10	N	10
R	0.52	r	0.24	R	0.71
SDx	1.02	SDx	0.87	SDx	1.26
SDy	1.62	SDy	0.79	SDy	1.55
SEMx	0.24	SEMx	0.29	SEMx	0.42
SEMy	0.37	SEMy	0.26	SEMy	0.52
SED	0.108	SED	0.115	SED	0.14
t-value	0.01	t-value	8.42	t-value	20.16
Sig	0.01	Sig	0.01	Sig	0.01

Figure 26. The graph shows the alpha EEG for subjects recorded after stress relief exercises

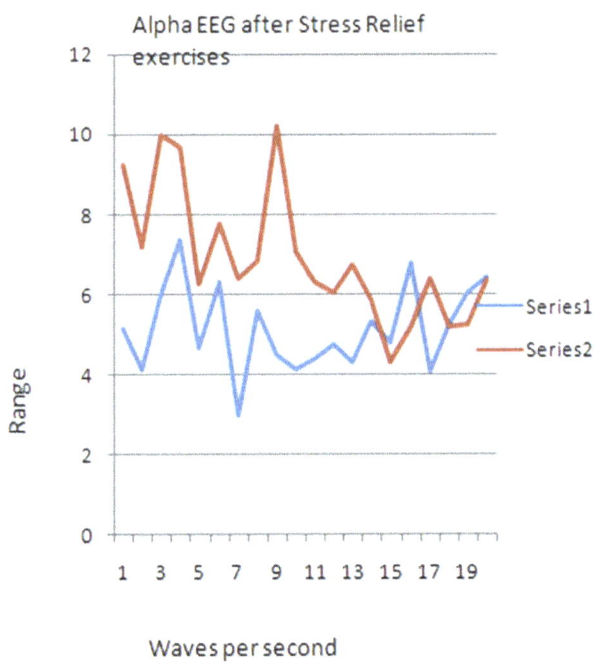

Figure 27. Bar graph showing alpha EEG after for subjects after stress relief exercises
Analysis (Fig. 26, 27):

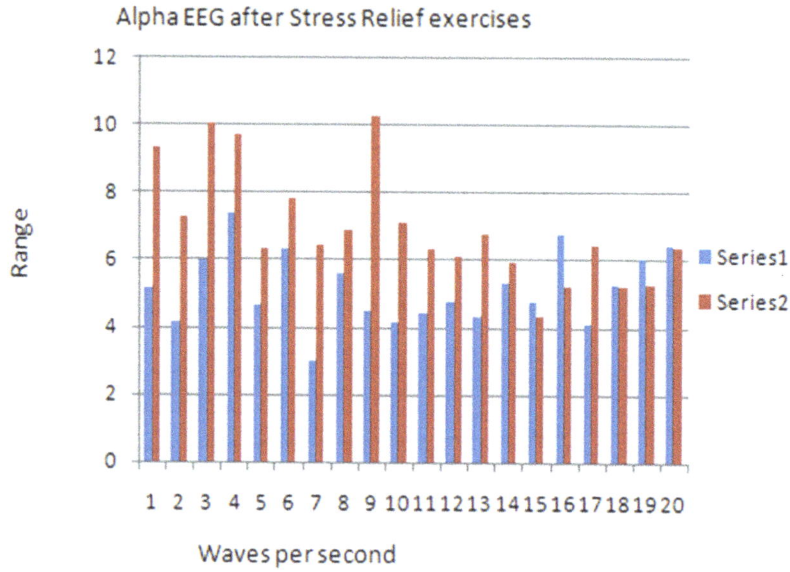

other medications).Except for control group, other groups were treated in a session for 20 minutes in isolated chambers. The results were recorded over a specific period of time say 1 month, 6 months or 12 months.

In this study, authors have also tried their best to check the effect of TTH over age and gender. TTH is one of harmful headache, TTH is produced by stress, it may start at any stage of life. Subjects usually suffer from two types of TTH i.e. for a short time and for a long time. When subjects suffer from a long time, then it affects both mind and body. So, one may check at which age it started and how gender is affected by this problem.

Another study similar to ours in terms of methodology, in which EMG and GSR BF were used for relaxation training. In this study the subjects were randomly assigned to four groups: 1) group receiving EMG-GSR audio BF with eyes closed; 2) group receiving EMG-GSR audio BF with eyes open; 3) group receiving EMG-GSR visual BF; and 4) control group which received no feedback. It was reported that group which received EMG audio BF with eyes closed showed a better decrease in frontalis muscle activity as compared to other groups. However, integrated feedback was not used in this study.

RECOMMENDATIONS

Till date the field of tension-type headache (stress) was less covered area, the time, a systematic study has been conducted to show the effect of other than medication therapies like BFB therapy and comparing the results of EMG and GSR techniques for the effect of positive thinking to manage daily life stress and increase the capacity of problem-solving. The study also shows the betterment of Bio-Feedback mechanism in a long duration of 1 year, subsequently recorded the SF-36 scores in 4 quarters and ignites the path of alternative medication techniques to overcome stress, anxiety, and depression-like psycho challenges. That means we can use this term commonly but stress is not so easy to explain. Stress is a word means "to draw tight" and has been used to describe hardship, affliction, force, pressures, strain or strong effort. There are two higher mental processes. Problem-solving has been conceived by psychologists as the discovery of correct response to a problem or situation that is new and difficult for the individual, but decision-making refers to the selection of a correct response, out of several correct responses already brought out and had been found that as people are getting older and older their problem-solving ability is reducing. The paper has shown a clear path to find the relation of stress (headache), problem-solving, decision making and physical and mental well-being of an individual.

Nowadays, stress is associated with everyone's life and every person of any society at some levels is affected by stress problems and thus suffers TTH. The work in this research is unique as it aims at reducing the headache level and to control the analgesic and prophylactic medications. Based on results it was seen the transfer of people from one group to other. As the number of sufferings is increasing in the society and the world, these types of research provide a means to treat various disorders according to (Millea, and Brodie, 2002) and (Mullaly, 2009).

FUTURE RESEARCH DIRECTIONS, LIMITATIONS AND POSSIBLE APPLICATIONS

In our research work, the experiment was conducted on a limited and fixed number of patients. And depending on the needs, it may be experimented on various patients based on a different type of factors like age, gender, climate, etc. Biofeedback therapies provide a way to treat mental disorders with minimal use of medications and these therapies conducted on different age groups, genders of various countries. Biofeedback therapies help individuals to improve their physical and mental health by gaining control of their bodies and minds. These therapies increase awareness of these functions, so patients can control stress and physical ailments. Although it is a bit costly for common people and efforts have been made to make this therapy accessible to every group of society. These therapies are also useful in treating:

- Alcohol use disorder
- Drug addiction
- Insomnia
- Anxiety
- Chronic pains
- Migraines
- Nausea

Various scientists believe that these therapies will bring a revolution in the treatment of TTH. The patients will be able to control their own pains and can record their real-time reactions as per (Crystal, Robbins, 2010) and (Zanella et al., 2004).

Our study based on TTH and the IoT will be very useful for studying on this topic in the future coming projects. It will be very useful and will aim to find an effective solution to TTH in a tech effective manner. The development of this topic will prove very useful as each and everyone around this world is suffering from TTH in one way or the other. Hence future scope regarding this topic is not just limited to studying it but will result in effective applications in the coming future.

Development in the field of technology is growing with fast pace, mainly the IoT (Internet of Things), i.e. it is usually called as the internet. It is an interface between machine-to-machine, machine-to-human, machine-to-infrastructure as well as machine -to-environment. IoT helps us to connect each other i.e. it is known a smart connecting thing (a sort of "Universal Global Neural Network" in cloud). It comprises of smart connecting machine with other machine, object and a lot more. IoT helps us in a way that the machine should judge on its own and can interact or judge some future information. Its data is being stored in the form of cloud which is being taken properly so that data cannot be misguided by someone. In the modern era, the volume of sample or raw data has increased at a rapid rate. This data may be used for evaluation in many fields. Big Data refers to huge sets of data which are also large enough in terms of variety and velocity. Due to this, it becomes more difficult to handle, organise, store, process and manipulate such data using traditional techniques of storage and processing.

Limitation

There have been several studies regarding TTH and use of IoT in such a field, but the studies have been limited merely to writings. The solution to TTH and its perfect cure is not yet found. With such a high prevalence rate, it becomes a necessity for researchers to have a discussion over this topic and come to a final conclusion rather than relating to its symptoms and their cures. Thus, important information must be derived to plan the optimal treatment for TTH patients.

Significance

This study covers all possible aspects of TTH, IoT and big data and their applications to the field of a medical study. It is done in a very short period of time but covers. As a large area of population suffers from TTH thus it becomes a necessity to have a worthy and fruitful discussion and research on this topic. Topics like the causes, effects, cures, biofeedback therapies, future scope, etc. have all been covered by the researchers but its effective application is yet to come. These studies will prove to be useful at the time of its application. This study needs to be done on a large scale in order to prove useful and bring out a solution.

More than half of the world experiences TTH in one form or the other. It has been called by different names over the years for example: tension headache, muscle contraction etc. Many biofeedback experiments are being conducted to reduce this tension, so our team has conducted an experiment where we have collected data on the study of the people; we have studied their tension level and helped them to cure it. In today's world, people know so much about the world around them but most of them know so little about their own selves. The world gets more mysterious and enigmatic as one tries to know it. The reach and scope of the human mind may be infinite, but the mental complexities generated result in the hampering of improvement and elevation in the personality. There are many cases of lack of knowledge of inner self and emotional instability in boys and girls of pre-adult age of 20-25 years which lead to various psychological imbalances. One can switch to proper meditation with positive attitude to find cure from all possible issues. It has been reflected by researchers that the complete personal effectiveness, social success, pleasant attitude and work style efficiency of an individual is governed by the imaginations, emotions and mental fitness.

CONCLUSION

From the above experimentation, we may conclude that EEG, audio-visual EMG-BF and GSR-BF are effective in the treatment of stress (TTH), with facts of EMG-BF being more effective than GSR-BF. In this study, the experimental group showed a significant reduction in the level of stress. Hence, it can be proven by EMG and GSR biofeedback therapy concluded that continuous positive thinking has the capacity to reduce stress among students and increase their working performance.

In EMG and GSR, a prophylactic is a treatment used to prevent diseases from occurring. "Prevention is better than cure"; these treatments work on this principle. They are used to prevent something from happening, for example, a prophylactic hepatitis vaccine prevents the patient from getting hepatitis. These are also called anti-depressants as they help to reduce headaches. Results show that there is a significant effect of the GSR therapy on the prophylactic treatment.

ACKNOWLEDGMENT

Our Sincere thanks to all direct and indirect supporters and well-wishers. Esteem gratitude to Management of Dev Sanskriti Vishwavidyalaya Hardwar and Shantikunj where the image processing experiments and study were conducted. We are especially thankful for ABESEC, Ghaziabad management and staff for their time contribution to be part of this study. We also convey gratitude to officers of DayalBagh Educational Institute for their mentorship and timely valuable suggestions.

This research received no specific grant from any funding agency in the public, commercial, or not-for-profit sectors.

REFERENCES

Arora, N., Rastogi, R., Chaturvedi, D. K., Satya, S., Gupta, M., Yadav, V., . . . Sharma, P. (2019b), Chronic TTH Analysis by EMG & GSR Biofeedback on Various Modes and Various Medical Symptoms Using IoT. In Big Data Analytics for Intelligent Healthcare Management (Ch. 5, pp. 87-149). Academic Press. doi:10.1016/B978-0-12-818146-1.00005-2

Arora, N., Trivedi, P., Chauhan, S., Rastogi, R., & Chaturvedi, D. K. (2017a). Framework for Use of Machine Intelligence on Clinical Psychology to study the effects of Spiritual tools on Human Behavior and Psychic Challenges. In *Proceedings of NSC-2017*. Academic Press.

Binder, H., & Blettner, M. (2015). Big Data in Medical Science—a Biostatistical View. Deutsches Ärzteblatt International, 112(9), 137. doi:10.3238/arztebl.2015.0137

Boureau, F., Luu, M., & Doubrere, J. F. (2001). Study of experimental pain measures and nociceptive reflex in Chronic pain patients and normal subjects. *Pain*, *44*(3), 131–138. PMID:2052379

Carlson, N. (2013). *Physiology of Behavior*. New Jersey: Pearson Education, Inc.

Cassel, R. N. (1997). Biofeedback for developing self-control of tension and stress in one's hierarchy of psychological states. *Psychology: A Journal of Human Behavior, 22*(2), 50-57.

Chaturvedi, D. K., Rastogi, R., Arora, N., Trivedi, P., & Mishra, V. (2017b). Swarm Intelligent Optimized Method of Development of Noble Life in the perspective of Indian Scientific Philosophy and Psychology. In *Proceedings of NSC-2017*. Academic Press.

Chaturvedi, D.K., Rastogi, R., Satya, S., Arora, N., Saini, H., Verma, H., Mehlyan K., Varshney Y, (2018b). Statistical Analysis of EMG and GSR Therapy on Visual Mode and SF-36 Scores for Chronic TTH. In *Proceedings of UPCON-2018*. Academic Press.

Chauhan, S., Rastogi, R., Chaturvedi, D. K., Satya, S., Arora, N., Yadav, V., & Sharma, P. (2018d). Analytical Comparison of Efficacy for Electromyography and Galvanic Skin Resistance Biofeedback on Audio-Visual Mode for Chronic TTH on Various Attributes. In Proceedings of the ICCIDA-2018. Academic Press.

Costa, F. F. (2014). *'Big Data in Biomedicine'*. *Drug Discovery Today, 19*(4), 433–440. doi:10.1016/j.drudis.2013.10.012 PMID:24183925

Crystal, S. C., & Robbins, M. S. (2010). Epidemiology of tension-type headache. *Current Pain and Headache Reports, 14*(6), 449–45. doi:10.100711916-010-0146-2 PMID:20865353

Fumal, A., & Scohnen, J. (2008). Tension-type headache: current research and clinical management. *Lancet Neurology, 7*(2), 70–83. doi:10.1016/S1474-4422(07)70325-3 PMID:18093564

Gulati, M., Rastogi, R., Chaturvedi, D. K., Sharma, P., Yadav, V., Chauhan, S., . . . Singhal, P. (2019e). Statistical Resultant Analysis of Psychosomatic Survey on Various Human Personality Indicators: Statistical Survey to Map Stress and Mental Health. In *Handbook of Research on Learning in the Age of Transhumanism* (Ch. 22, pp. 363-383). Hershey, PA: IGI Global. doi:10.4018/978-1-5225-8431-5.ch022

Gupta, M., Rastogi, R., Chaturvedi, D. K., & Satya, S. (2019a). Comparative study of trends observed during different medications by subjects under EMG & GSR biofeedback. *IJITEE, 8*(6S), 748-756. Retrieved from https://www.ijitee.org/download/volume-8-issue-6S/

Haddock, C. K., Rowan, A. B., Andrasik, F., Wilson, P. G., Talcott, G. W., & Stein, R. J. (1997). Home- based behavioral Treatments for chronic benign headache: A meta-analysis of controlled trials. *Cephalalgia, 17*(1), 113–118. doi:10.1046/j.1468-2982.1997.1702113.x PMID:9137849

Haynes, S. N., Griffin, P., Mooney, D., & Parise, M. (2005). Electromyographic BF and Relaxation Instructions in the Treatment of Muscle Contraction Headaches. *Behavior Therapy, 6*(1), 672–678.

Kropotov, J. D. (2009). *Quantitative EMG, event-related potentials and neurotherapy*. San Diego, CA: Academic Press.

Lee, C. H., & Yoon, H. J. (2017). '*Medical big data: Promise and challenges'. Kidney Research and Clinical Practice, 36*(1), 461–475. doi:10.23876/j.krcp.2017.36.1.3

Millea, J.P., Brodie, J.J. (2002). Tension type headache. *American Family Physician, 66*(5), 797- 803.

Mouradian, C., Naboulsi, D., Yangui, S., Glitho, R. H., Morrow, M. J., & Polakos, P. A. (2017). A comprehensive survey on fog computing: State-of-the-art and research challenges. IEEE Communications Surveys & Tutorials, 20(1), 416-464. Retrieved from https://ieeexplore.ieee.org/abstract/document/8100873/authors#authors

Mullaly, J. W., Hall, K., & Goldstein, R. (2009, November/December). Efficacy of BF in the Treatment of Migraine and Tension Type Headaches. *Pain Physician, 12*(1), 1005–1011. PMID:19935987

Rastogi, R., Chaturvedi, D. K., Satya, S., Arora, N., & Chauhan, S. (2018a). An optimized biofeedback therapy for chronic TTH between electromyography and galvanic skin resistance biofeedback on audio, visual and audio visual modes on various medical symptoms. In *Proceedings of the national Conference on 3rd MDNCPDR-2018*. Academic Press.

Rastogi, R., Chaturvedi, D. K., Satya, S., Arora, N., Singhal, P., & Gulati, M. (2018f). Statistical Resultant Analysis of Spiritual & Psychosomatic Stress Survey on Various Human Personality Indicators. In *Proceedings of ICCI 2018*. Academic Press. doi:10.1007/978-981-13-8222-2_25

Rastogi, R., Chaturvedi, D. K., Satya, S., Arora, N., Yadav, V., Chauhan, S., & Sharma, P. (2018c). SF-36 Scores Analysis for EMG and GSR Therapy on Audio, Visual and Audio Visual Modes for Chronic TTH. In Proceedings of the ICCIDA-2018. Academic Press.

Rubin, A. (1999). Biofeedback and binocular vision. *Journal of Behavioral Optometry*, *3*(4), 95–98.

Saini, H., Rastogi, R., Chaturvedi, D. K., Satya, S., Arora, N., Gupta, M., & Verma, H. (2019c). An Optimized Biofeedback EMG and GSR Biofeedback Therapy for Chronic TTH on SF-36 Scores of Different MMBD Modes on Various Medical Symptoms. In Hybrid Machine Intelligence for Medical Image Analysis (Ch. 8). Springer Nature. doi:10.1007/978-981-13-8930-6_8

Satya, S., Arora, N., Trivedi, P., Singh, A., Sharma, A., Singh, A., Rastogi, R., Chaturvedi, D.K. (2019a). Intelligent Analysis for Personality Detection on Various Indicators by Clinical Reliable Psychological TTH and Stress Surveys. In *Proceedings of CIPR 2019*. Academic Press.

Satya, S., Rastogi, R., Chaturvedi, D. K., Arora, N., Singh, P., & Vyas, P. (2018e). Statistical Analysis for Effect of Positive Thinking on Stress Management and Creative Problem Solving for Adolescents. In *Proceedings of the 12th INDIA-Com* (pp. 245-251). Academic Press.

Scott, D. S., & Lundeen, T. F. (2004). Myofascial pain involving the masticatory muscles: An experimental model. *Pain*, *8*(2), 207–215. doi:10.1016/0304-3959(88)90008-5 PMID:7402684

Sharma, S., Rastogi, R., Chaturvedi, D. K., Bansal, A., & Agrawal, A. (2018g). Audio visual EMG & GSR Biofeedback analysis for effect of spiritual techniques on human behavior and psychic challenges. In *Proceedings of the 12th INDIACom* (pp. 252-258). Academic Press.

Singh, A., Rastogi, R., Chaturvedi, D. K., Satya, S., Arora, N., Sharma, A., & Singh, A. (2019d). Intelligent Personality Analysis on Indicators inIoT-MMBD Enabled Environment. In Multimedia Big Data Computing for IoT Applications: Concepts, Paradigms, and Solutions (Ch. 7). Springer Nature. doi:10.1007/978-981-13-8759-3_7

Singhal, P., Rastogi, R., Chaturvedi, D. K., Satya, S., Arora, N., Gupta, M., … Gulati, M. (2019b). Statistical Analysis of Exponential and Polynomial Models of EMG & GSR Biofeedback for Correlation between Subjects Medications Movement & Medication Scores. *IJITEE*, *8*(6S), 625-635. Retrieved from https://www.ijitee.org/download/volume-8-issue-6S/

Wenk-Sormaz, H. (2005). Meditation can reduce habitual responding. *Advances in Mind-Body*, *3*(4), 34–39.

Yadav, V., Rastogi, R., Chaturvedi, D. K., Satya, S., Arora, N., Yadav, V., ... Chauhan, S. (2018j). Statistical Analysis of EMG & GSR Biofeedback Efficacy on Different Modes for Chronic TTH on Various Indicators. *Int. J. Advanced Intelligence Paradigms*, *13*(1), 251–275. doi:10.1504/IJAIP.2019.10021825

Zanella, A., Bui, N., Castellani, A., Vangelista, L., & Zorzi, M. (2004). Internet of things for smart cities. *IEEE Internet Things J.*, *1*(1), 22–32. doi:10.1109/JIOT.2014.2306328

KEY TERMS AND DEFINITIONS

Biofeedback Therapy: the process of collecting knowledge about the different psychological functions using some specific instruments. The major objective is to control and manipulate these functions. Some of these controllable functions or processes are important body functions like skin conductance, brainwaves, heart rate, pain perception, and muscle tone. It may also be used to rectify psychological changes related to altering emotions, thoughts, and human behaviour. This therapy is useful for treating migraines and headaches.

IoT: a technology that has made the non-connecting appliance as a connectivity appliance. The appliances that contain technology that helps us to communicate with human and technology. Let us take some example like the GPS is the latest technology that is inbuilt in car help the driver to make it easy to travel within the road, i.e. it is that technology in which we require internet base technique.

Sensor Modalities: are very high accurate instruments to record physiological activity through body functions like brainwaves, heart function, breathing, muscle activity, and skin temperature.

Section 7
Depression

Chapter 11
Depression:
An Overview and Management

Ndapewa Nehale Shifiona
University of Namibia, Namibia

Daniel Opotamutale Ashipala
University of Namibia, Namibia

ABSTRACT

This chapter provides a broad overview of depression in adults. Depression is one of the leading causes of disability globally. It is a syndrome with central features of low mood, lack of enjoyment, reduced energy, negative thinking, poor sleep and appetite, lack of concentration, and suicidal ideation. It affects everyone. The purpose of this chapter is to outline the link between various contributory factors and depression among the adult population. Optimal management processes, including self-care, reduce the risk of relapse and improve the quality of life.

INTRODUCTION

Some people feel down, some feel sad at times. This is a normal reaction to loss or life's struggle. But when intense sadness-including feelings of helplessness, hopelessness and worthlessness last for many days or weeks and keep you from living your life, it may be something more than sadness – this is called clinical depression. According to Shifiona, Poggenpoel, and Myburgh (2006), being clinically depressed is very different from the dejected feelings that all people experience from time to time. Occasional feelings of sadness are a normal part of life and it is unfortunate that such feelings are often colloquially referred to as "depression." There are things in

DOI: 10.4018/978-1-7998-2139-7.ch011

everyone's life that are possible causes of sadness, but people who are not depressed manage to cope with these things without becoming incapacitated. As one might expect, depression can present itself as feeling sad or having the "blues". However, sadness may not always be the dominant feelings of a depressed person.

BACKGROUND

Despite noticeable transformation in the healthcare system of different countries in the world, mental health and wellness still receives low priority with efforts directed mainly towards addressing communicable and life-threatening diseases (Ashipala, Wilkinson, & van Dyk, 2016). Depressive disorder has significant potential morbidity and mortality, contributing to suicide, the incidence and adverse outcomes of medical illness, disruption in interpersonal relations, and lost work time and productivity. Halverson (2019) states that as many as two-thirds of people with depression do not realise that they have a treatable illness and therefore do not seek professional help. In addition, persistent ignorance and misperceptions of the disease by the public as a personal weakness or failing that can be willed or wished away, leads to painful stigmas and avoidance of the diagnosis by many of those affected. Thus, an understanding about "depressive disorder" is necessary, not only by the sufferer, but also by the caretaker and the public at large.

What is Depression?

There are various explanations of the meaning of the term "depression." The American Psychiatric Association (2013) describes depression as a common and serious medical illness that negatively affects the way a person feels, thinks and acts. Depression causes feelings of sadness and/or a loss of interest in activities that were previously enjoyed. It can lead to a variety of emotional and physical problems and can decrease a person's ability to function at work and at home. Kaplan and Saddock (1994) attributed depression to a psychopathological feeling of sadness, while Townsend (1996) described depression as a disorder that is characterised by a depressed mood or loss of interest or pleasure in usual activities. Before a medical diagnosis may be made, evidence of impaired social and occupational functioning should have existed for at least two weeks. From the descriptions above, there are similarities in the way various authors describe and present depression, namely, sadness, loss of interest and pleasure in the activities a person used to enjoy before. As reported in a study by Thapa, Martinez, and Clausen (2014), depression is a common mental health problem and an increasingly common cause for morbidity and disability in lower income countries, including those in Africa. It is common among middle-aged and older adults, and can increase the likelihood of negative outcomes when suffered concurrently with other mental, physical, and somatic disorders. Globally, depression is the leading cause of ill health and disability. According to the latest estimates from the World Health Organisation (WHO, 2017), more than 300 million people are now living with depression, an increase of more than 18% between 2005 and 2015. Chentosova-Dutton, Ryder, and Tsai (2014) proposed further that diagnosable major depression is observed across cultural context, with varying prevalence rates. It disrupts lives worldwide, posing significant threats to people's productivity and well-being. Depression (Chentosova et al., 2014) is projected to become a leading contributor to the global burden of disease by 2030. Lack of support for people with mental disorders (depression included), coupled with a fear of stigma, prevent many people from accessing the treatment they need to live healthier and more productive lives.

Chisholm (2017) reported that, from a list of different mental disturbances that affect human beings, depression tops the list and can affect all people; young or old, rich or poor, and people of all races and ethnicities. It does not discriminate and causes great disability among those affected. The prevalence rates for depression peak among older adults, affecting 2%more women between the ages of 55 and 74 than men. However, Chand and Arif (2019) reported that across all age groups, depression is 1.5-3 times higher among females than males.

Different Types of Depression

When people think about depression, they generally regard it as one of two things: either clinical depression, which requires treatment or regular depression that almost anyone can go through. As a condition, depression can be a difficult concept to grasp since it is referred to as both the symptom of a condition and a condition in itself (Schimelpfening, 2019).

Wu (2018) points out the need to differentiate between situational depression and clinical depressive disorders. Clinical depression, which is also known as major depression or major depressive disorders, is more severe than situational depression and may interfere with daily function. The Diagnostic and Statistical Manual of Mental Disorders (DSM-5) classifies clinical depression as a mood disorder. However, according to Wu (2018), situational and clinical depression are similar but not the same. Situational depression is usually a short-term form of depression that occurs as a result of a traumatic event or change in a person's life. This mood state is also known as adjustment disorder with depressed mood. Triggers can include divorce, loss of a job, the death of a close friend, a serious accident as well as other major life changes such as retirement. Situational depression arises from a struggle to come to terms with dramatic life changes. Common noticeable changes include listlessness, feelings of hopelessness and sadness, sleeping difficulties, frequent episodes of crying, unfocused anxiety and worry, loss of concentration, withdrawal from normal activities and from family and friends, and suicidal thoughts.

How Does Situational Depression Differ from Clinical Depression?

Clinical depression is more severe than situational depression. In order to meet the criteria for clinically significant depression, an individual's distress level must impair their daily functioning. DiMaria (2019) expanded on this, stating that individuals with clinically significant depression experience sadness marked diminished interest in their activities, and several other symptoms to the extent that they struggle to function. The symptoms of clinically significant depression are persistent. An individual who feels down for an afternoon or a couple of days does not meet the diagnostic criteria for clinically significant depression if the symptoms resolve. If, however, symptoms persist for two weeks or longer and they represent a significant change from previous functioning, a person may have clinically significant depression.

In depression, certain chemicals, known as neurotransmitters, playa role. Animbalance of neurotransmitters such as serotonin and norepinephrine can cause clinical depression. However, other factors are likely to play a role, for example, genetic factors may influence an individual's response to an experience or event; major life events can trigger negative emotions such as anger, disappointment, or frustration; and alcohol and drug dependence also have links to depression(Schimelpfening, 2019).

Additionally, major depressive disorders are characterised by sadness, loss of interest or pleasure, feelings of guilt or low self-worth, disturbed sleep or appetite, feelings of tiredness, and poor concentration. Depression can be long lasting or recurrent, substantially impairing an individual's ability to function at work or school or cope with daily life. At its most severe, depression can lead to suicide.

Depressive disorders include two main sub-categories: major depressive disorder/ depressive episode, which involves symptoms such as depressed mood, loss of interest and enjoyment, and decreased energy; depending on the number and severity of the symptoms, a depressive episode can be categorized as mild, moderate (WHO, 2017). Depending on the number and severity of symptoms, a depressive episode can be categorised as mild, moderate, or severe. The other subcategory is dysthymia, a persistent or chronic form of mild depression, of which the symptoms are similar to depressive episode, but tend to be less intense and last longer. (WHO, 2017).

Types of Clinically Significant Depression

- There are different types of depression that may vary in duration, timing, presumed causes, or may involve different types of symptoms. The treatment for different types of depression varies too. The following sections discuss the most common types of depression which are categorised in the DSM-5as "depressive disorders" (American Psychiatric Association, 2013).

Major Depressive Disorder (MDD)

When people use the term clinical "depression", they are generally referring to major depressive disorder (MDD). This is characterised by a number of key features:

- Depressed mood
- Lack of interest in activities normally enjoyed
- Changes in weight
- Changes in sleep
- Fatigue
- Feelings of worthlessness and guilt
- Difficulty concentrating
- Thoughts of death and suicide

If a person experiences at least five or more of these symptoms for longer than atwo-week period, she/he will often be diagnosed with MDD.

Persistent Depressive Disorder

This type of depression is also known as dysthymia. It is a type of chronic depression that is present for more days than not for at least two years. It can be mild, moderate or severe.

Bipolar Disorder

Bipolar disorder is a mood disorder characterised by periods of abnormally elevated mood known as mania. These periods can be mild (hypomania) or they can be so extreme as to cause marked impairment with a person's life, require hospitalisation, and affect a person's reality. People with bipolar disorder often have a range of physical and emotional symptoms which may include;

- Fatigue, insomnia, and lethargy

- Unexplained aches, pain, and psychomotor agitation
- Hopelessness and loss of self-esteem
- Instability and anxiety
- Indecision and disorganisation.

During a manic episode, a person has a sustained and abnormally elevated, expansive, or irritable mood for at least one week, and at least three of the following symptoms: grandiosity, or an inflated sense of self. The person displays little need for sleep, feeling pressured to speak, talking loudly and rapidly (Purse, 2019). The risk of suicide in bipolar illness is 15 times greater than in the general population.

Postpartum Depression

This type of depression has its onset during pregnancy or following the birth of a child. Symptoms can range from persistent lethargy and sadness to postpartum psychosis, a condition in which the mood episode is accompanied by confusion, hallucinations or delusions. It is also important to note that postpartum depression is more common in women with a history of depression and that symptoms tend to become more intense with subsequent children.Women experience specific forms of depression-related illness, such as premenstrual dysphoric disorder, postpartum depression and postmenopausal depression and anxiety, that are associated with changes in ovarian hormones and could contribute to the increased prevalence in women (Albert, 2015). Risk factors for getting postpartum depression include; a history of depression prior to becoming pregnant, or during pregnancy, age and time of pregnancy-the risk is higher when the women is young, having a history of depression or premenstrual dysphoric disorder (PMDD), limited social support, and living alone (Johnson, 2019).

Premenstrual Dysphoric Disorder (PMDD)

Premenstrual dysphoric disorder (PMDD) is a cyclic, hormone-based mood disorder, that causes a variety of psychological symptoms around the time of menstruation (Truschel, 2019). It is a more severe and disabling form of premenstrual syndrome (PMS). This condition is characterised by irritability, fatigue, anxiety, mood swings, increased appetite, food craving or binging, aches, inability to concentrate, and breast tenderness.

Seasonal Affective Disorder (SAD)

Parekh (2017) described seasonal affective disorder (SAD) as a form of depression whereby an individual experiences mood changes and symptoms similar to depression. The symptoms usually occur during fall and winter months when there is less sunlight and usually improve with the arrival of spring. The symptoms can be distressing and overwhelming and can interfere with daily functioning. SAD is believed to be triggered by a disturbance in the normal circadian rhythm of the body. Light entering through the eyes influences this rhythm, and any seasonal variation in the night/day pattern can cause a disruption leading to depression.

Atypical Depression

Atypical depression refers to a depressive state where individuals experience improved mood when encountering pleasurable events (Lieber, 2017). With atypical depression, mood improvements from positive situations do not typically manifest in affected individuals. An increased risk of suicide and anxiety disorders is present with atypical depression. Atypical depression is characterised by a specific set of symptoms related to;

- Extreme eating or weight gain
- Excessive sleep
- Fatigue, weakness, and feeling "weighed down"
- Intense sensitivity to rejection
- Strongly reactive moods.

Symptoms of Depression

Doctors use the criteria outlined in the DSM-5to make a diagnosis. You should have at least five of the following symptoms, including no. 1 and no. 2 for at least two weeks in order to be diagnosed with depression:

- Depressed mood (can mean feeling down, sad, apathetic, irritable, pessimistic, hopeless, negative guilty, anxious, and empty etc.)
- Loss of interest or pleasure in almost all activities (sex, sports, hobbies, going out with friends, etc.)
- Changes in appetite or weight
- Disturbed sleep (sleeping too much or too little)
- Headaches, stomach aches or otherwise inexplicable aches and pains
- Neglecting responsibilities and personal appearance

- Slowed or restless movement
- Fatigue and loss of energy
- Feeling hopeless and helpless
- Feelings of worthlessness or excessive guilt
- Difficulty thinking, concentrating and making decisions
- Recurrent thoughts of death or suicide

Of course, having these symptoms does not necessarily mean that the person suffers from depression.

Everyone experiences some of these symptoms at some time. It is when they persist for weeks, months, or even years that they are not normal, for example thyroid dysfunction. The thyroid is a gland that produces hormones and when it is not working properly, it may be associated with symptoms of depression. Scientists are not sure exactly what causes depression. There are many theories, but they are not all agreed upon. There may also be other factors that people are not aware of yet (German Technical Cooperation, 2009).

So far, research has identified the following factors:

- **Genetics "It Runs in the Family":** In other words, having close relatives who have had depression makes you more likely to become depressed. People with a genetic predisposition may be more vulnerable to depression when something stressful or upsetting happens.
- **Physiology or Biochemistry**: An imbalance of brain chemicals, called neurotransmitters (messenger chemicals that carry signals from one nerve cell to the next) can result in depression. The neurotransmitters thought to be involved are serotonin (which helps regulate emotion, sleep and appetite), noradrenalin (which is linked to arousal and alertness) and dopamine (which is associated with pleasure and reward). People with depression are known to have lower brain levels of these chemicals. With the anti-depressant medications that elevate these brain chemicals can help to lift mood.
- **Environmental or External Events:** Events such as relationship problems or break-ups, conflict with parents or family members, death of a significant person in your life, and the anniversary of a loss can contribute to depression. So can financial worries, legal problems, retirement and other stresses.
- **Medical Conditions:** Certain medical conditions can also cause depression, such as an under-active thyroid, which can either contribute to depression on its own or through the stress that comes with being ill. People who have had a heart attack, stroke, cancer or diabetes, for example, have higher than average rates of depression. Some prescription medications can also increase your risk of depression.

Factors Contributing to Depression

Mental illness is socially defined – major disorders like depression and schizophrenia appear to be universal, while other disorders appear to be tied to specific cultures. In South Africa, especially among the African communities, important factors which contribute to vulnerability to mental illness include socioeconomic status, unemployment, lack of confiding relationships, and societal violence. While conditions such as depressive illness and states of anxiety were formerly thought to be rare among Africans, there are certain factors that can predispose someone to developing depression, such as high amount of environmental stress and a lower socioeconomic level. Although there are a number of other factors that are implicated, these two alone, according to the South African Depression and Anxiety Group (SADAG, 2006), could account for much of the elevated prevalence of depression in the black community. There are also certain cultural barriers that tend to predispose the black population, in particular, to depression. These include a mistrust of medical health professionals and community reliance on the support of family during periods of emotional distress (SADAG, 2006). Depression is often a result of interdependent physiologically and genetically based causes that can be triggered by certain life events such as familial discord or parental divorce and personal stresses such as academic problems, grief or the end of a significant relationship (Austin et al., 2017). Depression does not discriminate; it affects everybody, from all cultural backgrounds, rich or poor, illiterate or educated, as well as children and adults. However, in this chapter, the focus of the discussion is specifically on adult depression.

Depression can be attributed to the following causes, namely, biological influences, psychosocial influences and socio-cultural influences. These three factors interact with each other and there is no distinct separation between them. This interaction is shown in Figure 1.

With any psychological problem, it is necessary to understand the client's past major occurrences of depression, social situation, biological or family history and their economic and social status. In their study, Nemade, Staats Reiss, and Dombeck (2015) proposed that there are many factors that contribute to depression, and the relationship between one factor and another is often complex. Several models have also been developed by mental health professionals to describe the way that various factors that contribute to health and illness interrelate.

Figure 1. Schematic representation of the interactions between factors

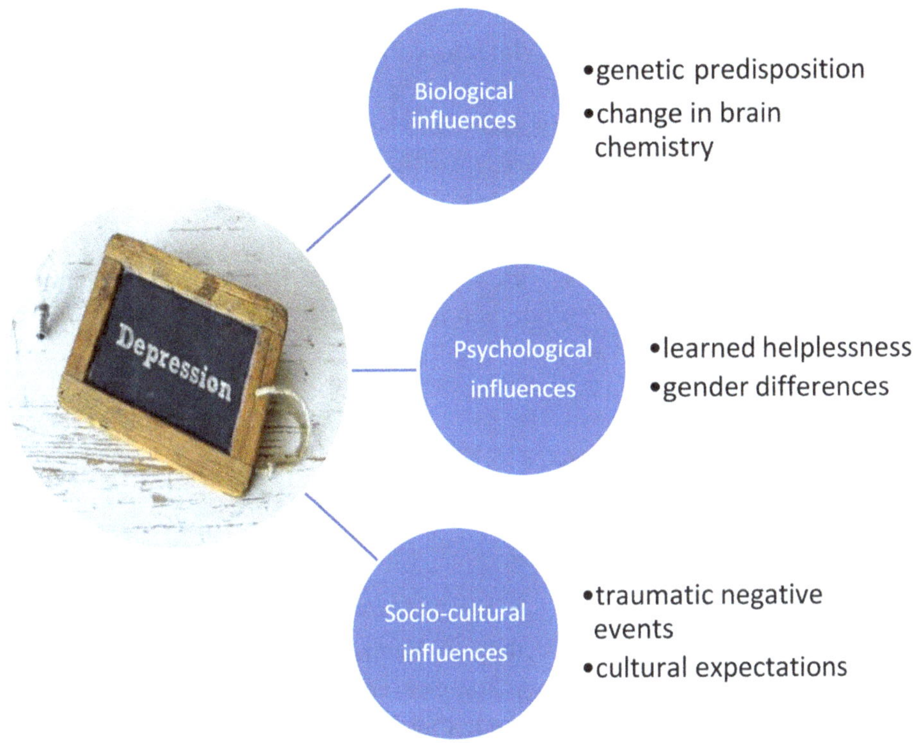

Case Example

Mr. Vitu is 38 years old from a rural village, where he has been living with a partner for the past five years. Mr. Vitu does not know his father. His grandmother from the maternal side raised him. He does not have any contact with other family members from the paternal side. Few days after birth, his mother dumped him at the dumping site where he was picked up by a cattle herder. The cattle herder took the "unidentified baby" to a local hospital while police investigations continues. After some days, his mother was found but she refused to accept him. She was locked up in prison and charged. Mr. Vitu has two half-sisters and one half-brother.

During adolescence, he was described as shy, withdrawn and timid. He attended a local school up to grade seven but left school because there was no money to pay for his school fees. He does casual work to earn an income for himself and his partner. About two years ago, his partner became pregnant, but she was very unfaithful to him. One day when he came back from work, he found his partner with another man and confronted the man right away. The argument ended up in a heavy fight and left Mr. Vitu with a broken arm. During the argument, the other man used vulgar language towards Mr. Vitu and was shouting, stating that Mr. Vitu is "useless, ugly and dumping-site garbage". Mr. Vitu was very devastated. He felt there was no alternative but to take his own life, so he took a rope, but was found before the act. The neighbors took him to the hospital where he was diagnosed with depression.

Since then, he has been hospitalized three times with major depression combined with suicidal ideation. He prefers being alone and does not take care of himself. His sex drive has severely diminished. Mr. Vitu very often complains of fatigue and low appetite. He cries very often for no apparent reasons and blame himself for being unemployed with no future in life. He regards himself as a burden to his grandmother, as well as his partner.

HOW DOES THE INTERACTION BETWEEN THESE FACTORS TAKE PLACE?

Biopsychosocial Model

The biopsychosocial model, according to Nemade, Staats Reiss, and Dombeck (2015) suggested that biological, psychological and social factors are all interlinked and are important with regard to promoting health or causing disease. In other words, the mind and the body are not independent and separate things but rather are connected and interdependent. What affects the body will often affect the mind and what affects the mind will also often end up affecting the body. Wellness or illness is not simply a matter of someone's physical state, but is also influenced by that person's psychological and social status.

With regard to biological factors, depressed individuals are often significantly disturbed with regard to functioning of the endocrine (hormone), immune and neurotransmitter system. In addition, depression can make a person more vulnerable to developing a range of physical disorders. Additionally, a person who has a physical disorder such as diabetes or hypertension is often more likely to develop depression. Genetic inheritance also has an influence on the development of depression.

Psychological factors influencing depression include characteristic negative patterns of thinking, deficits in coping skills, judgement problems, and impaired ability to perceive, understand and express the emotions that depressed people tend to exhibit. In turn, psychological factors mayalso be influenced by biological factors, for example an individual's personality traits can influence a person to be more or less likely to act in ways characteristic of depression.

People can also become depressed because of social factors such as experiencing traumatic situations, early separation, lack of social support, or harassment like in the case of Mr Vetu. Research has shown that stressful social events are capable of serving as triggers for turning genes on and off, causing changes in brain functioning. A social stressor can trigger a physical cause of depression. Environmental and social causes of depression can also be far more subtle than actual trauma (Nemade, Staats Reiss, & Dombeck, 2015).

Learned Helplessness in Depression

When humans or other animals come to understand (or believe) that they have no control over what happens to them, they begin to think, feel and act as if they are helpless. This is referred to as learned helplessness. It is not an inborn trait, no one is born believing that they have absolutely no control over what happens to them and that it is fruitless to even try to gain control. This behaviour is common among depressed individuals because they believe they are worthless, they have lost hope in life and they look down upon themselves. This is a learned behaviour, which was identified by Martin Seligman and Steven Maier's experiments in the 1960s and 70s (Cherry, 2019). They had initially observed helpless behaviours in dogs that were classically conditioned to expect an electrical shock after hearing a tone. Research on what is known as learned helplessness has shown that when people feel that they have no control over what happens, they tend to simply give up and accept their fate. Learned helplessness has been associated with several psychological disorders such as depression, anxiety, loneliness and shyness. These conditions are said to be exacerbated by learned helplessness. Sherman (2016) further defines learned helplessness as the "giving up reaction" or "quitting response" that follows from the belief that whatever you do does not matter or does not change things. In a depressed person, learned helplessness can result from the perceived absence of control over personal situations.

Gender Differences

Research, according to Schimelpfening (2019) has repeatedly indicated that women are twice as likely as men to be diagnosed with depression. One possible explanation is that hormonal changes that are specific to the female body could influence the onset of depression. Other reasons may include stressful life events in women's lives, victimisation and chronic stress. Women's lack of social power makes them more vulnerable than men to specific major traumas, particularly sexual abuse (Nolen-Hoeksema, 2001). According to Nolen-Hoeksema (2001), trauma may contribute directly to depression by making women feel they are helpless to control their lives, and may contribute indirectly by increasing women's reactivity to stress. Women's social roles also carry a number of chronic strains that might contribute directly or indirectly to depression.

Women are also victims of sexual assault at least twice often as men. Sexual assault during childhood has been more consistently linked with the gender difference in depression than sexual assault that first occurs during adulthood. Women are also facing a number of chronic burdens in everyday life because of their social status and roles relative to men, and these strains could contribute to their higher rates of depression. Women are more likely than men to be sexually harassed on the job. Women often have full-time jobs and undertake nearly all the childcare and domestic work in the home. When there is a sick person in the family, women take on the role of the caregiver on top of all the other female roles and responsibilities. This role overload contributes to a sense of burnout and general distress, including depressive symptoms, in women.

Many people with a depressive illness never seek treatment. However, the vast majority, even those with the most severe depression, could get better with treatment. Intensive research into the illness has resulted in the development of medication, psychotherapies and other methods to treat people with this disabling disorder.

Cultural Influences on Depression

Many of the risk factors for depression are similar across cultures. These include gender, unemployment, traumatic events and loss of significant others. The themes of depression according to Pogosyan (2017) tend to revolve around loss. However, what people make of their losses and how they interpret their distress differ tremendously across cultures. How Africans perceive depressive disorders differs from other races. Siebers (2016) states in this regard that culture can shape the development of complex and diverse personal feelings in a population and can influence the way people understand and express distress. While serious distress is understood as a diagnosable medical problem in some cultural context, it is recognised as a normal part of being human in others (Chentsova-Dutton, Ryder, & Tsai, 2014). Distress can be expressed in emotional and/or in physical terms. DSM-5highlights change in mood and decreased interest in activities as the core symptoms of a major depressive episode, playing down the physical symptoms that accompany the disorder. Other cultures may mediate their distress to a much greater extent through their bodies, expressing it in terms of physical symptoms such as pain, tiredness or fatigue.

Culture also influences health-seeking behaviour. Few societies encourage the open expression of mental health problems and anti-stigma campaigns have only limited success. Where mental health disorders are associated with high stigma and loss of reputation, people are even less likely to have these recorded in their medical history or acknowledge them on their application forms for employment.

Depression and anxiety are normal emotional responses to some life events, but any response is refracted through the culture of the person experiencing those events, and bereavement is a classic example of these events. It is often said that anything beyond six months represents an abnormal grief response but there are cultures where this would be thought of as a disrespectfully short period. Depression, as an expression of psychological distress, is the result of a complex interaction between genetic, biological and socio-cultural factors (Siebers, 2016). The psycho-social difficulties constitute the impairment on psychological and social daily functioning of individuals, linked with their particular health condition. Kamenov, Mellor-Marsa, Leal, Ayuso-Mateos, and Cabello (2014) elaborated further that, the broad range of psychosocial difficulties encompasses not only the personal, but also the economic and social impacts of the disorder. Therefore, according to Kamenov et al. (2014), it is of extreme importance that psychosocial difficulties and their related variables are analysed accordingly. More qualitative methodologies need to be undertaken to provide deeper, richer and elaborated data on patients' needs and stand points about psychosocial difficulties and its impact on the day-to-day functions of an individual client.

Who is at Risk for Depression?

Depression affects people of all ages, races and ethnic groups. Martin (2018) stated that a person's risk for depression might be related to a combination of genetic, physical, psychological, and environmental factors. It is the interaction between these factors that may determine the level and the type of depression that may affect the person. For unknown reasons, women are almost twice as likely as men to suffer from depression, although this may be misleading, since women may just seek help more readily than men, which would distort the statistics. Negative or stressful life events in women's lives according to Small, Lumley, and Yelland (2003), have been associated with maternal depression.

Management of Depression in Adults

Living with depression is like carrying a backpack full of boulders around all day. It weighs a person down, saps an individual's energy, hopes and drives and leaves a person with little motivation to get out of bed in the morning. This makes it difficult to take the steps that will help someone feeling better. Nevertheless, while overcoming depression is not easy or quick, it is far from impossible. The discussion below provides some guide on how to cope with depression and will help an individual with depression to live a better life without depression being the defining characteristic of it.

Tips for Overcoming Depression One-Step at a Time

Dealing with depression requires action; however, taking action when a person is depressed can be difficult. Sometimes, just thinking about the things an individual should do to feel better, like exercising or spending time with friends, can seem exhausting or impossible to put into action.

Taking the first step is always the hardest. However, going for a walk or getting up and dancing to favourite music, for example, is something a person can try to do. Such actions can substantially boost the mood and energy for several hours – long enough to put a second recovery step into action, such as preparing a mood-boosting meal or arranging to meet an old friend. By taking the following small but positive steps day by day, a person struggling with depression may lift the heavy fog of the illness from the shoulder and find him/herself feeling better and more hopeful again.

Coping with Depression

Robinson, Smith, Shubin and Segal (2019) provide the following tips on how to cope with depressive episodes on a daily basis.

Tip 1: Reach Out and Stay Connected

Getting support plays an essential role in overcoming depression. On your own, it can be difficult to maintain a healthy perspective and sustain the effort required to beat depression. At the same time, the very nature of depression makes it difficult to reach out for help. When you are depressed, the tendency is to withdraw and isolate yourself so that connecting to even close family members and friends can be tough.

You may feel too exhausted to talk, ashamed of your situation, or guilty for neglecting certain relationships. Nevertheless, this is just the depression talking. Staying connected to other people and taking part in social activities will make a world of difference to your mood and outlook. Reaching out is not a sign of weakness and it will not mean you are a burden to others. Your loved one care about you and want to help. In addition, if you do not feel that you have anyone to turn to, it is never too late to build new friendships and improve your support network.

How to Reach out for Depression Support

Look for support from trusted people, someone who listens attentively and compassionately without being distracted or being judgmental. Try to keep up with social activities even if you do not feel like it. Often when you are depressed, it feels more comfortable to retreat into your shell, but being around other people might help you feeling less depressed. It is good to receive support but giving support to others may boost your morale; hence, do something good for somebody. Join a support group for depression. Being with others dealing with depression can go a long way in reducing your sense of isolation. You can also encourage each other, give and receive advice on how to cope, and share the experiences.

Tip 2: Do Things that Make you Feel Good

In order to overcome depression, additional positive coping skills to manage depression involve activities that are relaxing and energizing. This includes following a healthy lifestyle, learning how to manage stress better, setting limits on what you are able to do, and scheduling fun activities into your day. Express yourself creatively through music, art or writing.

Support your health. Have enough sleep, at least eight hours per night. Get on a better sleep schedule by learning healthy sleep habits. Practice relaxation techniques on a daily basis because they can help relieve symptoms of depression, reduce stress and boost feelings of joy and well-being.

Tip 3: Get Moving

Regular exercise can be as effective as medication for relieving the symptoms of depression. It also helps prevent a relapse once you are well. To get the most benefit, aim for at least 30 minutes of exercise per day. This does not have to be all at once – and it is okay to start small. A 10-minute walk can improve your mood for two hours. Exercise is something you can do right now to boost your mood, your fatigue will improve if you stick with it. Starting to exercise can be difficult when you are depressed and feeling exhausted. However, research shows that your energy levels will improve if you keep with it. Exercise will help you to feel energised and less fatigued, not more. Find exercises that are continuous and rhythmic. The most benefits for depression come from rhythmic exercise such as walking, weight training, swimming, martial arts and dancing – where you move both your arms and legs.

Tip 4: Eat a Healthy, Depression-Fighting Diet

What you eat has a direct impact on the way you feel. Reduce your intake of foods that can adversely affect your brain and mood such as caffeine, alcohol, trans fats, and foods with high levels of chemical preservatives or hormones (such as certain meats). Do not skip meals. Going too long between meals can make you feel irritable and tired, so aim to eat something at least every three to four hours. Minimise sugar and refined carbs. You may crave sugary snacks, baked goods, or comfort foods such as pasta or French fries, but these "feel-good" foods quickly lead to a crash in mood and energy. Aim to cut out as much of these foods as possible. Boost your B vitamins. Deficiencies in B vitamins such as folic acid and B-12 can trigger depression. To get more, take a B-complex vitamin supplement or eat more citrus fruit, leafy greens, beans, chicken and eggs. Boost your mood with foods rich in omega-3 fatty acids. Omega-3 fatty acids play an essential role in stabilising mood. The best sources are fatty fish such as salmon, herring, mackerel, anchovies, sardines, tuna, and some cold-water fish oil supplements.

Tip 5: Challenge Negative Thinking

Do you feel like you are powerless or weak? That bad things happen and there is not much you can do about it? That your situation is hopeless? Depression puts a negative spin on everything, including the way you see yourself and your expectations for the future.

When these types of thoughts overwhelm you, it is important to remember that this is a symptom of your depression and these irrational, pessimistic attitudes – known as cognitive distortions – are not realistic. When you really examine them, they do not hold. Even so, they can be tough to give up. You cannot break out of this pessimistic frame of mind by telling yourself to "just think positive." Often, it is part of a lifelong pattern of thinking that has become so automatic you are not even completely aware of it. Rather, the trick is to identify the type of negative thoughts that are fuelling your depression and replace them with a more balanced way of thinking.

Negative, unrealistic ways of thinking that fuel depression include the following:

- **All-or-Nothing Thinking:** Looking at things in black or white categories, with no middle ground ("If I fall short of perfection, I am m a total failure.")
- **Overgeneralisation:** Generalising from a single negative experience, expecting it to hold true forever ("I can't do anything right.")
- **The Mental Filter:** Ignoring positive events and focusing on the negatives. Noticing the one thing that went wrong, rather than all the things that went right. ("Performance evaluation provides 9 scores of above average, but you only focus on the 1 score that is below average.")
- **Diminishing the Positive:** Coming up with reasons why positive events do not count ("She said she had a good time on our date, but I think she was just being nice.")
- **Jumping to Conclusions:** Making negative interpretations without actual evidence.

("My best friend was dismissive when I called—she must not like me any more… when actually she was overwhelmed by a work project deadline")

- Acting like a mind reader ("He must think I am pathetic") or a fortune-teller ("I will be stuck in this dead-end job forever.")
- **Emotional Reasoning:** Believing that the way you feel reflects reality ("I feel like such a loser. I really am no good.")
- **Labelling:** Classifying yourself based on mistakes and perceived shortcomings ("I am a failure; an idiot; a loser.")

Once the destructive thought patterns that contribute to depression have been identified, a person may start to challenge them with questions such as:

- What is the evidence that the thought is true or not true?
- What would I tell a friend who had negative thought?
- Is there another way of looking at the situation or an alternative explanation?
- How might I look at the situation if I did not have depression?

When cross-examining the negative thoughts, one may be surprised at how quickly they crumble. In the process, the person will develop a more balanced perspective, and that may help to relieve the depression. Often times, people struggling with re-occurring negative thoughts find writing the thinking errors down and working through why the thoughts are incorrect insightful and helpful with future bouts negative thinking.

When to get Professional Help for Depression

If a person has taken the self-help steps and made positive lifestyle changes and still find depression getting worse, it is recommended to look for professional help. Treatment usually involves medication or psychotherapy. Research indicates a combination of the two is most effective.

Antidepressants work to normalize the naturally occurring brain chemicals or neurotransmitters, notably serotonin and norepinephrine. Han (2018) described neurotransmitters as natural chemicals that help facilitate communication between nerve cells. An imbalance in norepinephrine and/or serotonin may lead to the development of depression. However, it should be stated that mental disorders such as depression are not simply caused by chemical imbalances in the brain. There is a lot more to them. Genetics, environmental, and social factors may play a role. Antidepressant medications work by increasing the amount of serotonin and other neurotransmitters in the brain (Han, 2018).

Scientists studying depression have found that these neurotransmitters are involved in regulating mood, but they are unsure of the exact ways in which they work. The three neurotransmitters implicated in depression are; norepinephrine, serotonin, and dopamine (Schimelpfening, 2019). When there is too little concentration of norepinephrine in certain brain circuits, depression may occur in some people. Serotonin act by regulating the mood, and low level of serotonin may also lead to a down fall in norepinephrine levels whereas dopamine is believed to create positive feelings associated with rewards and reduced levels of dopamine may contribute to depression in some people.

Several types of psychotherapy, or talk therapy, can also help people with depression. Some regimens are short (10–20weeks) and other regimens are longer term, depending on the needs of the individuals involved (German Technical Cooperation, 2009).For mild to moderate depression, psychotherapy may be the best treatment option. However, for major depression or for certain people, psychotherapy may not be enough. Studies (Cuijpers, Sijbrandij, Koole, Andersson, Beekman, and Reynolds, 2014) have indicated that a combination of antidepressant medication and psychotherapy maybe an effective approach to treating major depression thereby reducing the likelihood of a recurrence, other than treating with antidepressant medication alone.

In cases, where medication and psychotherapy do not help to alleviate a person's resistance to depression, electro convulsion therapy (ECT) maybe useful. This has shown to be effective with highly resistive depression that does not improve with other treatments. If depression is left untreated, it can have devastating effects on the individual and his/her family. Finally, depression may lead to suicide.

Role of Counselling in Overcoming Depression

During a depressive episode, a person's behaviour towards work, life and others may change dramatically. A person's self-esteem may be at its lowest ebb, creating feelings of worthlessness. At these moments, counselling may bring the sufferer up to a level where he/she is able to think practically, yet positively. The counselling technique associated with interpersonal therapy should focus on how social interactions will affect depression in a person and what can be done to help with that. Interpersonal therapy looks to understand how people react to social situations and the development of depressive symptoms that are associated with interpersonal behaviours.

Below are some of the benefits of counselling for depression.

- Counselling offers practical help for those who are suffering from depression.
- Counselling provides an opportunity for those affected to talk about their feelings openly and in a safe environment to help them find their way out.

- Counselling techniques can teach a person how to relax and respond effectively if feelings of depression surface.
- Counselling techniques can help teach a person the skills needed to overcome depressive thinking, as well as looking into its causes and reasons for the onset.

An understanding of the cultural background of a patient struggling with depression and how illness behaviour is understood and interpreted by the counsellor may enable the latter to assist depressed individuals when they are in dire need of their services.

Helping Someone who is Struggling with Depression

When a friend or a family member suffers from depression, your support and encouragement can play an important role in their recovery. You can help them to cope with depression symptoms, overcome negative thoughts, and regain their energy, optimism, and enjoyment of life. However, your loved one's depression can also wear you down if you neglect your own needs. If someone you love is struggling with depression, you may be experiencing any number of difficult emotions, including helplessness, frustrations, anger, fear, guilt, and sadness. These feelings are all normal. It is not easy dealing with a friend or family member who is struggling with depression. Remember that neglecting your own health can become overwhelming. Your companionship and support can be crucial to your loved one's recovery.

Helping someone who is struggling with depression is a process, which follows a pattern of actions and behaviors to be taken by the helper. For many family members and friends, communication with someone who is struggling with depression remains a problem. Sometimes it is hard to know what to say when speaking to someone about depression. You might fear that if you bring up your worries, the person will get angry, feel insulted, or ignore your concerns. You may be unsure what questions to ask or how to be supportive. If you do not know where to start, the following suggestions may help. Remember that being a compassionate listener is much more important than giving advice. You do not have to try to "fix" your friend or family member; you just have to be a good listener. Often, the simple act of talking face to face can be an enormous help to someone struggling with depression. Encourage the depressed person to talk about their feelings, and be willing to listen without judgment. Do not expect a single conversation to be the end of it. A person who is struggling with tend to withdraw from others and isolate themselves. You may need to express your concern and willingness to listen over and over again. Be gentle, yet persistent.

Below are some examples of statements to make when you start a conversation with a person struggling with depression.

- "I have been feeling concerned about you lately"
- "Recently, I have noticed some differences in you and wondered how you are doing"
- "I wanted to check in with you because you have seemed pretty down lately"

Following are examples of possible questions to ask:

- "When did you begin feeling like this?"
- "Did something happen that made you start feeling this way?"
- " How can I best support you right now?"
- "Have you thought about getting help?"

Remember, being supportive involves offering encouragement and hope. Very often, this is a matter of talking to the person in a language that they will understand and can respond to while in a depressed state of mind.

What you can say that helps:

- "You are not alone in this, I am here for you"
- "I may not be able to understand exactly how you feel, but I care about you and want to help"
- "When you want to give up, tell yourself you will hold on for just one more day, hour, and minute, whatever you can manage"
- "You are important to me. Your life is important to me"
- "Tell me what I can do now to help you"

What you should AVOID saying:

- "We all go through times like this"
- "Look on the bright side"
- "You have so much to live for, why do you want to die?"
- "What is wrong with you?"
- "I cannot do anything about your situation" (Smith, Robinson & Segal, 2019).

Taking Care of Yourself (Caretaker)

Smith, Robinson and Segal (2019) pointed out that there is a natural impulse to want to solve the problems of the people we care about, but one cannot control someone else's depression. However, one can control how well you take care of yourself. It is just as important for you to stay healthy as it is for the depressed person to get treatment, therefore, make your own well-being a priority. Make sure your own health and happiness are solid before you try to help someone who is depressed. When your own needs are taken care of, you will have the energy you need to lend a helping hand.

Set Boundaries

Your own health will suffer if you let your life be controlled by your loved one's depression. You cannot be a caretaker round the clock without paying a psychological price. To avoid burnout and resentment, set clear limits on what you are willing and able to do.

Seek support. You are not betraying your depressed relative or friend by turning to others for support. Joining a support group, talking to a counselor or clergyman, or confiding in a trusted friend will help you get through this tough time. Focus on your emotions and feelings about having and helping a relative through depression. Make sure you are honest with the person you turn to-choose someone who will listen without interruption and without judging you.

Depression and Suicide: What is the Link Between the Two Phenomena?

Most people who commit suicide are likely to be depressed during the time of this act. However, it should be remembered that not all individuals who commit suicide are struggling with depression. There are also other contributing factors to this phenomenon. Suicide is the second leading cause of death, especially in young people, aged 15-29-years-old (WHO, 2019). A major cause of suicide is mental illness, very commonly depression. People feeling suicidal are overwhelmed by painful emotions and see death as the only way out, losing sight of the fact that suicide is a permanent "solution" to a temporary state – most people who tried to kill themselves but live later say they are glad they did not die. Most people who die by suicide could have been helped. An individual considering suicide frequently confides in a friend, who may be able to convince them to seek treatment. When the risk is high, concerned friends and relatives should seek professional guidance.

According to WHO (2019), every year close to 800 000 worldwide people take their own life and there are many more people who attempt suicide. Every suicide is a tragedy that affects families, communities and entire countries and has long-lasting effects on the people left behind. Suicide is a global phenomenon (WHO, 2019) in all regions of the world, of which 79% of global suicides occurred in low-and middle-income countries in 2016. It is a serious public health problem; however, suicides are preventable with timely, evidence-based and often low-cost interventions. For national responses to be effective, a comprehensive multi-sectoral suicide prevention strategy is needed.

Who is at Risk?

While the link between suicide and mental disorders (in particular, depression and alcohol use disorders) is well established in high-income countries, many suicides happen impulsively in moments of crisis with a breakdown in the ability to deal with life stresses, such as financial problems, relationship break-up or chronic pain and illness (WHO, 2019).

In addition, experiencing conflict, disaster, violence, abuse or loss and a sense of isolation are strongly associated with suicidal behaviour. Suicide rates are also high among vulnerable groups who experience discrimination, such as refugees and migrants; indigenous peoples; lesbian, gay, bisexual, transgender, intersex (LGBTI) persons; and prisoners. By far the strongest risk factor for suicide is a previous suicide attempt (WHO, 2019)

Suicide Warning Signs

Not all people who struggle with suicidal ideation move forward with a plan to attempt self-harm, however, a commonality of suicidal ideation is the presence of depression. Signs may include

- Depressed mood
- Agitated behaviour and sleeplessness
- Change in appetite or weight
- Speaking or moving with unusual speed or slowness
- Fatigue or loss of energy
- Feelings of worthlessness, self-reproach or quilt.
- Feelings of loneliness and isolation
- Thoughts of death and suicide
- Neglect of personal welfare, deteriorating physical experience.

Note that the presence of one of these signs does not necessarily mean the person is suicidal. These signs are common in distressed people, and many people have some of these symptoms at one point in their life.

Impact of Depression in the Workplace

Employees who struggle with depression are vulnerable to adverse work outcomes. The increasing incidence of depression is a growing concern for many companies. Depression, if left untreated, may have a significant impact on work performance. It contributes to presenteeism, or employees at work but not engaged and absenteeism, or employees missing days of work. It may also adversely impact multiple areas of employee performance, including focus and decision making, time management, completing physical tasks, social interactions, and communications (American Psychiatric Association, 2019).

SOLUTIONS AND RECOMMENDATIONS

Individuals struggling with depression need the support from significant others, family, colleagues and community members to enable them to cope with the illness. People need to know the facts about the nature and course of depression to enable them to seek help. People struggling with depression should be encouraged to talk about depression. Written information about depression need to be made available and it should be provided to people struggling with depression. Such information should be relevant and appropriate to their level of understanding to maximise their understanding of the illness. Patients and their supporters need to be encouraged to join and participate in local self-help and support groups (if available) to enhance feelings of belongingness and sharing of experiences. Glen-Spyron and Jacobs (2019) expanded the notion further that there is a need to educate family, friends on mental health issues and by so-doing, the stigma attached to mental health issues may be broken down. To the family or carer of someone struggling with depression, they need to be advised to be vigilant for mood changes, negativity, hopelessness, and suicidal ideations in a person, and to contact healthcare providers for assistance. Individuals struggling with depression need to be encouraged and motivated to embark on a number of lifestyle changes that may be beneficial to his/her mental health. Lifestyle changes could be in the form of adequate sleep, eating habits, refrain from alcohol abuse, engaging in physical activities and exercises.

Depression according to Kamenov, Mellor-Marsa, Leal, Ayuso-Mateos, and Cabello (2014) is regarded as one of the main causes of disability in the life of the sufferer, together with ischemic heart diseases. The latter conclusion is based on the functional limitations caused by depression which are equal to or even sometimes greater than the ones engendered by many other chronic medical conditions. Therefore, because of a broad range of attributing factors to depression, future management strategies need to address all relevant areas that have personal, psychological, cultural, economic, social and spiritual impact on the development of the disorder.

FUTURE RESEARCH DIRECTIONS

Holistic approaches towards the management of depression deserve researchers' attention. Depression is not only a biological disease, nor is it only a set of cognitive distortions, nor is it only a culturally sanctioned way of communicating social sufferings. It is a profoundly distressing set of experiences involving disruptions within the single complex system that encompasses culture, mind and brain (Chentsova-Dutton, Ryder & Tsai, 2014). Hence, future research directions need to evolve around cross-cultural research on depression from a non-Western cultural context, involving more qualitative approaches, in order to obtain rich descriptions of the phenomenon from the participants, and to complement findings from existing quantitative studies on depression. Chentsova-Dutton, et al (2014) further proposed that future work on depression should aim to better understand the ways in which culture interacts with biological and psychological factors in shaping serious distress in an individual. More research examining cultural similarities and differences in experiences of sadness in various cultural contexts is needed (Chentsova-Dutton, Choi, Ryder & Reyes, 2015), because findings from the latter may guide clinicians in the assessment of depression and on the choice of management strategies. According to Chang (2017),we are all profoundly influenced by the broader cultural frame in which we live, and yet, it is easy to overlook these influences in the context of one's own culture, hence there is need to explore ways in which expression of depression is culturally shaped among communities. Future work should also be embarked upon examining help-seeking intentions (Taylor, 2018),more specifically among black African communities to ensure that the needs of this communities can be effectively and comprehensively addressed.

CONCLUSION

In this chapter, an overview of depression in adults was given. A wider explanation of the interconnectedness between biological, psychological and socio-cultural influences of depression was provided. Furthermore, highlights on the types of self-care intervention strategies as well as medical and other treatment options were included. The necessity for seeking out for professional help once self-help actions failed yielding desirable results was pointed out. Future research efforts should be made to further expand the knowledge of the biological bases for depression and will likely contribute to appropriate and helpful intervention strategies that may benefit people struggling with depression.

REFERENCES

Albert, P. R. (2015). Why is depression more prevalent in women? *Journal of Psychiatry & Neuroscience*, *40*(4), 219–221. doi:10.1503/jpn.150205

American Psychiatric Association. (2013). Diagnostic and statistical manual of mental disorders (DSM-5) (5th ed.). Washington, DC: APA.

American Psychiatric Association. (2019). Depression: A costly condition for business. Retrieved from https://www.workplacementalhealth.org

Ashipala, D. O., Wilkinson, W., & van Dyk, A. (2016). Mental health policy implementation as an integral part of primary health care services in Oshana region, *Namibia. Journal of Nursing Education and Practice*, *6*(11), 53–60. doi:10.5430/jnep.v6n11p53

Austin, T., Bezuidenhout, C., Botha, K., Du Plessis, E., Du Plessis, L., Jordaan, E., ... Vorster, A. (2017). *Abnormal psychology: A South African perspective*. Cape Town: Oxford University Press.

Barlow, D. H., & Durand, V. M. (2012). *Abnormal psychology: An integrative approach* (6th ed.). Belmont, CA: Cengage Learning.

Chand, S. P., & Arif, H. (2019). *Depression*. Treasure Island, FL: StatPearls Publishing.

Chang, M. X. L. (2017). Understanding depression across cultures: A social identity perspective [Doctor's thesis]. School of Psychology, University of Queensland. Retrieved from https://www.espace.library.uq.edu.au

Chentsova-Dutton, Y. E., Choi, E., Ryder, A. G., & Reyes, J. (2015). "I felt sad and did not enjoy life": Cultural context and the associations between anhedonia, depressed mood, and momentary emotions. *Transcultural Psychiatry*, *52*(5), 616–635. doi:10.1177/1363461514565850 PMID:25603917

Chentsova-Dutton, Y. E., Ryder, A. G., & Tsai, J. (2014). Understanding depression across cultural context. In I. H. Gotlib & C. L. Hammen (Eds.), *Handbook of depression* (pp. 337-354). New York: Guilford Press.

Cherry, K. (2019). What is learned helplessness and why does it happen? *VeryWellMind.* Retrieved from https://www.verywellmind.com/what-is-learned-helplessness-2795326

Chisholm, D. (2017). Depression: Let's talk. Retrieved from https://www.who.int/

Cowan, P. (2010). Depression will be the second leading cause of disease by 2010: WHO. *Calgary Herald*. Retrieved from http://www.calgaryherald.com/health/

Cuijpers, P., Sijbrandij, M., Koole, S. L., Andersson, G., Beekman, A. T., & Reynolds, C. F. (2014). Adding Psychotherapy to antidepressant medication in depression and anxiety disorders: a meta-analysis. World Psychiatry Association. Retrieved from https://www.ncbi.nlm.gov

DiMaria, L. (2019). *Clinically significant depression overview. VeryWellMind.* Retrieved from https://www.verywellmind.com/clinically-significant-depression-1067143

German Technical Cooperation Agency. (2009). Health and wellness: Peer educator handbook. Windhoek. Namibia.

Glen-Spyron, C., & Jacobs, A. (2019). Striking a healthy balance between studies and mental health. *The Namibian*. Retrieved from https://www.namibian.com.na

Grohol, G. M. (2018). Living with depression: A guide for coping with depressive feelings. Psychcentral. Retrieved from https://psychcentral.com/

Halverson, J. I. (2019). Depression. *Medscape*. Retrieved from https://emedicine.medscape.com/article/286759-overview

Jezard, A. (2018). *World Economic Forum 2018: Depression is the no. 1 cause of ill-health and disability worldwide*. WEForum. Retrieved from https://www.weforum.org/agenda/2018/05/d

Johnson, T. C. (2019). Postpartum Depression. *WebMD*. Retrieved from http://www.webmd.com

Kamenov, K., Mellor-Marsa, B., Leal, I., Ayuso-Mateos, J. L., & Cabello, M. (2014). Analysing psychosocial difficulties in depression: A content comparison between systematic literature review and patient perspective. Biomed Research International. Retrieved from https://www.ncbi.nlm.nih.gov/

Kaplan, H. I., Sadock, B. J., & Grebb, J. A. (1994). *Kaplan and Sadock's synopsis of psychiatry* (8th ed.). Baltimore, ML: Williams & Wilkins.

Kessler, R. C., Berglund, P., Demler, O., Jin, R., Merikangas, K. R., & Walters, E. E. (2005). Lifetime prevalence and age-of-onset distributions of DSM-IV disorders in the National Co- morbidity Survey Replication. *Archives of General Psychiatry*, *62*(6), 593–602. doi:10.1001/archpsyc.62.6.593 PMID:15939837

Lieber, A. (2017). Understanding Atypical Depression: Symptoms & Treatment. Psycom. Retrieved from https://www.psycom.net

Martin, B. (2018). What are the risk factors for depression? Psych Central. Retrieved from https://www.com

Nemade, R., Staats Reiss, N., & Dombeck, M. (2015b). *Sociology of depression: Effects of culture.* Retrieved from https://www.mentalhelp.net/

Nemade, R., Staats Reiss, N. S., & Dombeck, M. (2015a). Current understanding of major depression: Biopsychosocial model. *MentalHelp.net.* Retrieved from https://www.mentalhelp.net

Nolen-Hoeksema, S. (2001). Gender differences in depression. *Current Directions in Psychological Science.*

Parekh, R. (2017). Seasonal Affective Disorder (SAD). American Psychiatric Association. Retrieved from https://www.psychiatry.org

Pogosyan, M. (2017). How culture affects depression. *Psychology today.* Retrieved from https://www.psychologytoday.com/

Psychiatric Mental Health. (n.d.). Retrieved from https://www.ncbi.nlm.nih.gov

Purse, M. (2019). Types of bipolar episodes according to DSM-5. *Verywellmind.* Retrieved from https://www.verywellmind.com

Robinson, L., Smith, M., Shubin, J., & Segal, J. (2019). Depression in Men. *HelpGuide.* Retrieved from https://www.helpguide.org

Rush, A. J., Fava, M., Wisniewski, S. R., Lavori, P. W., Trivedi, M. H., Sackeim, H. A., ... Niederehe, G.STAR*D Investigators Group. (2004). Sequenced treatment alternatives to relieve depression (STAR*D): Rationale and design. *Controlled Clinical Trials, 25*(1), 119–142. doi:10.1016/S0197-2456(03)00112-0 PMID:15061154

Schimelpfening, N. (2019). Common types of depression. *VeryWellMind.* Retrieved from https://www.verywellmind.com/common-types-of-depression-1067313

Schimelpfening, N. (2019). Is depression different in males and females? Understanding the subtle differences. *VeryWellMind.* Retrieved from https://www.verywellmind.com/common-types-of-depression-1067313

Sherman, A. (2016). Learned helplessness and depression: Dysfunction interrupted. *PsychCentral.* Retrieved from https://www.blogs.psychcentral.com

Shifiona, N. N., Poggenpoel, M., & Myburgh, C. P. H. (2006). Life stories of depressed adult women in peri-urban Namibia. *Curationis*, *29*(2), 5–11. doi:10.4102/curationis.v29i2.1063 PMID:16910128

Siebers, A. (2016). Does culture influence our response to depression? *Perspective*. Retrieved from https://www.genre.com/knowledge/blog/

Small, R., Lumley, J., & Yelland, J. (2003). Cross-cultural experiences of maternal depression: Associations and contributing factors for Vietnamese, Turkish and Fillipino Immigrant women in Victoria, Australia. *Ethnicity & Health*, *8*(3), 189–206. doi:10.1080/1355785032000136416 PMID:14577995

Smith, M., Robinson, L., & Segal, J. (2019). *Coping with Depression: Tips for overcoming depression one step at a time. HelpGuide.org* Retrieved from https://www.helpguide.org/

South African Depression and Anxiety Group (SADAG). (2006). *Depression in black South Africans.* Retrieved from https://www.sadag.com

Taylor, R. (2018). Explaining intentions to seek mental health services among black Canadians. Retrieved from https://www.scholar.uwindsor.ca/

Thapa, S. B., Martinez, P., & Clausen, T. (2014). Depression and its correlates in South Africa and Ghana among people aged 50 and above: Findings from the WHO study on Global AGEing and adult health. *Journal of Psychiatry*, *17*(6). PMID:25914902

Townsend, M. C. (1996). *Psychiatric-mental health nursing: Concepts of care.* Philadelphia, PA: F. A. Davis.

Truschel, J. (2019). PMDD: Premenstrual Dysphoric Disorder Symptoms, Causes, Treatment. Psycom.net. Retrieved from https://www.psycom.net

World Health Organization (WHO). (2017a). *Depression and other common mental disorders: Global health estimates.* Geneva: World Health Organization. Retrieved from https://apps.who.int/iris/bitstream/handle/10665/254610/WHO-MSD-MER-2017.2-eng.pdf?sequence=1

World Health Organization (WHO). (2017b). *Depression: Let's talk [News release].* Retrieved from https://www.who.int/

World Health Organization (WHO). (2017c). *Depression: Largest cause of disability worldwide.* Retrieved from https://www.voanews.com/a/who-depression-statistics/3737024.html

World Health Organization (WHO). (2018). *Suicide*. Retrieved from https://www.who.int/news-room/fact-sheets/detail/suicid

World Health Organization (WHO). (2019). *Suicide Data*. Retrieved from https://www.who.int/

Wu, B. (2018). Situational depression or clinical depression. *Medical News Today*. Retrieved from https://www.medicalnewstoday.com

ADDITIONAL READING

Antai-Otong, D. (2008). *Psychatric Nursing: Biological and Behavioural Concepts* (2nd ed.). New York: Thomas Delmar Learning.

Baumann, S. E. (1998). *Psycahiatry and Primary Health Care: A practical guide for Health Care Workers in Southern Africa.* Cape Town: Juta & Co. Ltd.

Caspi, A., Sugden, K., Moffitt, T. E., Taylor, A., Craig, I. W., Harrington, H., ... Poulton, R. (2006). Influence of life stress on depression: Moderation by a polymorphism in the 5-HTT gene. *Science*, *301*(5631), 386–389. doi:10.1126cience.1083968 PMID:12869766

Frisch, N. C., & Frisch, L. E. (2006). *Psychatric Mental Health Nursing* (3rd ed.). New York: Thomas Delmar Learning.

Holtzheimer, P. E., & Nemeroff, C. B. (2006). Future prospects in depression research. *Dialogues in Clinical Neuroscience*, *8*(2), 175–189. PMID:16889104

Karp, J. F., Dew, M. A., Wahed, A. S., Fitzgerald, K., Bolon, C. A., Weiner, D. K., … Reynolds, C. F. (2016). Challenges and Solutions for Depression Prevention Research: Methodology for a Depression Prevention Trial for Older Adults with Knee Arthritis and Emotional Distress. *The American journal of geriatric psychiatry: official journal of the American Association for Geriatric Psychiatry*, *24*(6), 433–443. doi:10.1016/j.jagp.2015.10.012

Middleton, L., & Uys, L. (2014). *Mental Health Nursing: A South African Perspective* (6th ed.). Cape Town: Juta& Co. Ltd.

Ministry of Health and Social Services. (2005). *National Policy for Mental Health.* Windhoek, Namibia.

Sackeim, H. A. (2001). The definition and meaning of treatment-resistant depression. *The Journal of Clinical Psychiatry*, *62*(16), 10–17. PMID:11480879

KEY TERMS AND DEFINITIONS

Biopsychosocial Model: An interdisciplinary model that looks at the interconnection between biology, psychology, and socio-environmental factors. The model specifically examines how these aspects play a role in topics ranging from health and disease models to human development.

Corticotrophin-Releasing Factor: A peptide hormone involved in the stress response.

Counselling: A therapy that involves a trained therapist listening to you and helping you find ways to deal with emotional issues. Sometimes the term "counseling "is used to refer to talking therapies in general, but counseling.

Electro Convulsion Therapy: A medical treatment most commonly used in patients with severe major depression or bipolar disorder that has not responded to other treatments. ECT involves a brief electrical stimulation of the brain while the patient is under anesthesia.

Persistent Depressive Disorder: Also called dysthymia is a form of chronic depression, with symptoms that are less severe but longer lasting than other forms of depression.

Psychotherapy: The treatment of mental disorder by psychological rather than medical means.

Suicide: Ending one's own life. It is sometimes a way for people to escape pain or suffering.

Compilation of References

Abu Seman, S. A., & Ramayah, T. (2017). Are We Ready to App?: A Study on mHealth Apps, Its Future, and Trends in Malaysia Context. In J. Pelet (Ed.), *Mobile Platforms, Design, and Apps for Social Commerce* (pp. 69–83). Hershey, PA: IGI Global. doi:10.4018/978-1-5225-2469-4.ch005

Abuyassin, B., & Laher, I. (2015). Obesity-linked diabetes in the Arab world: A review. *Eastern Mediterranean Health Journal, 21*(6), 420–439. doi:10.26719/2015.21.6.420

Achwoka, D., Waruru, A., Chen, T.-H., Masamaro, K., Ngugi, E., Kimani, M., ... De Cock, K. M. (2019). Noncommunicable disease burden among HIV patients in care: A national retrospective longitudinal analysis of HIV-treatment outcomes in Kenya, 2003-2013. *BMC Public Health, 19*(1), 372. doi:10.118612889-019-6716-2 PMID:30943975

Adato, M., & Bassett, L. (2009). Social protection to support vulnerable children and families: The potential of cash transfers to protect, health and nutrition. *AIDS Care, 21*(1), 60–75. doi:10.1080/09540120903112351 PMID:22380980

Adedotun, A. A., Morenikeji, O. A., & Odaibo, A. B. (2010). Knowledge, attitudes and practices about malaria in an urban community in south-western Nigeria. *Journal of Vector Borne Diseases, 47*(3), 155–159. PubMed

Adeniyi, A., Idowu, O., Ogwumike, O., & Adeniyi, C. (2012). Comparative influence of self-efficacy, social support and perceived barriers on low physical activity development in patients with type 2 diabetes, hypertension or stroke. *Ethiopian Journal of Health Sciences, 22*(2), 113–119.

Aggarwal, S., & Azad, V. (2017). A Hybrid System Based on FMM and MLP to Diagnose Heart Disease. In S. Bhattacharyya, S. De, I. Pan, & P. Dutta (Eds.), *Intelligent Multidimensional Data Clustering and Analysis* (pp. 293–325). Hershey, PA: IGI Global. doi:10.4018/978-1-5225-1776-4.ch011

Akaichi, J., & Mhadhbi, L. (2016). A Clinical Decision Support System: Ontology-Driven Approach for Effective Emergency Management. In J. Moon & M. Galea (Eds.), *Improving Health Management through Clinical Decision Support Systems* (pp. 270–294). Hershey, PA: IGI Global. doi:10.4018/978-1-4666-9432-3.ch013

Akerkar, R. (2016). Towards an Intelligent Integrated Approach for Clinical Decision Support. In A. Aggarwal (Ed.), *Managing Big Data Integration in the Public Sector* (pp. 187–205). Hershey, PA: IGI Global. doi:10.4018/978-1-4666-9649-5.ch011

Al Kareh, T., & Thoumy, M. (2018). The Impact of Health Information Digitization on the Physiotherapist-Patient Relationship: A Pilot Study of the Lebanese Community. *International Journal of Healthcare Information Systems and Informatics, 13*(2), 29–53. doi:10.4018/IJHISI.2018040103

Albert, P. R. (2015). Why is depression more prevalent in women? *Journal of Psychiatry & Neuroscience, 40*(4), 219–221. doi:10.1503/jpn.150205

Al-Busaidi, S. S. (2018). Interdisciplinary Relationships Between Medicine and Social Sciences. In M. Al-Suqri, A. Al-Kindi, S. AlKindi, & N. Saleem (Eds.), *Promoting Interdisciplinarity in Knowledge Generation and Problem Solving* (pp. 124–137). Hershey, PA: IGI Global. doi:10.4018/978-1-5225-3878-3.ch009

Aldemi, S., Dalbudak, E., & Topcu, M. (2015). Relationship of posttraumatic stress symptoms with depression, anxiety, childhood trauma and personality characteristics. *Klinik Psikofarmakoloji Bülteni, 25*, S98.

Alenzuela, R. (2017). Research, Leadership, and Resource-Sharing Initiatives: The Role of Local Library Consortia in Access to Medical Information. In S. Ram (Ed.), *Library and Information Services for Bioinformatics Education and Research* (pp. 199–211). Hershey, PA: IGI Global. doi:10.4018/978-1-5225-1871-6.ch012

Ali, S., Stone, M. A., Peters, J. L., Davies, M. J., & Khunti, K. (2006). The prevalence of co-morbid depression in adults with type 2 diabetes: A systematic review and meta-analysis. *Diabetic Medicine, 23*(11), 1165–1173. doi:10.1111/j.1464-5491.2006.01943.x

Allen, N. A. (2004). Social cognitive theory in diabetes exercise research: An integrative literature review. *The Diabetes Educator, 30*(5), 805–819. doi:10.1177/014572170403000516

Almeida, O. P., McCaul, K., Hankey, G. J., Yeap, B. B., Golledge, J., Norman, P. E., & Flicker, L. (2016). Duration of diabetes and its association with depression in later life: The Health In Men Study (HIMS). *Maturitas, 86*, 3–9. doi:10.1016/j.maturitas.2016.01.003

Amakali, K., Haoses-Gorases, L., & Taukuheke, L. (2013). Tobacco smoking among University of Namibia students: Behaviours, reasons, attitudes, awareness and knowledge of associated health risks. *Online Journal of Medicine and Medical Science Research, 2*(3), 30–37.

Amer, F. A., Mohamed, M. S., Elbur, A. I., Abdelaziz, S. I., & Elrayah, Z. A. (2018). Influence of self-efficacy management on adherence to self-care activities and treatment outcome among diabetes mellitus type 2. *Pharmacy Practice, 16*(4), 1274. doi:10.18549/PharmPract.2018.04.1274

American Diabetes Association. (2018). Classification and diagnosis of diabetes: Standards of medical care in diabetes. *Diabetes Care, 41*(Supplement 1), S13–S27. doi:10.2337/dc18-S002

American Lung Association. (2019). Be prepared for challenges when quiting smoking. Retrieved from https://www.lung.org/stop-smoking/i-want-to-quit/be-prepared-for-challenges.html

American Psychiatric Association. (1994). Task Force on DSM-IV. Diagnostic and Statistical Manual of Mental Disorders: DSM-IV. American Psychiatric Association.

American Psychiatric Association. (2013). Diagnostic and statistical manual of mental disorders (DSM-5) (5th ed.). Washington, DC: APA.

American Psychiatric Association. (2019). Depression: A costly condition for business. Retrieved from https://www.workplacementalhealth.org

Ameri, H., Alizadeh, S., & Noughabi, E. A. (2017). Application of Data Mining Techniques in Clinical Decision Making: A Literature Review and Classification. In E. Noughabi, B. Raahemi, A. Albadvi, & B. Far (Eds.), *Handbook of Research on Data Science for Effective Healthcare Practice and Administration* (pp. 257–295). Hershey, PA: IGI Global. doi:10.4018/978-1-5225-2515-8.ch012

Amin, S. & Khan, A,W. (2009). Life in conflict: characteristics of Depression in Kashmir. Retrieved from www.ncbi.nlm.nih.gov/pmc/articles/PMC3068807/

Amir, A., & Beyene, P. (2018). Knowledge, attitudes and practices of malaria transmission and preventive measures in Woreta town, Northwest Ethiopia. Bio Medical Central Research Notes, 11, 491. doi:10.118613104-018-3607-z

Anand, S. (2017). Medical Image Enhancement Using Edge Information-Based Methods. In B. Singh (Ed.), *Computational Tools and Techniques for Biomedical Signal Processing* (pp. 123–148). Hershey, PA: IGI Global. doi:10.4018/978-1-5225-0660-7.ch006

Anda, R. F., Croft, J. B., Felitti, V. J., Norenberg, D., Giles, W. H., Williamson, D. R., & Giovino, G. A. (1999). Adverse childhood events and smoking during adolescence and adulthood. *American Medical Association, 282*(17), 1652-1658.

Andover, M. S., & Morris, B. W. (2014). Expanding and clarifying the role of emotional regulation in nonsuicidal self-injury. *Canadian Journal of Psychiatry, 59*(11), 569–575. doi:10.1177/070674371405901102

Angjellari-Dajci, F., Sapienza, C., Lawless, W. F., & Kavanagh, K. (2016). Human Capital Accumulation in Medical Simulated Learning Environments: A Framework for Economic Evaluation. In M. Russ (Ed.), *Quantitative Multidisciplinary Approaches in Human Capital and Asset Management* (pp. 65–88). Hershey, PA: IGI Global. doi:10.4018/978-1-4666-9652-5.ch004

Anil, M., Ayyildiz-Tamis, D., Tasdemir, S., Sendemir-Urkmez, A., & Gulce-Iz, S. (2016). Bioinspired Materials and Biocompatibility. In M. Bououdina (Ed.), *Emerging Research on Bioinspired Materials Engineering* (pp. 294–322). Hershey, PA: IGI Global. doi:10.4018/978-1-4666-9811-6.ch011

Ankrah, E. (1993). The impact of HIV/AIDS on the family and other significant relationships: The African clan revisited. *AIDS Care, 5*(1), 5–22. doi:10.1080/09540129308258580 PMID:8461361

Antolin-Fontes, B., Ables, J. L., Görlich, A., & Ibañez-Tallon, I. (2015).*The habenulo-interpeduncular pathway in nicotine aversion and withdrawal.* Neuropharmacology, *96*(Pt. B), 213–222.

Anton, J. L., Soriano, J. V., Martinez, M. I., & Garcia, F. B. (2018). Comprehensive E-Learning Appraisal System. In M. Khosrow-Pour, D.B.A. (Ed.), Encyclopedia of Information Science and Technology, Fourth Edition (pp. 5787-5799). Hershey, PA: IGI Global. doi:10.4018/978-1-5225-2255-3.ch503

Arabi, M. (2016). Redesigning the Organizational Structure to Reach Efficiency: The Case of Ministry of Health and Medical Education of Iran. In R. Gholipour & K. Rouzbehani (Eds.), *Social, Economic, and Political Perspectives on Public Health Policy-Making* (pp. 257–294). Hershey, PA: IGI Global. doi:10.4018/978-1-4666-9944-1.ch012

Ardington, C. A., Case, A., Islam, M., Lam, D., Leibbrandt, M., Menendez, A., & Olgiati, A. (2010). The impact of AIDS on intergenerational support in South Africa: Evidence form the Cape Area Panel Study. *Research on Aging*, *32*(1), 91–121. doi:10.1177/0164027509348143 PMID:20161477

Arkell, C., & Harrigan, M. (2018). *HIV treatment and an undetectable viral load to prevent HIV transmission.* Retrieved from https://www.catie.ca/en/factsheets/transmission/hiv-viral-load-hiv-treatment-and-sexual-hiv-transmission

Arora, N., Rastogi, R., Chaturvedi, D. K., Satya, S., Gupta, M., Yadav, V., . . . Sharma, P. (2019b), Chronic TTH Analysis by EMG & GSR Biofeedback on Various Modes and Various Medical Symptoms Using IoT. In Big Data Analytics for Intelligent Healthcare Management (Ch. 5, pp. 87-149). Academic Press. doi:10.1016/B978-0-12-818146-1.00005-2

Arora, N., Trivedi, P., Chauhan, S., Rastogi, R., & Chaturvedi, D. K. (2017a). Framework for Use of Machine Intelligence on Clinical Psychology to study the effects of Spiritual tools on Human Behavior and Psychic Challenges. In *Proceedings of NSC-2017*. Academic Press.

Ashalata, P. R., & Deepa, G. (2015). *Textbook of Anatomy and Physiology for Nurses* (4th ed.). New Delhi, India: Jaypee Brothers Medical Publishers.

Ashipala, D. O., Wilkinson, W. & Van Dyk, A. (2016). Mental health policy implementation as an integral part of primary health care services in Oshana region, Namibia. *Journal of Nursing Education and Practice*, *11*(6), 53–59. doi:10.5430/jnep.v6n11p53

Ashraf, M. (2008). *Kashmir First- Kashmir Story, A collection of commentaries, Politics & History* (Vol. I). India: Gulshan Books.

Ashton, R. A., Kefyalew, T., Tesfaye, G., Pullan, R. L., Yadeta, D., Reinthinger, R., & Brooker, S. (2011). School-based surveys of malaria in Oromia regional State, Ethiopia: A rapid survey method for malaria in low transmission settings. *Malaria Journal*, *10*(1), 25. doi:10.1186/1475-2875-10-25 PubMed

Asok, A., Bernard, K., Roth, T. L., Rosen, J. B., & Dozier, M. (2013). Parental responsiveness moderates the association between early-life stress and reduced telomere length. *Development and Psychopathology*, *25*(3), 577–585. doi:10.1017/S0954579413000011

Assis-Hassid, S., Heart, T., Reychav, I., & Pliskin, J. S. (2016). Modelling Factors Affecting Patient-Doctor-Computer Communication in Primary Care. *International Journal of Reliable and Quality E-Healthcare*, *5*(1), 1–17. doi:10.4018/IJRQEH.2016010101

Atulomah, E. T., Farotimi, A. A., & Atulomah, N. O. (2014). Knowledge, attitudes and practices of malaria prevention among expectant mothers attending antenatal clinic at OOUTH, Sagamu, Ogun State, Nigeria. *Acta Satech*, *5*(1), 9–25.

Atzori, B., Hoffman, H. G., Vagnoli, L., Messeri, A., & Grotto, R. L. (2018). Virtual Reality as Distraction Technique for Pain Management in Children and Adolescents. In M. Khosrow-Pour, D.B.A. (Ed.), Encyclopedia of Information Science and Technology, Fourth Edition (pp. 5955-5965). Hershey, PA: IGI Global. doi:10.4018/978-1-5225-2255-3.ch518

Aubin, H. J., Luquiens, A., & Berlin, I. (2013). Pharmacotherapy for smoking cessation: Pharmacological principles and clinical practice. *British Journal of Clinical Pharmacology*, *77*(2), 324–336. doi:10.1111/bcp.12116 PMID:23488726

Audibert, M., Mathonnat, J., Pélissier, A., & Huang, X. X. (2018). The Impact of the New Rural Cooperative Medical Scheme on Township Hospitals' Utilization and Income Structure in Weifang Prefecture, China. In I. Management Association (Ed.), Health Economics and Healthcare Reform: Breakthroughs in Research and Practice (pp. 109-121). Hershey, PA: IGI Global. doi:10.4018/978-1-5225-3168-5.ch007

Austin, T., Bezuidenhout, C., Botha, K., Du Plessis, E., Du Plessis, L., Jordaan, E., ... Vorster, A. (2017). *Abnormal psychology: A South African perspective*. Cape Town: Oxford University Press.

Auvert, B., Taljaard, D., Lagarde, E., Sobngwi-Tambekou, J., Sitta, R., & Puren, A. (2005). Randomized controlled intervention trial of male circumcision for reduction of HIV infection risk: The ANRS 1265 Trial. *PLoS Medicine*, *2*(11), e298. doi:10.1371/journal.pmed.0020298 PMID:16231970

AVERT. (2015). *Children and HIV/AIDS*. Sussex, Brighton: AVERT.

Awolola, T. S. (2017). *Malaria, Mosquitoes and Man: The Battle Continues* (7th ed.). Nigerian Institute of Medical Research.

Ayyachamy, S. (2016). Analysis and Comparison of Developed 2D Medical Image Database Design using Registration Scheme, Retrieval Scheme, and Bag-of-Visual-Words. In N. Dey & A. Ashour (Eds.), *Classification and Clustering in Biomedical Signal Processing* (pp. 149–168). Hershey, PA: IGI Global. doi:10.4018/978-1-5225-0140-4.ch007

Babalola, A. C. (2016). Literacy and Decision Making on Health Issues among Married Women in Southwest Nigeria. In V. Wang (Ed.), *Handbook of Research on Advancing Health Education through Technology* (pp. 191–212). Hershey, PA: IGI Global. doi:10.4018/978-1-4666-9494-1.ch009

Babalola, E., Ross, N., & White, R. (2017). The biopsychosocial approach and global mental health: Synergies and opportunities. *Indian Journal of Social Psychiatry*, *33*(4), 291–296. doi:10.4103/ijsp.ijsp_13_17

Babu, A., & Ayyappan, S. (2017). A Methodological Evaluation of Crypto-Watermarking System for Medical Images. In C. Bhatt & S. Peddoju (Eds.), *Cloud Computing Systems and Applications in Healthcare* (pp. 189–217). Hershey, PA: IGI Global. doi:10.4018/978-1-5225-1002-4.ch010

Baek, R. N., Tanenbaum, M. L., & Gonzalez, J. S. (2014). Diabetes burden and diabetes distress: The buffering effect of social support. *Annals of Behavioral Medicine*, *48*(2), 145–155. doi:10.100712160-013-9585-4

Bahrmann, A., Abel, A., Zeyfang, A., Petrak, F., Kubiak, T., Hummel, J., & Bahrmann, P. (2014). Psychological insulin resistance in geriatric patients with diabetes mellitus. *Patient Education and Counseling*, *94*(3), 417–422. doi:10.1016/j.pec.2013.11.010

Bakke, A. (2017). Ethos in E-Health: From Informational to Interactive Websites. In M. Folk & S. Apostel (Eds.), *Establishing and Evaluating Digital Ethos and Online Credibility* (pp. 85–103). Hershey, PA: IGI Global. doi:10.4018/978-1-5225-1072-7.ch005

Bali, S. (2018). Enhancing the Reach of Health Care Through Telemedicine: Status and New Possibilities in Developing Countries. In U. Pandey & V. Indrakanti (Eds.), *Open and Distance Learning Initiatives for Sustainable Development* (pp. 339–354). Hershey, PA: IGI Global. doi:10.4018/978-1-5225-2621-6.ch019

Bansal, V., Gassenhuber, J., Phillips, T., Oliveira, G., Harbaugh, R., Villarasa, N., ... Boehm, B. O. (2017). Spectrum of mutations in monogenic diabetes genes identified from high-throughput DNA sequencing of 6888 individuals. *BMC Medicine*, *15*(1), 213. doi:10.118612916-017-0977-3

Barlow, D. H., & Durand, V. M. (2012). *Abnormal psychology: An integrative approach* (6th ed.). Belmont, CA: Cengage Learning.

Barrett, T. E. (2018). Essentials for Education and Training for Tomorrow's Physicians. In C. Smith (Ed.), *Exploring the Pressures of Medical Education From a Mental Health and Wellness Perspective* (pp. 230–252). Hershey, PA: IGI Global. doi:10.4018/978-1-5225-2811-1.ch010

Barrett, T. J. (2016). Knowledge in Action: Fostering Health Education through Technology. In V. Wang (Ed.), *Handbook of Research on Advancing Health Education through Technology* (pp. 39–62). Hershey, PA: IGI Global. doi:10.4018/978-1-4666-9494-1.ch003

Beegle, K., Filmer, D., Strokes, A., & Tiererova, L. (2008). *Orphanhood and living arrangements of children in sub-Saharan Africa*. New York, NY: World Bank.

Bell, R., & Louw, A. (2002). Improving equity in the provision of primary health care: Lessons from decentralized planning and management in Namibia. *Bulletin of the World Health Organization*. doi:10.1590/S0042-96862002000800013 PMID:12219160

Benjamin, R. M. (2010). *A Report of the Surgeon General: How tobacco smoke causes disease*. CDC. Retrieved from https://www.cdc.gov/tobacco/data_statistics/sgr/2010/consumer_booklet/pdfs/consumer.pdf

Ben-Porat, A. (2015). Vicarious post-traumatic growth: Domestic violence therapists versus social service department therapists in Israel. *Journal of Family Violence*, *30*(7), 923–933. doi:10.100710896-015-9714-x

Berhan, Y. T., Eliasson, M., Möllsten, A., Waernbaum, I., & Dahlquist, G. (2015). Swedish Childhood Diabetes Study Group 2013. Impact of parental socioeconomic status on excess mortality in a population-based cohort of subjects with childhood-onset type 1 diabetes. *Diabetes Care*, *38*(5), 827–832. doi:10.2337/dc14-1522

Bernstein, C. M., Stockwell, M. S., Gallagher, M. P., Rosenthal, S. L., & Soren, K. (2013). Mental health issues in adolescents and young adults with T1D prevalence and impact on glycemic control. *Clinical Pediatrics*, *52*, 10–15. doi:10.1177/0009922812459950

Berrahal, S., & Boudriga, N. (2017). The Risks of Wearable Technologies to Individuals and Organizations. In A. Marrington, D. Kerr, & J. Gammack (Eds.), *Managing Security Issues and the Hidden Dangers of Wearable Technologies* (pp. 18–46). Hershey, PA: IGI Global. doi:10.4018/978-1-5225-1016-1.ch002

Better Health Channel. (2019). *Smoking – effects on your body*. Retrieved from https://www.betterhealth.vic.gov.au/healthyliving/smoking-effects-onyour-body

Bhagat, A. P., & Atique, M. (2016). Medical Image Mining Using Fuzzy Connectedness Image Segmentation: Efficient Retrieval of Patients' Stored Images. In W. Karâa & N. Dey (Eds.), *Biomedical Image Analysis and Mining Techniques for Improved Health Outcomes* (pp. 184–209). Hershey, PA: IGI Global. doi:10.4018/978-1-4666-8811-7.ch009

Bhargava, P. (2018). Blended Learning: An Effective Application to Clinical Teaching. In S. Tang & C. Lim (Eds.), *Preparing the Next Generation of Teachers for 21st Century Education* (pp. 302–320). Hershey, PA: IGI Global. doi:10.4018/978-1-5225-4080-9.ch018

Biggar, R. J., Chaturvedi, A. K., Goedert, J. J., & Engels, E. A. (2007). AIDS-related cancer and severity of immunosuppression in persons with AIDS. *Journal of the National Cancer Institute*, *99*(12), 962–972. doi:10.1093/jnci/djm010 PMID:17565153

Binder, H., & Blettner, M. (2015). Big Data in Medical Science—a Biostatistical View. Deutsches Ärzteblatt International, 112(9), 137. doi:10.3238/arztebl.2015.0137

Binh, N. T., & Tuyet, V. T. (2016). The Combination of Adaptive Filters to Improve the Quality of Medical Images in New Wavelet Domain. In N. Dey & A. Ashour (Eds.), *Classification and Clustering in Biomedical Signal Processing* (pp. 46–76). Hershey, PA: IGI Global. doi:10.4018/978-1-5225-0140-4.ch003

Bird, J. L. (2017). Writing Healing Narratives. In V. Bryan & J. Bird (Eds.), *Healthcare Community Synergism between Patients, Practitioners, and Researchers* (pp. 1–28). Hershey, PA: IGI Global. doi:10.4018/978-1-5225-0640-9.ch001

Blockmeyer, B. (2012). The health system in Namibia: Deliberation about an affordable national health insurance for the low workforce in Namibia. Retrieved from http://cms.my.na/assets/documents/p19p2lof2lsi2moqo2tsjfbp5a.pdf

Blosnich, J. R., & Anderson, J. P. (2015). Thursday's child: The role of adverse childhood experiences in explaining mental health disparities among lesbian, gay, and bisexual U.S. adults. *Social Psychiatry and Psychiatric Epidemiology*, *50*(2), 335–338. doi:10.100700127-014-0955-4

Bock, B. C., Thind, H., Fava, J. L., Dunsiger, S., Guthrie, K. M., Stroud, L., ... Wu, W. (2019). Feasibility of yoga as a complementary therapy for patients with type 2 diabetes: The Healthy Active and in Control (HA1C) study. *Complementary Therapies in Medicine*, *42*, 125–131. doi:10.1016/j.ctim.2018.09.019

Boga, D. (2014). No Juvenile Court in J&K. Retrieved from http://infochangeindia.org/children/features/no-juvenile-courts-in –j&k/

Bohman, D. M., Vasuthevan, S., van Wyk, N. C., & Ekman, L. (2007). "We clean our houses, prepare for weddings and go to funerals": Daily lives of elderly Africans in Majaneng, South Africa. *Journal of Cross-Cultural Gerontology*, *22*(4), 323–337. doi:10.100710823-007-9040-8 PMID:17616794

Boon, H., James, S., Ruiter, R. A. C., van den Borne, B., Williams, E., & Reddy, P. (2010). Explaining the perceived ability among older people to provide care as a result of HIV and AIDS in South Africa. *AIDS Care*, *22*(4), 399–408. doi:10.1080/09540120903202921 PMID:20140795

Borus, J. S., & Laffel, L. (2010). Adherence challenges in the management of type 1 diabetes in adolescents: Prevention and intervention. *Current Opinion in Pediatrics*, *22*(4), 405–411. doi:10.1097/MOP.0b013e32833a46a7

Boskey, E. (2019). What is an HIV test?: What to expect when undergoing this test. Verywell Health. Retrieved from https://www.verywellhealth.com/everything-you-need-to-know-about-getting-an-hiv-test-3132731

Bottrighi, A., Leonardi, G., Piovesan, L., & Terenziani, P. (2016). Knowledge-Based Support to the Treatment of Exceptions in Computer Interpretable Clinical Guidelines. *International Journal of Knowledge-Based Organizations*, *6*(3), 1–27. doi:10.4018/IJKBO.2016070101

Bougoulias, K., Kouris, I., Prasinos, M., Giokas, K., & Koutsouris, D. (2017). Ob/Gyn EMR Software: A Solution for Obstetricians and Gynecologists. In A. Moumtzoglou (Ed.), *Design, Development, and Integration of Reliable Electronic Healthcare Platforms* (pp. 101–111). Hershey, PA: IGI Global. doi:10.4018/978-1-5225-1724-5.ch006

Bouldin, E. D., Trivedi, R. B., Reiber, G. E., Rosland, A. M., Silverman, J. B., Krieger, J., & Nelson, K. M. (2017). Associations between having an informal caregiver, social support, and self-care among low-income adults with poorly controlled diabetes. *Chronic Illness, 13*(4), 239–250. doi:10.1177/1742395317690032

Boulé, N. G., Haddad, E., Kenny, G. P., Wells, G. A., & Sigal, R. J. (2001). Effects of exercise on glycemic control and body mass in type 2 diabetes mellitus: A meta-analysis of controlled clinical trials. *Journal of the American Medical Association, 286*(10), 1218–1227. doi:10.1001/jama.286.10.1218

Boureau, F., Luu, M., & Doubrere, J. F. (2001). Study of experimental pain measures and nociceptive reflex in Chronic pain patients and normal subjects. *Pain, 44*(3), 131–138. PMID:2052379

Bouslimi, R., Ayadi, M. G., & Akaichi, J. (2018). Medical Image Retrieval in Healthcare Social Networks. *International Journal of Healthcare Information Systems and Informatics, 13*(2), 13–28. doi:10.4018/IJHISI.2018040102

Bouzaabia, O., Bouzaabia, R., & Mejri, K. (2017). Role of Internet in the Development of Medical Tourism Service in Tunisia. In A. Capatina & E. Rancati (Eds.), *Key Challenges and Opportunities in Web Entrepreneurship* (pp. 211–241). Hershey, PA: IGI Global. doi:10.4018/978-1-5225-2466-3.ch009

Boyer, S., March, L., Kouanfack, C., Laborde-Balen, G., Marino, P., Aghokeng, A. F., ... Moatti, J.-P. (2013). Monitoring of HIV viral load, CD4 cell count, and clinical assessment versus clinical monitoring alone for antiretroviral therapy in low-resource settings (Stratall ANRS 12110/ESTHER): A cost-effectiveness analysis. *The Lancet. Infectious Diseases, 13*(7), 577–586. doi:10.1016/S1473-3099(13)70073-2 PMID:23602084

Branson, D. C., Radu, M. B., & Loving, J. D. (in press). Adverse Childhood Experiences (ACE) scores: When social work students and trauma mix. *The Journal of Baccalaureate Social Work.*

Breckenridge, T. N., Black-Hughes, C., Rautenbach, J., & McKinley, M. (2019). HIV/AIDS orphans in South Africa: NGO interventions supporting transitions to alternative care. *International Social Work, 62*(2), 502, 517.

Briz-Ponce, L., Juanes-Méndez, J. A., & García-Peñalvo, F. J. (2016). A Research Contribution to the Analysis of Mobile Devices in Higher Education from Medical Students' Point of View. In L. Briz-Ponce, J. Juanes-Méndez, & F. García-Peñalvo (Eds.), *Handbook of Research on Mobile Devices and Applications in Higher Education Settings* (pp. 196–221). Hershey, PA: IGI Global. doi:10.4018/978-1-5225-0256-2.ch009

Briz-Ponce, L., Juanes-Méndez, J. A., & García-Peñalvo, F. J. (2016). The Role of Gender in Technology Acceptance for Medical Education. In M. Cruz-Cunha, I. Miranda, R. Martinho, & R. Rijo (Eds.), *Encyclopedia of E-Health and Telemedicine* (pp. 1013–1027). Hershey, PA: IGI Global. doi:10.4018/978-1-4666-9978-6.ch079

Bronte-Tinkew, J., Moore, K. A., Matthews, G., & Carrano, J. (2007). Symptoms of Major Depression in a Sample of Fathers of Infants. *Journal of Family Issues*, *28*(1), 61–99. doi:10.1177/0192513X06293609

Brown-Jackson, K. L. (2018). Telemedicine and Telehealth: Academics Engaging the Community in a Call to Action. In S. Burton (Ed.), *Engaged Scholarship and Civic Responsibility in Higher Education* (pp. 166–193). Hershey, PA: IGI Global. doi:10.4018/978-1-5225-3649-9.ch008

Burguet, A., Kaminski, M., Abraham-Lerat, L., Schaal, J. P., Cambonie, G., Fresson, J., ... Larroque, B. (2004). The complex relationship between smoking in pregnancy and very preterm delivery. Results of the Epipage study. *BJOG*, *111*(3), 258–265. doi:10.1046/j.1471-0528.2003.00037.x PMID:14961888

Burke-Harris, N. (2018). *The deepest well: Healing the long-term effects of childhood adversity*. London, England: Bluebird.

Bursch, B. (2016). Pain and the biopsychosocial model. *Journal of the American Academy of Child and Adolescent Psychiatry*, *55*(10), S34. doi:10.1016/j.jaac.2016.07.565

Bwalya, K. J. (2017). Next Wave of Tele-Medicine: Virtual Presence of Medical Personnel. In K. Moahi, K. Bwalya, & P. Sebina (Eds.), *Health Information Systems and the Advancement of Medical Practice in Developing Countries* (pp. 168–180). Hershey, PA: IGI Global. doi:10.4018/978-1-5225-2262-1.ch010

Camacho, R. C., Galassetti, S. N., Davis, S. N., & Wasserman, D. H. (2005). Gluco-regulation during and after exercise in health and insulin dependent diabetes. *Exercise and Sport Sciences Reviews*, *33*(1), 17–23.

Carlson, N. (2013). *Physiology of Behavior*. New Jersey: Pearson Education, Inc.

Carlton, E. L., Holsinger, J. W. Jr, & Anunobi, N. (2016). Physician Engagement with Health Information Technology: Implications for Practice and Professionalism. *International Journal of Computers in Clinical Practice*, *1*(2), 51–73. doi:10.4018/IJCCP.2016070103

Casale, M., Wild, L., Cluver, L., & Kuo, C. (2015). Social support as a protective factor for depression among women caring for children in HIV-endemic South Africa. *Journal of Behavioral Medicine*, *38*(1), 17–27. doi:10.100710865-014-9556-7 PMID:24510353

Cassel, R. N. (1997). Biofeedback for developing self-control of tension and stress in one's hierarchy of psychological states. *Psychology: A Journal of Human Behavior, 22*(2), 50-57.

Castillo-Page, L., Eliason, J., Conrad, S. S., & Nivet, M. A. (2016). Diversity in Undergraduate Medical Education: An Examination of Organizational Culture and Climate in Medical Schools. In C. Scott & J. Sims (Eds.), *Developing Workforce Diversity Programs, Curriculum, and Degrees in Higher Education* (pp. 304–326). Hershey, PA: IGI Global. doi:10.4018/978-1-5225-0209-8.ch016

Cebeci, H. I., & Hiziroglu, A. (2016). Review of Business Intelligence and Intelligent Systems in Healthcare Domain. In N. Celebi (Ed.), *Intelligent Techniques for Data Analysis in Diverse Settings* (pp. 192–206). Hershey, PA: IGI Global. doi:10.4018/978-1-5225-0075-9.ch009

Celik, G. (2018). Determining Headache Diseases With Genetic Algorithm. In U. Kose, G. Guraksin, & O. Deperlioglu (Eds.), *Nature-Inspired Intelligent Techniques for Solving Biomedical Engineering Problems* (pp. 249–262). Hershey, PA: IGI Global. doi:10.4018/978-1-5225-4769-3.ch012

Çelik, S., Kayar, Y., Önem Akçakaya, R., Türkyılmaz Uyar, E., Kalkan, K., Yazısız, V., ... Yücel, B. (2015). Correlation of binge eating disorder with level of depression and glycemic control in type 2 diabetes mellitus patients. *General Hospital Psychiatry*, *37*(2), 116–119. doi:10.1016/j.genhosppsych.2014.11.012

Cemeroglu, A., Can, A., Davis, A., Cemeroglu, O., Kleis, L., Daniel, M., & Koehler, T. (2015). Fear of needles in children with type 1 diabetes mellitus on multiple daily injections and continuous subcutaneous insulin infusion. *Endocrine Practice*, *21*(1), 46–53. doi:10.4158/EP14252.OR

Centers for Disease Control and Prevention. (2017). Understanding the HIV care continuum. Retrieved from https://www.cdc.gov/hiv/pdf/library/factsheets/cdc-hiv-care-continuum.pdf

Centre for Disease Control (CDC). 2019). Saving lives, protecting people: Malaria impact worldwide (Social and Economic toll). Retrieved from https://www.cdc.gov/parasites/malaria/index.html

Chakraborty, C., Gupta, B., & Ghosh, S. K. (2016). Mobile Telemedicine Systems for Remote Patient's Chronic Wound Monitoring. In A. Moumtzoglou (Ed.), *M-Health Innovations for Patient-Centered Care* (pp. 213–239). Hershey, PA: IGI Global. doi:10.4018/978-1-4666-9861-1.ch011

Chakraborty, S., Chatterjee, S., Ashour, A. S., Mali, K., & Dey, N. (2018). Intelligent Computing in Medical Imaging: A Study. In N. Dey (Ed.), *Advancements in Applied Metaheuristic Computing* (pp. 143–163). Hershey, PA: IGI Global. doi:10.4018/978-1-5225-4151-6.ch006

Chand, S. P., & Arif, H. (2019). *Depression*. Treasure Island, FL: StatPearls Publishing.

Chang, M. X. L. (2017). Understanding depression across cultures: A social identity perspective [Doctor's thesis]. School of Psychology, University of Queensland. Retrieved from https://www.espace.library.uq.edu.au

Chaturvedi, D. K., Rastogi, R., Arora, N., Trivedi, P., & Mishra, V. (2017b). Swarm Intelligent Optimized Method of Development of Noble Life in the perspective of Indian Scientific Philosophy and Psychology. In *Proceedings of NSC-2017*. Academic Press.

Chaturvedi, D.K., Rastogi, R., Satya, S., Arora, N., Saini, H., Verma, H., Mehlyan K., Varshney Y, (2018b). Statistical Analysis of EMG and GSR Therapy on Visual Mode and SF-36 Scores for Chronic TTH. In *Proceedings of UPCON-2018*. Academic Press.

Chauhan, S., Rastogi, R., Chaturvedi, D. K., Satya, S., Arora, N., Yadav, V., & Sharma, P. (2018d). Analytical Comparison of Efficacy for Electromyography and Galvanic Skin Resistance Biofeedback on Audio-Visual Mode for Chronic TTH on Various Attributes. In Proceedings of the ICCIDA-2018. Academic Press.

Chavez, A., & Kovarik, C. (2017). Open Source Technology for Medical Practice in Developing Countries. In K. Moahi, K. Bwalya, & P. Sebina (Eds.), *Health Information Systems and the Advancement of Medical Practice in Developing Countries* (pp. 33–59). Hershey, PA: IGI Global. doi:10.4018/978-1-5225-2262-1.ch003

Chazan, M. (2008). Seven 'deadly' assumptions: Unraveling implications of HIV/AIDS among grandmothers in South Africa and beyond. *Aging and Society*, *28*(7), 935–958. doi:10.1017/S0144686X08007265

Chen, E. T. (2016). Examining the Influence of Information Technology on Modern Health Care. In P. Manolitzas, E. Grigoroudis, N. Matsatsinis, & D. Yannacopoulos (Eds.), *Effective Methods for Modern Healthcare Service Quality and Evaluation* (pp. 110–136). Hershey, PA: IGI Global. doi:10.4018/978-1-4666-9961-8.ch006

Chentsova-Dutton, Y. E., Ryder, A. G., & Tsai, J. (2014). Understanding depression across cultural context. In I. H. Gotlib & C. L. Hammen (Eds.), *Handbook of depression* (pp. 337-354). New York: Guilford Press.

Chentsova-Dutton, Y. E., Choi, E., Ryder, A. G., & Reyes, J. (2015). "I felt sad and did not enjoy life": Cultural context and the associations between anhedonia, depressed mood, and momentary emotions. *Transcultural Psychiatry*, *52*(5), 616–635. doi:10.1177/1363461514565850 PMID:25603917

Chepngeno-Langat, G., Falking, J., Madise, N. J., & Evandrou, M. (2010). Socioeconomic differentials between HIV caregivers and non-caregivers: Is there a selection effect? A case of older people living in Nairobi city slums. *Research on Aging*, *32*(1), 67–96. doi:10.1177/0164027509348116 PMID:21552461

Cherry, K. (2019). What is learned helplessness and why does it happen? *VeryWellMind*. Retrieved from https://www.verywellmind.com/what-is-learned-helplessness-2795326

Chew, B. H., Shariff-Ghazali, S., & Fernandez, A. (2014). Psychological aspects of diabetes care: Effecting behavioral change in patients. *World Journal of Diabetes*, *5*(6), 796–808. doi:10.4239/wjd.v5.i6.796

Chew, B. H., Vos, R., Mohd-Sidik, S., & Rutten, G. E. (2016). Diabetes-related distress, depression and distress-depression among adults with type 2 diabetes mellitus in Malaysia. *PLoS One*, *11*(3), e0152095. doi:10.1371/journal.pone.0152095

Chimwaza, A. F., & Watkins, S. C. (2004). Giving care to people with symptoms of AIDS in rural sub-Saharan Africa. *AIDS Care*, *16*(7), 795–807. doi:10.1080/09540120412331290211 PMID:15385234

Chin, S. (2016). Surviving Sandy: Recovering Collections after a Natural Disaster. In E. Decker & J. Townes (Eds.), *Handbook of Research on Disaster Management and Contingency Planning in Modern Libraries* (pp. 366–388). Hershey, PA: IGI Global. doi:10.4018/978-1-4666-8624-3.ch016

Chisholm, D. (2017). Depression: Let's talk. Retrieved from https://www.who.int/

Chojnacki, M., & Wójcik, A. (2016). Security and the Role of New Technologies and Innovation in Medical Ethics. In A. Rosiek & K. Leksowski (Eds.), *Organizational Culture and Ethics in Modern Medicine* (pp. 52–77). Hershey, PA: IGI Global. doi:10.4018/978-1-4666-9658-7.ch003

Cılız, N., Yıldırım, H., & Temizel, Ş. (2016). Structure Development for Effective Medical Waste and Hazardous Waste Management System. In U. Akkucuk (Ed.), *Handbook of Research on Waste Management Techniques for Sustainability* (pp. 303–327). Hershey, PA: IGI Global. doi:10.4018/978-1-4666-9723-2.ch016

Ciufudean, C. (2018). Innovative Formalism for Biological Data Analysis. In M. Khosrow-Pour, D.B.A. (Ed.), Encyclopedia of Information Science and Technology, Fourth Edition (pp. 1814-1824). Hershey, PA: IGI Global. doi:10.4018/978-1-5225-2255-3.ch158

Ciufudean, C., & Ciufudean, O. (2016). Tele-Monitoring for Medical Diagnosis Availability. In M. Cruz-Cunha, I. Miranda, R. Martinho, & R. Rijo (Eds.), *Encyclopedia of E-Health and Telemedicine* (pp. 401–411). Hershey, PA: IGI Global. doi:10.4018/978-1-4666-9978-6.ch032

Colaguori, R., & Danesi, M. (2017). Medical Semiotics: A Revisitation and an Exhortation. *International Journal of Semiotics and Visual Rhetoric*, *1*(1), 11–18. doi:10.4018/IJSVR.2017010102

Cole, A. W., & Salek, T. A. (2017). Adopting a Parasocial Connection to Overcome Professional Kakoethos in Online Health Information. In M. Folk & S. Apostel (Eds.), *Establishing and Evaluating Digital Ethos and Online Credibility* (pp. 104–120). Hershey, PA: IGI Global. doi:10.4018/978-1-5225-1072-7.ch006

Contreras, E. C., & Puente, G. J. (2016). How to Identify Rheumatic Diseases by General Physicians. In T. Gasmelseid (Ed.), *Advancing Pharmaceutical Processes and Tools for Improved Health Outcomes* (pp. 136–166). Hershey, PA: IGI Global. doi:10.4018/978-1-5225-0248-7.ch006

Coons, M. J., Greiver, M., Aliarzadeh, B., Meaney, C., Moineddin, R., Williamson, T., ... Kane, J. J. (2016). Is glycemia control in Canadians with diabetes individualized? A cross-sectional observational study. *BMJ Open Diabetes Research & Care*, *5*(1), e000316. doi:10.1136/bmjdrc-2016-000316

Corbin, T. J., Purtle, J., Rich, L. J., Rich, J. A., Adams, E. J., Yee, G., & Bloom, S. L. (2013). The prevalence of trauma and childhood adversity in an urban, hospital-based violence intervention program. *Journal of Health Care for the Poor and Underserved*, *24*(3), 1021–1030. doi:10.1353/hpu.2013.0120

Costa, F. F. (2014). *'Big Data in Biomedicine'. Drug Discovery Today*, *19*(4), 433–440. doi:10.1016/j.drudis.2013.10.012 PMID:24183925

Cowan, P. (2010). Depression will be the second leading cause of disease by 2010: WHO. *Calgary Herald*. Retrieved from http://www.calgaryherald.com/health/

Cross, D., Fani, N., Powers, A., & Bradley, B. (2017). Neurobiological development in the context of childhood trauma. *Clinical Psychology: Science and Practice*, *24*(2), 111–124. doi:10.1111/cpsp.12198

Crystal, S. C., & Robbins, M. S. (2010). Epidemiology of tension-type headache. *Current Pain and Headache Reports*, *14*(6), 449–45. doi:10.100711916-010-0146-2 PMID:20865353

Cuijpers, P., Sijbrandij, M., Koole, S. L., Andersson, G., Beekman, A. T., & Reynolds, C. F. (2014). Adding Psychotherapy to antidepressant medication in depression and anxiety disorders: a meta-analysis. World Psychiatry Association. Retrieved from https://www.ncbi.nlm.gov

D'Andrea, A., Ferri, F., & Grifoni, P. (2016). RFID Technologies in Healthcare Setting: Applications and Future Perspectives. *International Journal of Computers in Clinical Practice*, *1*(1), 15–27. doi:10.4018/IJCCP.2016010102

D'Andrea, W., Ford, J., Stolbach, B., Spinazzola, J., & van der Kolk, B. A. (2012). Understanding interpersonal trauma in children: Why we need a developmentally appropriate trauma diagnosis. *The American Journal of Orthopsychiatry*, *82*(2), 187–200. doi:10.1111/j.1939-0025.2012.01154.x

Damianakis, A., Kallonis, P., Loudos, G., Tsatsos, D., & Tsoukalis, A. (2016). Exploiting 3D Medical Equipment Simulations to Support Biomedical Engineering Academic Courses: Design Methodology and Implementation in a Small Scale National Project. In B. Khan (Ed.), *Revolutionizing Modern Education through Meaningful E-Learning Implementation* (pp. 277–295). Hershey, PA: IGI Global. doi:10.4018/978-1-5225-0466-5.ch015

Danese, A., & McEwen, B. S. (2012). Adverse childhood experiences, allostasis, allostatic load, and age-related disease. *Physiology & Behavior*, *106*(1), 29–39. doi:10.1016/j.physbeh.2011.08.019

Dar, M. M. (Ed.). (2016). Presentation on mental health work at the Institute of Mental Health and Neurosciences, Srinagar. In *Symposium on the results of the Kashmir Mental Health Survey*. Academic Press.

Davies, M. A., & Pinto, J. (2015). Targeting 90-90-90 – don't leave children and adolescents behind. *Journal of the International AIDS Society*, *18*(7 Suppl. 6), 20745. doi:10.7448/IAS.18.7.20745 PMID:26639121

Dayton, J., & Ainsworth, M. (2004). The elderly and AIDS: Coping with the impact of adult death in Tanzania. *Social Science & Medicine*, *59*(10), 2161–2172. doi:10.1016/j.socscimed.2004.03.013 PMID:15351481

De Bellis, M. D., Keshavan, M. S., Shifflett, H., Iyengar, S., Beers, S. R., Hall, J., & Moritz, G. (2006). Cerebellar volumes in pediatric maltreatment-related posttraumatic stress disorder: A sociodemographically matched study. *Biological Psychiatry*, *52*(11), 1066–1078. doi:10.1016/S0006-3223(02)01459-2

de Groot, M., Crick, K. A., Long, M., Saha, C., & Shubrook, J. H. (2016). Lifetime duration of depressive disorders in patients with type 2 diabetes. *Diabetes Care*, *39*(12), 2174–2181. doi:10.2337/dc16-1145

de Groot, M., Golden, S. H., & Wagner, J. (2016). Psychological conditions in adults with diabetes. *The American Psychologist*, *71*(7), 552–562. doi:10.1037/a0040408

De Jong, A. R. (2016). Domestic violence, children, and toxic stress. *Widener Law Review*, *22*(2), 201–213.

De Jong, K., Van de Kam, S., Ford, N., Lokuge, K., Fromm, S., Van de Galen, R., & ... (2008). Conflict in the Indian Kashmir Valley II: Psychosocial impact. *Conflict and Health*, *2*(11), 11. doi:10.1186/1752-1505-2-11 PMID:18854027

Deaton, A. S., & Tortora, R. (2014). People in sub-Saharan Africa rate their health and health care among lowest in the world. *Health Affairs (Project Hope)*, *34*(3), 519–527. doi:10.1377/hlthaff.2014.0798 PubMed

Deida, J., Tahar, R., Khalef, Y. O., Khadijetou, M. L., Hmeyade, A., Khairu, M. L., & Boukhary, A. (2019). Oasis malaria in North Mauritania. *Emerging Infectious Diseases*, *25*(2), 282–289. doi:10.3201/eid2502.180732 PubMed

Delahanty, L.M., Conroy, M.B., & Nathan, D.M. (2006). The diabetes prevention program research group psychological predictors of physical activity in the diabetes prevention program. *J. Am. Diabetic. Assoc.*, *l06*, 698-705.

Demiroz, E. (2016). Principles of Instructional Design for E-Learning and Online Learning Practices: Implications for Medical Education. In V. Wang (Ed.), *Handbook of Research on Advancing Health Education through Technology* (pp. 419–451). Hershey, PA: IGI Global. doi:10.4018/978-1-4666-9494-1.ch018

Demmer, C. (2011). Experiences of families caring for HIV-infected child in KwaZulu-Natal, South Africa. *AIDS Care*, *23*(7), 873–879. doi:10.1080/09540121.2010.542123 PMID:21400305

Deperlioglu, O. (2018). Intelligent Techniques Inspired by Nature and Used in Biomedical Engineering. In U. Kose, G. Guraksin, & O. Deperlioglu (Eds.), *Nature-Inspired Intelligent Techniques for Solving Biomedical Engineering Problems* (pp. 51–77). Hershey, PA: IGI Global. doi:10.4018/978-1-5225-4769-3.ch003

Dey, N., & Ashour, A. S. (2018). Meta-Heuristic Algorithms in Medical Image Segmentation: A Review. In N. Dey (Ed.), *Advancements in Applied Metaheuristic Computing* (pp. 185–203). Hershey, PA: IGI Global. doi:10.4018/978-1-5225-4151-6.ch008

Dey, N., Ashour, A. S., & Althoupety, A. S. (2017). Thermal Imaging in Medical Science. In V. Santhi (Ed.), *Recent Advances in Applied Thermal Imaging for Industrial Applications* (pp. 87–117). Hershey, PA: IGI Global. doi:10.4018/978-1-5225-2423-6.ch004

Di Battista, A. M., Hart, T. A., Greco, L., & Gloizer, J. (2009). Type 1 diabetes mellitus among adolescents reduced diabetes self-care caused by social fear and fear of hypoglycemia. *The Diabetes Educator*, *35*, 465–475. doi:10.1177/0145721709333492

Di Virgilio, F., Camillo, A. A., & Camillo, I. C. (2017). The Impact of Social Network on Italian Users' Behavioural Intention for the Choice of a Medical Tourist Destination. *International Journal of Tourism and Hospitality Management in the Digital Age*, *1*(1), 36–49. doi:10.4018/IJTHMDA.2017010103

Diallo, N., Akweongo, P., Maya, E., Aikins, M., & Safo, B. (2017). Burden of malaria in mobile populations in the Greater Accra region, Ghana: A cross- sectional study. *Malaria Journal*, *16*(1), 109. doi:10.1186/s12936-017-1751-x PubMed

Dias, C. M., Ribeiro, A. G., & Furtado, S. F. (2016). An Overview about the Use of Healthcare Applications on Mobile Devices. In M. Cruz-Cunha, I. Miranda, R. Martinho, & R. Rijo (Eds.), *Encyclopedia of E-Health and Telemedicine* (pp. 285–298). Hershey, PA: IGI Global. doi:10.4018/978-1-4666-9978-6.ch024

Dias, P. C., & Cadime, I. (2017). Protective factors and resilience in adolescents: The mediating role of self-regulation. *Psicologia dell'Educazione*, *23*(1), 37–43. doi:10.1016/j.pse.2016.09.003

Diiro, G. M., Hippolyte, D., Affognon, B. W., Muriithi, S. K., Mbogo, W. C., & Clifford, M. (2016). The role of gender on malaria preventive behaviour among rural households in Kenya. *Malaria Journal*, *15*, 14. doi:10.118612936-015-1039y

DiMaria, L. (2019). *Clinically significant depression overview. VeryWellMind.* Retrieved from https://www.verywellmind.com/clinically-significant-depression-1067143

Dogra, A. K., & Dogra, P. (2017). The Medical Tourism Industry in the BRIC Nations: An Indian Analysis. In M. Dhiman (Ed.), *Opportunities and Challenges for Tourism and Hospitality in the BRIC Nations* (pp. 320–336). Hershey, PA: IGI Global. doi:10.4018/978-1-5225-0708-6.ch020

Dooley, L. N., Slavich, G. M., Moreno, P. I., & Bower, J. E. (2017). Strength through adversity: Moderate lifetime stress exposure is associated with psychological resilience in breast cancer survivors. *Stress and Health*, *33*(5), 549–557. doi:10.1002mi.2739

Drowos, J. L., & Wood, S. K. (2017). Preparing Future Physicians to Adapt to the Changing Health Care System: Promoting Humanism through Curricular Design. In V. Bryan & J. Bird (Eds.), *Healthcare Community Synergism between Patients, Practitioners, and Researchers* (pp. 106–125). Hershey, PA: IGI Global. doi:10.4018/978-1-5225-0640-9.ch006

Dube, S. R., Anda, R. F., Felitti, V. J., Chapman, D. P., Williamson, D. F., & Giles, W. H. (2001). Childhood abuse, household dysfunction, and the risk of attempted suicide throughout the life span: Findings from the Adverse Childhood Experiences study. *American Medical Association, 286*(24), 3089-3095.

Dulam, K. (2017). Medical Patents and Impact on Availability and Affordability of Essential Medicines in India. In R. Aggarwal & R. Kaur (Eds.), *Patent Law and Intellectual Property in the Medical Field* (pp. 41–57). Hershey, PA: IGI Global. doi:10.4018/978-1-5225-2414-4.ch003

Duros, P., & Crowley, D. (2014). The body comes to therapy too. *Clinical Social Work Journal, 42*(3), 237–246. doi:10.100710615-014-0486-1

Dutta, P. (2017). Decision Making in Medical Diagnosis via Distance Measures on Interval Valued Fuzzy Sets. *International Journal of System Dynamics Applications, 6*(4), 63–83. doi:10.4018/IJSDA.2017100104

Dutton, G. R., Tan, F., Provost, B. C., Sorenson, J. L., Allen, B., & Smith, D. (2009). Relationship between self-efficacy and physical activity among patients with type 2 diabetes. *Journal of Behavioral Medicine, 32*(3), 270–277. doi:10.100710865-009-9200-0

Edoh, T. O., Pawar, P. A., Brügge, B., & Teege, G. (2016). A Multidisciplinary Remote Healthcare Delivery System to Increase Health Care Access, Pathology Screening, and Treatment in Developing Countries: The Case of Benin. *International Journal of Healthcare Information Systems and Informatics, 11*(4), 1–31. doi:10.4018/IJHISI.2016100101

Egede, L. E., & Dismuke, C. E. (2012). Serious psychological distress and diabetes: A review of the literature. *Current Psychiatry Reports, 14*(1), 15–22. doi:10.100711920-011-0240-0

Eisinger, R.W., Dieffenbach, C.W., & Fauci, A.S. (2019). HIV viral load and transmissibility of HIV infection: Undetectable equals untrasmittable. *Journal of American Association*, E1-E2.

El Guemhioui, K., & Demurjian, S. A. (2017). Semantic Reconciliation of Electronic Health Records Using Semantic Web Technologies. *International Journal of Information Technology and Web Engineering, 12*(2), 26–48. doi:10.4018/IJITWE.2017040102

Ellouze, N., Rekhis, S., & Boudriga, N. (2016). Forensic Investigation of Digital Crimes in Healthcare Applications. In O. Isafiade & A. Bagula (Eds.), *Data Mining Trends and Applications in Criminal Science and Investigations* (pp. 169–210). Hershey, PA: IGI Global. doi:10.4018/978-1-5225-0463-4.ch007

Eneanya, A. N. (2016). Health Policy Implementation and Its Barriers: The Case Study of US Health System. In R. Gholipour & K. Rouzbehani (Eds.), *Social, Economic, and Political Perspectives on Public Health Policy-Making* (pp. 42–63). Hershey, PA: IGI Global. doi:10.4018/978-1-4666-9944-1.ch003

Enlow, M. B., Blood, E., & Egeland, B. (2013). Sociodemographic risk, developmental competence, and PTSD symptoms in young children exposed to interpersonal trauma in early life. *Journal of Traumatic Stress, 26*(6), 686–694. doi:10.1002/jts.21866

Entico, G. J. (2016). Knowledge Management and the Medical Health Librarians: A Perception Study. In J. Yap, M. Perez, M. Ayson, & G. Entico (Eds.), *Special Library Administration, Standardization and Technological Integration* (pp. 52–77). Hershey, PA: IGI Global. doi:10.4018/978-1-4666-9542-9.ch003

Erkie, M., Feleke, Y., Desalegne, F., Anbessie, J., & Shibre, T. (2013). Magnitude, clinical and sociodemographic correlate of depression in diabetic patients, Addis Ababa, Ethiopia. *Ethiopian Medical Journal*, *51*(4), 249–259.

Ernst, K. C., Hayden, M. H., Olsen, H., Cavanaugh, J. L., Ruberto, I., Agawo, M., & Munga, S. (2016). Comparing ownership and use of bed nets at two sites with differential malaria transmission in western Kenya. *Malaria Journal*, *15*(1), 217. doi:10.1186/s12936-016-1262-1 PubMed

Es, M., & Boyle, B. (2002). Excess and access: The continuing controversy regarding HIV and health care in Africa. *The AIDS Reader*, *12*(7), 288–292. PMID:12161849

Farkas, J. (2015, September). *Recognizing and managing paradoxical reactions from benzodiazepines and propofol*. Retrieved from https://emcrit.org/pulmcrit/recognizing-and-managing-paradoxical-reactions-from-benzodiazepines-propofol/

Federal Ministry of Health, Nigeria. (2015). FMoHN document: National Guidelines for Diagnosis and Treatment of Malaria, 2015.

Felitti, V. J., Anda, R. F., Nordenberg, D., Williamson, D. F., Spitz, A. M., Edwards, V., ... Marks, J. S. (1998). Relationship of childhood abuse and household dysfunction to many of the leading causes of death in adults: The Adverse Childhood Experience (ACE) study. *American Journal of Preventive Medicine*, *14*(4), 245–258. doi:10.1016/S0749-3797(98)00017-8

Ferradji, M. A., & Zidani, A. (2016). Collaborative Environment for Remote Clinical Reasoning Learning. *International Journal of E-Health and Medical Communications*, *7*(4), 62–81. doi:10.4018/IJEHMC.2016100104

Festinger, L. (1962). *A theory of cognitive dissonance*. Stanford, CA: Stanford University Press.

Fisher, J. (2018). Sociological Perspectives on Improving Medical Diagnosis Emphasizing CAD. In M. Khosrow-Pour, D.B.A. (Ed.), Encyclopedia of Information Science and Technology, Fourth Edition (pp. 1017-1024). Hershey, PA: IGI Global. doi:10.4018/978-1-5225-2255-3.ch088

Fisher, L., Skaff, M. M., Mullan, J. T., Arean, P., Glasgow, R., & Masharani, U. (2008). A longitudinal study of affective and anxiety disorders, depressive affect and diabetes distress in adults with Type 2 diabetes. *Diabetic Medicine*, *25*(9), 1096–1101. doi:10.1111/j.1464-5491.2008.02533.x

Flores, C. D., Respício, A., Coelho, H., Bez, M. R., & Fonseca, J. M. (2016). Simulation for Medical Training. In M. Cruz-Cunha, I. Miranda, R. Martinho, & R. Rijo (Eds.), *Encyclopedia of E-Health and Telemedicine* (pp. 827–842). Hershey, PA: IGI Global. doi:10.4018/978-1-4666-9978-6.ch064

Foster, G. (2000). The capacity of the extended family safety net for orphans in Africa. *Psychology & Health*, *346*, 1907–1910.

Francis, L., DePriest, K., Wilson, M., & Gross, D. (2018). Child poverty, toxic stress, and social determinants of health: Screening and care coordination. *Online Journal of Issues in Nursing*, *23*(3), 2. doi:10.3912/OJIN.Vol23No03Man02

Frank, E. M. (2018). Healthcare Education: Integrating Simulation Technologies. In V. Bryan, A. Musgrove, & J. Powers (Eds.), *Handbook of Research on Human Development in the Digital Age* (pp. 163–182). Hershey, PA: IGI Global. doi:10.4018/978-1-5225-2838-8.ch008

Freeman, J. (2015). Developing social skills and relationships. *Reclaiming Children and Youth*, *23*(4), 48–51.

Freeman, M., & Nkomo, N. (2006). Guardianship of orphans and vulnerable children: A survey of current and prospective South African caregivers. *AIDS Care*, *18*(4), 302–310. doi:10.1080/09540120500359009 PMID:16809107

Fumal, A., & Scohnen, J. (2008). Tension-type headache: current research and clinical management. *Lancet Neurology*, *7*(2), 70–83. doi:10.1016/S1474-4422(07)70325-3 PMID:18093564

Galobardes, B., Shaw, M., Lawlor, D. A., Lynch, J. W., & Davey Smith, G. (2006). Indicators of socioeconomic position (part 1). *Journal of Epidemiology and Community Health*, *60*(1), 7–12. doi:10.1136/jech.2004.023531

Gandhe, R. J. (2014). Positive stress: Review of relevant theories and an alternative conceptualization. *Indian Journal of Positive Psychology*, *5*(3), 260–266.

Gardner, R. M. (2002). *Psychology Applied to everyday life*. Belmont: C Thomson/Wadsworth.

Garner, E. M., McLees, M. P., Steiner, J. F., del Rio, C., & Burman, W. J. (2011). The spectrum of engagement in HIV care and its relevance to test and treat strategies for prevention of HIV infection. *Clinical Infectious Diseases*, *52*(6), 793–800. doi:10.1093/cid/ciq243 PMID:21367734

Garner, G. (2018). Foundations for Yoga Practice in Rehabilitation. In S. Telles & N. Singh (Eds.), *Research-Based Perspectives on the Psychophysiology of Yoga* (pp. 263–307). Hershey, PA: IGI Global. doi:10.4018/978-1-5225-2788-6.ch015

Gasmelseid, T. M. (2016). Improving Pharmaceutical Care through the Use of Intelligent Pharmacoinformatics. In T. Gasmelseid (Ed.), *Advancing Pharmaceutical Processes and Tools for Improved Health Outcomes* (pp. 167–188). Hershey, PA: IGI Global. doi:10.4018/978-1-5225-0248-7.ch007

Gates, S., Hegre, H., Nygård, H. M., & Strand, H. (2012). Development consequences of armed conflict. *World Development*, *40*(9), 1713-1722. Retrieved from https://www.sciencedirect.com/science/article/pii/s0305750x12001015

Gavurová, B., Kováč, V., & Šoltés, M. (2018). Medical Equipment and Economic Determinants of Its Structure and Regulation in the Slovak Republic. In M. Khosrow-Pour, D.B.A. (Ed.), Encyclopedia of Information Science and Technology, Fourth Edition (pp. 5841-5852). Hershey, PA: IGI Global. doi:10.4018/978-1-5225-2255-3.ch508

George, S., McGrath, N., & Oni, T. (2019). The association between a detectable HIV viral load and non-communicable diseases comorbidity in HIV positive adults on antiretroviral therapy in Western Cape, South Africa. *BMC Infectious Diseases*, *19*(1), 348. doi:10.118612879-019-3956-9 PMID:31029087

German Technical Cooperation Agency. (2009). Health and wellness: Peer educator handbook. Windhoek. Namibia.

German Technical Cooperation. (2009). *Health and wellness: Peer educator handbook.*

German Technical Cooperation. (2009). Health and wellness: Peer educator handbook. Windhoek.

Gewald, H., & Gewald, C. (2018). Inhibitors of Physicians' Use of Mandatory Hospital Information Systems (HIS). *International Journal of Healthcare Information Systems and Informatics*, *13*(1), 29–44. doi:10.4018/IJHISI.2018010103

Ge, X., Wang, Q., Huang, K., Law, V., & Thomas, D. C. (2017). Designing Simulated Learning Environments and Facilitating Authentic Learning Experiences in Medical Education. In J. Stefaniak (Ed.), *Advancing Medical Education Through Strategic Instructional Design* (pp. 77–100). Hershey, PA: IGI Global. doi:10.4018/978-1-5225-2098-6.ch004

Ghosh, D., & Dinda, S. (2017). Health Infrastructure and Economic Development in India. In R. Das (Ed.), *Social, Health, and Environmental Infrastructures for Economic Growth* (pp. 99–119). Hershey, PA: IGI Global. doi:10.4018/978-1-5225-2364-2.ch006

Ghosh, K., & Sen, K. C. (2017). The Potential of Crowdsourcing in the Health Care Industry. In N. Wickramasinghe (Ed.), *Handbook of Research on Healthcare Administration and Management* (pp. 418–427). Hershey, PA: IGI Global. doi:10.4018/978-1-5225-0920-2.ch024

Ghrab, S., & Saad, I. (2016). Identifying Crucial Know-How and Knowing-That for Medical Decision Support. *International Journal of Decision Support System Technology*, *8*(4), 14–33. doi:10.4018/IJDSST.2016100102

Gilks, C. F., Crowley, S., Ekpini, R., Gove, S., Perriens, J., Souteyrand, Y., ... De Cock, K. (2006). The WHO public-health approach to antiretroviral treatment against HIV in resource-limited settings. *Lancet*, *368*(9534), 505–510. doi:10.1016/S0140-6736(06)69158-7 PMID:16890837

Giokas, K., Tsirmpas, C., Anastasiou, A., Iliopoulou, D., Costarides, V., & Koutsouris, D. (2016). Contemporary Heart Failure Treatment Based on Improved Knowledge and Personalized Care of Comorbidities. In D. Fotiadis (Ed.), *Handbook of Research on Trends in the Diagnosis and Treatment of Chronic Conditions* (pp. 301–314). Hershey, PA: IGI Global. doi:10.4018/978-1-4666-8828-5.ch014

Glenn, C. R., Lanzillo, E. C., Esposito, E. C., Santee, A. C., Nock, M. K., & Auerbach, R. P. (2017). Examining the course of suicidal and nonsuicidal self-injurious thoughts and behaviors in outpatient and inpatient adolescents. *Journal of Abnormal Child Psychology*, *45*(5), 971–983. doi:10.100710802-016-0214-0

Glen-Spyron, C., & Jacobs, A. (2019). Striking a healthy balance between studies and mental health. *The Namibian*. Retrieved from https://www.namibian.com.na

Gnavi, R., Petrelli, A., Demaria, M., Spadea, T., Carta, Q., & Costa, G. (2004). Mortality and educational level among diabetic and non-diabetic population in the Turin Longitudinal Study: A 9-year follow-up. *International Journal of Epidemiology*, *33*(4), 864–871. doi:10.1093/ije/dyh089

Goetz, K., Szecseny, J., Campbell, S., Rosemann, T., Rueter, G., Raum, E., ... Miksch, A. (2012). The importance of social support for people with type 2 diabetes: A qualitative study with general practitioners, practice nurses and patients. *Psycho-Social Medicine*, *9*, 1–9.

Gonder-Frederick, L. A., Fisher, C. D., Ritterband, L. M., Cox, D. J., Hou, L., DasGupta, A. A., & Clarke, W. L. (2006). Predictors of fear of hypoglycemia in adolescents with type 1 diabetes and their parents. *Pediatric Diabetes*, *7*(4), 215–222. doi:10.1111/j.1399-5448.2006.00182.x

Gonzalez-Zacarias, A. A., Mavarez-Martinez, A., Arias-Morales, C. E., Stoicea, N., & Rogers, B. (2016). Impact of demographic, socioeconomic, and psychological factors on glycemic self-management in adults with type 2 diabetes mellitus. *Frontiers in Public Health*, *4*. doi:10.3389/fpubh.2016.00195

Gopalan, V., Chan, E., & Ho, D. T. (2018). Deliberate Self-Harm and Suicide Ideology in Medical Students. In C. Smith (Ed.), *Exploring the Pressures of Medical Education From a Mental Health and Wellness Perspective* (pp. 122–143). Hershey, PA: IGI Global. doi:10.4018/978-1-5225-2811-1.ch005

Goswami, S., Dey, U., Roy, P., Ashour, A., & Dey, N. (2017). Medical Video Processing: Concept and Applications. In N. Dey, A. Ashour, & P. Patra (Eds.), *Feature Detectors and Motion Detection in Video Processing* (pp. 1–17). Hershey, PA: IGI Global. doi:10.4018/978-1-5225-1025-3.ch001

Goswami, S., Mahanta, K., Goswami, S., Jigdung, T., & Devi, T. P. (2018). Ageing and Cancer: The Epigenetic Basis, Alternative Treatment, and Care. In B. Prasad & S. Akbar (Eds.), *Handbook of Research on Geriatric Health, Treatment, and Care* (pp. 206–235). Hershey, PA: IGI Global. doi:10.4018/978-1-5225-3480-8.ch012

Gouva, M. I. (2017). The Psychological Impact of Medical Error on Patients, Family Members, and Health Professionals. In M. Riga (Ed.), *Impact of Medical Errors and Malpractice on Health Economics, Quality, and Patient Safety* (pp. 171–196). Hershey, PA: IGI Global. doi:10.4018/978-1-5225-2337-6.ch007

Govender, K., Penning, S., George, G., & Quilan, T. (2012). Weighing up the burden of care on caregivers of orphan children: The Amajuba District Child Health and Wellbeing Project, South Africa. *AIDS Care Psychological and Socio-Medical Aspects of HIV/AIDS*, *24*(6), 712-721.

Government of India. (2012). 2011 Indian National Census Online: Census Organization of India. Retrieved from www.census2011.co.in

Grigsby, A. B., Anderson, R. J., Freedland, K. E., Clouse, R. E., & Lustman, P. J. (2002). Prevalence of anxiety in adults with diabetes: A systematic review. *Journal of Psychosomatic Research*, *53*(6), 1053–1060. doi:10.1016/S0022-3999(02)00417-8

Grohol, G. M. (2018). Living with depression: A guide for coping with depressive feelings. Psychcentral. Retrieved from https://psychcentral.com/

Gulati, M., Rastogi, R., Chaturvedi, D. K., Sharma, P., Yadav, V., Chauhan, S., . . . Singhal, P. (2019e). Statistical Resultant Analysis of Psychosomatic Survey on Various Human Personality Indicators: Statistical Survey to Map Stress and Mental Health. In *Handbook of Research on Learning in the Age of Transhumanism* (Ch. 22, pp. 363-383). Hershey, PA: IGI Global. doi:10.4018/978-1-5225-8431-5.ch022

Gul, E., & Karanci, A. N. (2017). What determines posttraumatic stress and growth following various traumatic events? A study in a Turkish community sample. *Journal of Traumatic Stress*, *30*(1), 54–62. doi:10.1002/jts.22161

Gupta, M., Rastogi, R., Chaturvedi, D. K., & Satya, S. (2019a). Comparative study of trends observed during different medications by subjects under EMG & GSR biofeedback. *IJITEE*, *8*(6S), 748-756. Retrieved from https://www.ijitee.org/download/volume-8-issue-6S/

Gürcü, M., & Tengilimoğlu, D. (2017). Health Tourism-Based Destination Marketing. In A. Bayraktar & C. Uslay (Eds.), *Strategic Place Branding Methodologies and Theory for Tourist Attraction* (pp. 308–331). Hershey, PA: IGI Global. doi:10.4018/978-1-5225-0579-2.ch015

Gurel, N. Z., Carek, A. M., Inan, O. T., Levantsevych, O., Abdelhadi, N., Hammadah, M., ... Shah, A. J. (2019). Comparison of autonomic stress reactivity in young healthy versus aging subjects with heart disease. *PLoS One*, *14*(5), 1–16. doi:10.1371/journal.pone.0216278

Gürsel, G. (2016). Mobility in Healthcare: M-Health. In A. Panagopoulos (Ed.), *Handbook of Research on Next Generation Mobile Communication Systems* (pp. 485–511). Hershey, PA: IGI Global. doi:10.4018/978-1-4666-8732-5.ch019

Gürsel, G. (2017). For Better Healthcare Mining Health Data. In S. Bhattacharyya, S. De, I. Pan, & P. Dutta (Eds.), *Intelligent Multidimensional Data Clustering and Analysis* (pp. 135–158). Hershey, PA: IGI Global. doi:10.4018/978-1-5225-1776-4.ch006

Guzman-Lugo, G., Lopez-Martinez, M., Lopez-Ramirez, B., & Avila-Vazquez, D. (2016). City-Driven Approach to Determine Health Services Based on Current User Location and Collaborative Information. *International Journal of Knowledge Society Research*, *7*(1), 53–62. doi:10.4018/IJKSR.2016010104

Gyaase, P. O., Darko-Lartey, R., William, H., & Borkloe, F. (2017). Towards an Integrated Electronic Medical Records System for Quality Healthcare in Ghana: An Exploratory Factor Analysis. *International Journal of Computers in Clinical Practice*, *2*(2), 38–55. doi:10.4018/IJCCP.2017070103

Habtewold, T. D., Islam, M. A., Radie, Y. T., & Tegegne, B. S. (2016). Comorbidity of depression and diabetes: An application of biopsychosocial model. *International Journal of Mental Health Systems*, *10*(1), 1–9. doi:10.118613033-016-0106-2

Haddock, C. K., Rowan, A. B., Andrasik, F., Wilson, P. G., Talcott, G. W., & Stein, R. J. (1997). Home- based behavioral Treatments for chronic benign headache: A meta-analysis of controlled trials. *Cephalalgia*, *17*(1), 113–118. doi:10.1046/j.1468-2982.1997.1702113.x PMID:9137849

Hagger, M. S., Leaver, E., Esser, K., Leung, C. M., Pas, N. T., Keatley, D. A., ... Chatzisarantis, N. L. D. (2013). Cue-induced urges deplete cigarette smoker's selfcontrol resources. *Annals of Behavioral Medicine*, *46*(3), 394–400. doi:10.100712160-013-9520-8 PMID:23720186

Haji M. (2018). Killing One Colonial Law at a Time – After Section 377, It's Time to Repeal AFSPA. The Wire.

Hall, K. K., Tambekou, J., Penn, L., Camara, A., Balde, N. M., & Sobngwi, E. (2017). Association between depression, glycaemic control and the prevalence of diabetic retinopathy in a diabetic population in Cameroon. *South African Journal of Psychiatry*, *23*, 983. doi:10.4102ajpsychiatry.v23i0.983

Halverson, J. I. (2019). Depression. *Medscape.* Retrieved from https://emedicine. medscape.com/article/286759-overview

Hammond, M. (2005). First Nations of Quebec and Labrador Health and Social Services Commission. (2005). *Healing from smoking.* Retrieved from https://www.nicotinedependenceclinic.com/English/teach/SiteAssets/Pages/Special-Populations/Healing%20From%20Smoking.pdf

Handayani, P. W., Sandhyaduhita, P. I., Hidayanto, A. N., Pinem, A. A., Fajrina, H. R., Junus, K. M., ... Ayuningtyas, D. (2016). Integrated Hospital Information System Architecture Design in Indonesia. In T. Iyamu & A. Tatnall (Eds.), *Maximizing Healthcare Delivery and Management through Technology Integration* (pp. 207–236). Hershey, PA: IGI Global. doi:10.4018/978-1-4666-9446-0.ch013

Hanel, P. (2017). Is China Catching Up?: Health-Related Applications of Biotechnology. In T. Bas & J. Zhao (Eds.), *Comparative Approaches to Biotechnology Development and Use in Developed and Emerging Nations* (pp. 465–520). Hershey, PA: IGI Global. doi:10.4018/978-1-5225-1040-6.ch016

Hanson, G. R., Venturelli, P. J., & Fleckenstein, A. E. (2018). *Drugs and society* (13th ed.). Burlington, MA: Jones & Bartlett Learning.

Harmsen, C. A., & Royle, R. N. (2016). St. Stephen's Hospital Hervey Bay: Study of Developing a Digital Hospital. In J. Moon & M. Galea (Eds.), *Improving Health Management through Clinical Decision Support Systems* (pp. 127–153). Hershey, PA: IGI Global. doi:10.4018/978-1-4666-9432-3.ch006

Harp, D., Shim, R. S., Johnson, J., Harp, J. A., Wilcox, W. C., & Wilcox, J. K. (2016). Race and Gender Inequalities in Medicine and Biomedical Research. In U. Thomas & J. Drake (Eds.), *Critical Research on Sexism and Racism in STEM Fields* (pp. 115–134). Hershey, PA: IGI Global. doi:10.4018/978-1-5225-0174-9.ch006

Hartman, A., & Brown, S. (2017). Synergism through Therapeutic Visual Arts. In V. Bryan & J. Bird (Eds.), *Healthcare Community Synergism between Patients, Practitioners, and Researchers* (pp. 29–48). Hershey, PA: IGI Global. doi:10.4018/978-1-5225-0640-9.ch002

Hassan, A., & Shafi, A. (2013). Impact of conflict situation on mental health in Srinagar, Kashmir. *Bangladesh e-Journal of Sociology*, *10*(1), 101–126.

Hassan, A., & Shafi, A. (2013). Impact of Conflict Situation on Mental Health in Srinagar, Kashmir. *Bangladesh e-Journal of Sociology*, *10*(1).

Hassan, K., Loar, R., Anderson, B. J., & Heptulla, R. A. (2006). The role of socioeconomic status, depression, quality of life, and glycemic control in type 1 diabetes mellitus. *The Journal of Pediatrics*, *149*(4), 526–531. doi:10.1016/j.jpeds.2006.05.039

Haynes, S. N., Griffin, P., Mooney, D., & Parise, M. (2005). Electromyographic BF and Relaxation Instructions in the Treatment of Muscle Contraction Headaches. *Behavior Therapy*, *6*(1), 672–678.

Hazra, J., Chowdhury, A. R., & Dutta, P. (2016). Cluster Based Medical Image Registration Using Optimized Neural Network. In S. Bhattacharyya, P. Banerjee, D. Majumdar, & P. Dutta (Eds.), *Handbook of Research on Advanced Hybrid Intelligent Techniques and Applications* (pp. 551–581). Hershey, PA: IGI Global. doi:10.4018/978-1-4666-9474-3.ch018

Hein, F. A., Qouta, S., Thabet, A., & El Sarraj, E. (1993). Trauma and mental health of children in Gaza. *BMJ: British Medical Journal*, *306*(6885), 1130.

Helleringer, S., Kohler, H. P., Frimpong, J. A., & Mkandawire, J. (2009). Increasing uptake of HIV testing and counseling among the poorest in sub-Saharan countries through home-based service provision. *Journal of Acquired Immune Deficiency Syndromes*, *51*(2), 185–193. doi:10.1097/QAI.0b013e31819c1726 PMID:19352202

HelpAge International (HAI). (2003). *Forgotten families: Older people as carers of orphans and vulnerable children*. London: Help Age International.

Herman, J. (1997). *Trauma and recovery: The aftermath of violence-from domestic abuse to political terror*. New York, NY: Basic Books.

Hertzman, C., Power, C., Matthew, S., & Manor, O. (2001). Using an interactive framework of society and lifecourse to explain self-rated health in early adulthood. *Social Science & Medicine*, *53*(12), 1575–1585. doi:10.1016/S0277-9536(00)00437-8 PMID:11762884

Herzer, M., & Hood, K. K. (2010). Anxiety symptoms in adolescents with Type 1 Diabetes: Association with blood glucose monitoring and glycemic control. *Journal of Pediatric Psychology*, *35*(4), 415–425. doi:10.1093/jpepsy/jsp063

Hill-Briggs, F., & Gemmell, L. (2007). Problem solving in diabetes self-management and control: A systematic review of the literature. *The Diabetes Educator*, *33*(6), 1032–1050. doi:10.1177/0145721707308412

Hilliard, M. E., Yi-Frazier, J. P., Hessler, D., Butler, A. M., Anderson, B. J., & Jaser, S. (2016). Stress and A1c Among People with Diabetes Across the Lifespan. *Current Diabetes Reports*, *16*(8), 67. doi:10.100711892-016-0761-3

Hillis, S. D., Mercy, J. A., & Saul, J. R. (2017). The enduring impact of violence against children. *Psychology Health and Medicine*, *22*(4), 393–405. doi:10.1080/13548506.2016.1153679

Hines, T. (April 2018). *Anatomy of the brain*. Mayfield Brain and Spine. Retrieved from https://mayfieldclinic.com/pe-anatbrain.htm

Hogg, R. (2018). Understanding the HIV care continuum. *The Lancet. HIV*, *3018*(18), 30102–30104. PMID:29893238

Holt, R. I. G., de Groot, M., & Golden, S. H. (2014). Diabetes and Depression. *Current Diabetes Reports*, *14*(6), 491. doi:10.100711892-014-0491-3

Hsu, Y. M., Su, L. T., Chang, H. M., Sung, F. C., Lyu, S. Y., & Chen, P. C. (2012). Diabetes mellitus and risk of subsequent depression: A longitudinal study. *International Journal of Nursing Studies*, *49*(4), 437–444. doi:10.1016/j.ijnurstu.2011.09.019

Hu, J., Amirehsani, K., Wallace, D. C., & Letvak, S. (2013). Perceptions of barriers in managing diabetes: Perspectives of Hispanic immigrant patients and family members. *The Diabetes Educator*, *39*(4), 494–503. doi:10.1177/0145721713486200

Human Rights Watch. (2006). *Everyone Lives in Fear: Patterns of Impunity in Jammu and Kashmir*. New York: Human Rights Watch.

Hung, S., Huang, W., Yen, D. C., Chang, S., & Lu, C. (2016). Effect of Information Service Competence and Contextual Factors on the Effectiveness of Strategic Information Systems Planning in Hospitals. *Journal of Global Information Management*, *24*(1), 14–36. doi:10.4018/JGIM.2016010102

Hyu, J. H., Sun-Young, K., Jeong, J. Y., & Jeong-Ho, C. (2014). Childhood trauma and adult interpersonal relationship problems in patients with depression and anxiety disorders. *Annals of General Psychiatry*, *13*(1), 1–23. doi:10.118612991-014-0026-y

Ice, G. H., Zidron, A., & Juma, E. (2008). Health and health perceptions among Kenyan grandmothers. *Journal of Cross-Cultural Gerontology*, *23*(2), 111–129. doi:10.100710823-008-9063-9 PMID:18437546

Iltchev, P., Śliwczyński, A., Szynkiewicz, P., & Marczak, M. (2016). Mobile Health Applications Assisting Patients with Chronic Diseases: Examples from Asthma Care. In A. Moumtzoglou (Ed.), *M-Health Innovations for Patient-Centered Care* (pp. 170–196). Hershey, PA: IGI Global. doi:10.4018/978-1-4666-9861-1.ch009

Imran, S. A., Agarwal, G., Harpreet, S. B., & Ross, S. (2018). Targets for glycemic control. *Canadian Journal of Diabetes*, *42*, S42–S46. doi:10.1016/j.jcjd.2017.10.030

Institute of Medicine. (2012). *Monitoring HIV care in the United States: Indicators and data systems*. Washington, DC: National Academies Press.

Inter-Agency Standing Committee. (2006). *IASC guidelines on mental health and psychosocial support in emergency settings*. Geneva, Switzerland: IASC.

Iqbal, S., Ahmad, S., & Willis, I. (2017). Influencing Factors for Adopting Technology Enhanced Learning in the Medical Schools of Punjab, Pakistan. *International Journal of Information and Communication Technology Education*, *13*(3), 27–39. doi:10.4018/IJICTE.2017070103

Isiugo-Abanihe, U. (1985). Child fosterage in West Africa. *Aging and Development*, 53-73.

Jacob, V., & Nuuyoma, V. (2019). Knowledge, attitudes and practices of University students on Malaria prevention in Kavango, East, Namibia. *Global Journal of Health Science*, *11*(2), 102–109. doi:10.5539/gjhs.v11n2p102

Jagan, J., Dalkiliç, Y., & Samui, P. (2016). Utilization of SVM, LSSVM and GP for Predicting the Medical Waste Generation. In G. Hua (Ed.), *Smart Cities as a Solution for Reducing Urban Waste and Pollution* (pp. 224–251). Hershey, PA: IGI Global. doi:10.4018/978-1-5225-0302-6.ch008

Jagiello, K., Sosnowska, A., Mikolajczyk, A., & Puzyn, T. (2017). Nanomaterials in Medical Devices: Regulations' Review and Future Perspectives. *Journal of Nanotoxicology and Nanomedicine*, *2*(2), 1–11. doi:10.4018/JNN.2017070101

Jaser, S. S. (2011). Family interaction in pediatric diabetes. *Current Diabetes Reports*, *11*(6), 480–485. doi:10.100711892-011-0222-y

Jayawardena, R., Ranasinghe, P., Chathuranga, T., Atapattu, P. M., & Misra, A. (2018). The benefits of yoga practice compared to physical exercise in the management of type 2 Diabetes Mellitus: A systematic review and meta-analysis. *Diabetes & Metabolic Syndrome*, *12*(5), 795–805. doi:10.1016/j.dsx.2018.04.008

Jena, T. K. (2018). Skill Training Process in Medicine Through Distance Mode. In U. Pandey & V. Indrakanti (Eds.), *Optimizing Open and Distance Learning in Higher Education Institutions* (pp. 228–243). Hershey, PA: IGI Global. doi:10.4018/978-1-5225-2624-7.ch010

Jesus, Â., & Gomes, M. J. (2016). Web 2.0 Tools in Biomedical and Pharmaceutical Education: Updated Review and Commentary. In T. Gasmelseid (Ed.), *Advancing Pharmaceutical Processes and Tools for Improved Health Outcomes* (pp. 52–78). Hershey, PA: IGI Global. doi:10.4018/978-1-5225-0248-7.ch003

Jezard, A. (2018). *World Economic Forum 2018: Depression is the no. 1 cause of ill-health and disability worldwide*. WEForum. Retrieved from https://www.weforum.org/agenda/2018/05/d

Johnson, T. C. (2019). Postpartum Depression. *WebMD*. Retrieved from http://www.webmd.com

Jombo, G. T., Mbaawuagu, E. M., Denen, A., Alao, O. O., Peters, E. J., Utsulo, S. J., & Etukumana, E. A. (2010). Sociocultural factors influencing the control of malaria in an endemic city in north central, Nigeria. *International Journal of Biological and Medical Research, 1*(4), 277–282.

Joseph, V., & Miller, J. M. (2018). Medical Students' Perceived Stigma in Seeking Care: A Cultural Perspective. In C. Smith (Ed.), *Exploring the Pressures of Medical Education From a Mental Health and Wellness Perspective* (pp. 44–67). Hershey, PA: IGI Global. doi:10.4018/978-1-5225-2811-1.ch002

Jose, S., Delpech, V., Howarth, A., Burns, F., Hill, T., Porter, K., ... Walsh, J.UK CHIC Study Steering Committee. (2018). A continuum of HIV care describing mortality and loss to follow-up: A longitudinal cohort study. *The Lancet. HIV*, *5*(6), e301–e308. doi:10.1016/S2352-3018(18)30048-1 PMID:29893243

Joyce, B. L., & Swanberg, S. M. (2017). Using Backward Design for Competency-Based Undergraduate Medical Education. In J. Stefaniak (Ed.), *Advancing Medical Education Through Strategic Instructional Design* (pp. 53–76). Hershey, PA: IGI Global. doi:10.4018/978-1-5225-2098-6.ch003

Kagotho, N., & Ssewamala, F. M. (2012). Correlates of depression among caregivers of children affected by HIV/AIDS in Uganda: Findings from the Suubi-Maka family study. *AIDS Care, 24*(10), 1226–1232. doi:10.1080/09540121.2012.658754 PMID:22375826

Kahiurika, N. (2019). *Tobacco plant approval draws criticism.* The Namibian Newspaper. Retrieved from https://www.namibian.com.na/189733/archive-read/Tobacco-plant-approval-draws-criticism

Kak, L., Chitsike, I., Luo, C., & Rollins, N. (2011). *Prevention of Mother-To-Child Transmission of HIV/AIDS programs, opportunities for Africa's newborns: Practical data, policy and programmatic support for newborn care in Africa.* Retrieved from www.who.int/pmnch/media/publications/oanfullreport.pdf

Kalichman, S. C., & Simbayi, L. C. (2003). HIV testing attitudes, AIDS stigma and voluntary HIV counseling and testing in a black township in Cape Town, South Africa. *Sexually Transmitted Infections*, *79*(6), 442–447. doi:10.1136ti.79.6.442 PMID:14663117

Kaljo, K., & Jacques, L. (2018). Flipping the Medical School Classroom. In M. Khosrow-Pour, D.B.A. (Ed.), Encyclopedia of Information Science and Technology, Fourth Edition (pp. 5800-5809). Hershey, PA: IGI Global. doi:10.4018/978-1-5225-2255-3.ch504

Kalomo, E.N., & Besthorn, F.H. (2018). Elderly grandmothers raising orphans and vulnerable children affected by HIV/AIDS in sub-Saharan Africa: A literature review and emerging efforts in Namibia. *GrandFamilies: The Contemporary Journal of Research, Practice and Policy, 5*(1).

Kalomo, E. N. (2017). Associations between HIV-related stigma, self-esteem, social support, and depressive symptoms in Namibia. *Aging & Mental Health*. PMID:29019412

Kalomo, E. N., Kyoung, H. L., & Besthorn, F. H. (2017). Depressive symptoms among older, female caregivers raising children affected by HIV/AIDS in the Omusati Region of Namibia. *Health Care for Women International*, *38*(12), 1327–1343. doi:10.1080/07399332.2017.1368514 PMID:28850326

Kalomo, E. N., & Liao, M. (2018). Burden of care among caregivers of persons living with HIV/AIDS in rural Namibia. *Social Work in Public Health*, *33*(1), 70–84. doi:10.1080/19371918.2017.1415180 PMID:29297790

Kamenov, K., Mellor-Marsa, B., Leal, I., Ayuso-Mateos, J. L., & Cabello, M. (2014). Analysing psychosocial difficulties in depression: A content comparison between systematic literature review and patient perspective. Biomed Research International. Retrieved from https://www.ncbi.nlm.nih.gov/

Kampala Dispatch. (2017). *Low HIV load suppression worries Kabarole medics*. Available online:http://dispatch.ug/2017/11/21/low-hiv-viral-load-suppression-worries-kabarole-medics/

Kampala, L. T. (2019). Explaining the World daily: What is sub-Saharan Africa? The Economist explains. Retrieved from http://www.economist.com

Kamya, H., & Poindexter, C. C. (2009). Mama Jaja: The stresses and strengths of HIV-affected Ugandan grandmothers. *Social Work in Public Health*, *24*(1-2), 4–21. doi:10.1080/19371910802569294 PMID:19229769

Kaplan, H. I., Sadock, B. J., & Grebb, J. A. (1994). *Kaplan and Sadock's synopsis of psychiatry* (8th ed.). Baltimore, ML: Williams & Wilkins.

Karon, R. (2016). Utilisation of Health Information Systems for Service Delivery in the Namibian Environment. In T. Iyamu & A. Tatnall (Eds.), *Maximizing Healthcare Delivery and Management through Technology Integration* (pp. 169–183). Hershey, PA: IGI Global. doi:10.4018/978-1-4666-9446-0.ch011

Kasina, H., Bahubalendruni, M. V., & Botcha, R. (2017). Robots in Medicine: Past, Present and Future. *International Journal of Manufacturing, Materials, and Mechanical Engineering*, *7*(4), 44–64. doi:10.4018/IJMMME.2017100104

Katehakis, D. G. (2018). Electronic Medical Record Implementation Challenges for the National Health System in Greece. *International Journal of Reliable and Quality E-Healthcare*, *7*(1), 16–30. doi:10.4018/IJRQEH.2018010102

Katz, A., & Shtub, A. (2016). Design and Build a Wizard of Oz (WOZ) Telemedicine Simulator Platform. In M. Cruz-Cunha, I. Miranda, R. Martinho, & R. Rijo (Eds.), *Encyclopedia of E-Health and Telemedicine* (pp. 128–141). Hershey, PA: IGI Global. doi:10.4018/978-1-4666-9978-6.ch011

Kaur, P. D., & Sharma, P. (2017). Success Dimensions of ICTs in Healthcare. In B. Singh (Ed.), *Computational Tools and Techniques for Biomedical Signal Processing* (pp. 149–173). Hershey, PA: IGI Global. doi:10.4018/978-1-5225-0660-7.ch007

Kaushik, P. (2018). Comorbidity of Medical and Psychiatric Disorders in Geriatric Population: Treatment and Care. In B. Prasad & S. Akbar (Eds.), *Handbook of Research on Geriatric Health, Treatment, and Care* (pp. 448–474). Hershey, PA: IGI Global. doi:10.4018/978-1-5225-3480-8.ch025

Kay, E. S., Batey, D. S., & Mugavero, M. J. (2016). The HIV treatment cascade and care continuum: Updates, goals, and recommendations for the future. *AIDS Research and Therapy*, *13*(1), 35. doi:10.118612981-016-0120-0 PMID:27826353

Kayono-Male, H., & Onyango, P. (1984). *The sociology of the African family*. London: Longman.

Kelly, S. J., Whitley, D. M., & Campos, P. E. (2013). Psychological distress in African American grandmothers raising grandchildren: The contribution of child behavior problems, physical health, and family resources. *Research in Nursing & Health*, *36*(4), 373–385. doi:10.1002/nur.21542 PMID:23606233

Kendzor, D. E., Chen, M., Reininger, B. M., Businelle, M. S., Stewart, D. W., Fisher-Hoch, S. P., & McCormick, J. B. (2014). The association of depression and anxiety with glycemic control among Mexican Americans with diabetes living near the U.S.-Mexico border. *BMC Public Health*, *14*(1), 176. doi:10.1186/1471-2458-14-176

Kessler, R. C., Berglund, P., Demler, O., Jin, R., Merikangas, K. R., & Walters, E. E. (2005). Lifetime prevalence and age-of-onset distributions of DSM-IV disorders in the National Comorbidity Survey Replication. *Archives of General Psychiatry*, *62*(6), 593–602. doi:10.1001/archpsyc.62.6.593 PMID:15939837

Kessler, R. C., Chiu, W. T., & Demler Walters, E. E. (2005). prevalence, severity, and comorbidity of 12- month DSM-IV disorders in the National comorbidity survey Replication. *Archives of General Psychiatry*, *62*(6), 617–627. doi:10.1001/archpsyc.62.6.617 PMID:15939839

Keulder, C. (2011). *Positive vibes. HIV/AIDS and stigma in Namibia: Results of a qualitative study among support group members*. Retrieved from https://www.positivevibes.org/02_Stigma%20report.pdf

Keyserling, T. C., Samuel-Hodge, C. D., Ammerman, A. S., Ainsworth, B. E., Henriquez-Roldan, C. F., Elasy, T. A., ... Bangdiwala, S. I. (2002). A randomized trial of an intervention to improve self-care behaviors of African-American women with type 2 diabetes: Impact on physical activity. *Diabetes Care*, *25*(9), 1576–1583. doi:10.2337/diacare.25.9.1576

Khachane, M. Y. (2017). Organ-Based Medical Image Classification Using Support Vector Machine. *International Journal of Synthetic Emotions*, *8*(1), 18–30. doi:10.4018/IJSE.2017010102

Khan, P., Qayyum, N., Malik, F., Khan, T., Khan, M., & Tahir, A. (2019). Incidence of anxiety and depression among patients with type 2 diabetes and the predicting factors. *Cureus*, *11*(3), e4254. doi:10.7759/cureus.4254

Kharsany, A. B. M., & Karim, Q. A. (2016). HIV infection and AIDS in sub-Saharan Africa: Current status, challenges and opportunities. *The Open AIDS Journal, 10*(1), 34–48. doi:10.2174/1874613601610010034 PMID:27347270

Khumbulani, W. H., Musawenkosi, L. H., Mabaso, S. K., Dayanandan, G., & Rajendra, M. (2009). Community knowledge, attitudes and practices (KAP) on malaria in Swaziland, a country earmarked for malaria elimination. *Malaria Journal, 8*(1), 29–36. doi:10.1186/1475-2875-8-29 PubMed

Kiggundu, E., & Oldewage-Theron, W. (2009). Coping: A challenge for guardians of children orphaned by HIV/AIDS in a South African Township. *Development Southern Africa, 26*(3), 383–397. doi:10.1080/03768350903086754

Kipp, W., Matukala, T., Laing, L., & Jhangri, G. S. (2006). Care burden and self-reported health status of informal women caregivers of HIV/AIDS patients in Kinshasa, Democratic Republic of Congo. *AIDS Care, 18*(7), 694–697. doi:10.1080/13548500500294401 PMID:16971277

Kirci, P. (2018). Intelligent Techniques for Analysis of Big Data About Healthcare and Medical Records. In N. Shah & M. Mittal (Eds.), *Handbook of Research on Promoting Business Process Improvement Through Inventory Control Techniques* (pp. 559–582). Hershey, PA: IGI Global. doi:10.4018/978-1-5225-3232-3.ch029

Kldiashvili, E. (2016). Cloud Computing as the Useful Resource for Application of the Medical Information System for Quality Assurance Purposes. *International Journal of Computers in Clinical Practice, 1*(2), 1–23. doi:10.4018/IJCCP.2016070101

Kldiashvili, E. (2018). Cloud Approach for the Medical Information System: MIS on Cloud. In M. Khosrow-Pour (Ed.), *Incorporating Nature-Inspired Paradigms in Computational Applications* (pp. 238–261). Hershey, PA: IGI Global. doi:10.4018/978-1-5225-5020-4.ch008

Kldiashvili, E., Burduli, A., Ghortlishvili, G., & Sheklashvili, I. (2016). Georgian Experience in Telecytology. In M. Cruz-Cunha, I. Miranda, R. Martinho, & R. Rijo (Eds.), *Encyclopedia of E-Health and Telemedicine* (pp. 62–71). Hershey, PA: IGI Global. doi:10.4018/978-1-4666-9978-6.ch006

Kline, M. W. (2006). Perspective on the pediatric HIV/AIDS pandemic: Catalyzing access of children to care and treatment. *Pediatrics, 117*(4), 1388–1393. doi:10.1542/peds.2005-1348 PMID:16585337

Ko, H., Mesicek, L., Choi, J., Choi, J., & Hwang, S. (2018). A Study on Secure Contents Strategies for Applications With DRM on Cloud Computing. *International Journal of Cloud Applications and Computing, 8*(1), 143–153. doi:10.4018/IJCAC.2018010107

Komendziński, T., Dreszer-Drogorób, J., Mikołajewska, E., Mikołajewski, D., & Bałaj, B. (2016). Interdisciplinary Education for Research and Everyday Clinical Practice: Lessons Learned from InteRDoCTor Project. In A. Rosiek & K. Leksowski (Eds.), *Organizational Culture and Ethics in Modern Medicine* (pp. 78–110). Hershey, PA: IGI Global. doi:10.4018/978-1-4666-9658-7.ch004

Komendziński, T., Mikołajewska, E., & Mikołajewski, D. (2018). Cross-Cultural Decision-Making in Healthcare: Theory and Practical Application in Real Clinical Conditions. In A. Rosiek-Kryszewska & K. Leksowski (Eds.), *Healthcare Administration for Patient Safety and Engagement* (pp. 276–298). Hershey, PA: IGI Global. doi:10.4018/978-1-5225-3946-9.ch015

Konecny, L. T. (2018). Medical School Wellness Initiatives. In C. Smith (Ed.), *Exploring the Pressures of Medical Education From a Mental Health and Wellness Perspective* (pp. 209–228). Hershey, PA: IGI Global. doi:10.4018/978-1-5225-2811-1.ch009

Konieczna, A., & Słomkowski, P. (2016). Confrontation of Human Rights in Daily Clinical Situations. In A. Rosiek & K. Leksowski (Eds.), *Organizational Culture and Ethics in Modern Medicine* (pp. 255–281). Hershey, PA: IGI Global. doi:10.4018/978-1-4666-9658-7.ch011

Korthuis, P. T., & Edelman, E. J. (2018). Substance use and the HIV care continuum: Important advances. *Addiction Science & Clinical Practice*, *13*(1), 13. doi:10.118613722-018-0114-4 PMID:29530080

Kromrei, H., Solomonson, W. L., & Juzych, M. S. (2017). Teaching Residents How to Teach. In J. Stefaniak (Ed.), *Advancing Medical Education Through Strategic Instructional Design* (pp. 164–185). Hershey, PA: IGI Global. doi:10.4018/978-1-5225-2098-6.ch008

Kropotov, J. D. (2009). *Quantitative EMG, event-related potentials and neurotherapy*. San Diego, CA: Academic Press.

Kruger, G., Burke, A., & Harper, M. (2006). *Psychology for nurses*. Pretoria: Van Schaik.

Kruse, J., Schmitz, N., & Thefeld, W. (2003). German National Health Interview and Examination Survey On the association between diabetes and mental disorders in a community sample: Results from the German National Health Interview and Examination Survey. *Diabetes Care*, *26*(6), 1841–1846. doi:10.2337/diacare.26.6.1841

Kulkarni, S., Savyanavar, A., Kulkarni, P., Stranieri, A., & Ghorpade, V. (2018). Framework for Integration of Medical Image and Text-Based Report Retrieval to Support Radiological Diagnosis. In M. Kolekar & V. Kumar (Eds.), *Biomedical Signal and Image Processing in Patient Care* (pp. 86–122). Hershey, PA: IGI Global. doi:10.4018/978-1-5225-2829-6.ch006

Kumar, A., & Sarkar, B. K. (2018). Performance Analysis of Nature-Inspired Algorithms-Based Bayesian Prediction Models for Medical Data Sets. In U. Singh, A. Tiwari, & R. Singh (Eds.), *Soft-Computing-Based Nonlinear Control Systems Design* (pp. 134–155). Hershey, PA: IGI Global. doi:10.4018/978-1-5225-3531-7.ch007

Kuo, C., & Operario, D. (2011). Health of adults caring for orphaned children in an HIV-endemic community in South Africa. *AIDS Care*, *23*(9), 1128–1135. doi:10.1080/09540121.2011.554527 PMID:21480009

Kurtz, R. S. (2016). Fortitude: A Study of African Americans in Surgery in New York City. In U. Thomas & J. Drake (Eds.), *Critical Research on Sexism and Racism in STEM Fields* (pp. 153–169). Hershey, PA: IGI Global. doi:10.4018/978-1-5225-0174-9.ch009

Kuyini, A. B., Alhassan, A. R., Tollerud, I., Weld, H., & Haruna, I. (2009). Traditional experiences and views of children and carers and adults in Tamle. *Child & Family Social Work*, *14*, 440–449. doi:10.1111/j.1365-2206.2009.00616.x

La Greca, A. M., Swales, T., Klemp, S., Madigan, S., & Skyler, J. (1995). Adolescents with diabetes: Gender differences in psychosocial functioning and glycemic control. *Children's Health Care*, *24*(1), 61–78. doi:10.120715326888chc2401_6

Labbadi, W., & Akaichi, J. (2017). Efficient Algorithm for Answering Fuzzy Medical Requests in Pervasive Healthcare Information Systems. *International Journal of Healthcare Information Systems and Informatics*, *12*(2), 46–64. doi:10.4018/IJHISI.2017040103

Lagumdzija, A., & Swing, V. K. (2017). Health, Digitalization, and Individual Empowerment. In F. Topor (Ed.), *Handbook of Research on Individualism and Identity in the Globalized Digital Age* (pp. 380–402). Hershey, PA: IGI Global. doi:10.4018/978-1-5225-0522-8.ch017

Lamey, T. W., & Davidson-Shivers, G. V. (2017). Instructional Strategies and Sequencing. In J. Stefaniak (Ed.), *Advancing Medical Education Through Strategic Instructional Design* (pp. 30–52). Hershey, PA: IGI Global. doi:10.4018/978-1-5225-2098-6.ch002

Lam, K. Y. (2015). Disclosure and psychological well-being of sexually abused adolescents in Hong Kong. *Journal of Child Sexual Abuse*, *24*(7), 731–752. doi:10.1080/10538712.2015.1077364

Laureate. (2014). *Smoking kills so why do people do it*. (Pt. 2).

Laxaminarayna, R., & Murthy, S. (2006). Mental Health Consequences of war: A Brief Review of Research Findings. *World Psychiatry; Official Journal of the World Psychiatric Association (WPA)*. PMID:16757987

Lee, C. H., & Yoon, H. J. (2017). *'Medical big data: Promise and challenges'. Kidney Research and Clinical Practice*, *36*(1), 461–475. doi:10.23876/j.krcp.2017.36.1.3

Lee, C. M., Chang, C. F., Pan, M. Y., Hsu, T. H., & Chen, M. Y. (2017). Depression and its associated factors among rural diabetic residents. *The Journal of Nursing Research*, *25*(1), 31–40. doi:10.1097/jnr.0000000000000143

Lee, P. G., & Halter, J. B. (2017). The pathophysiology of hyperglycemia in older adults: Clinical considerations. *Diabetes Care*, *40*(4), 444–452. doi:10.2337/dc16-1732

Lehman, B.J., David, D.M., & Gruber, J.A. (2017). Rethinking the biopsychosocial model of health: Understanding health as a dynamic system. *Social and Personality Psychology Compass*, *11*, 8.

LeMessurier, J., Traversy, G., Varsaneux, O., Weekes, M., Avey, M. T., Niragira, O., ... & Rodin, R. (2018). Risk of sexual transmission of human immunodeficiency viral load and condom use: A systematic review. *Canadian Medical Association Journal*, *190*(46), E1350–E1360. doi:10.1503/cmaj.180311 PMID:30455270

Leon, G. (2017). The Role of Forensic Medicine in Medical Errors. In M. Riga (Ed.), *Impact of Medical Errors and Malpractice on Health Economics, Quality, and Patient Safety* (pp. 144–170). Hershey, PA: IGI Global. doi:10.4018/978-1-5225-2337-6.ch006

Levine, K. A., Proulx, J., & Schwartz, K. (2018). Disconnected lives: Women with intellectual disabilities in conflict with the law. *Journal of Applied Research in Intellectual Disabilities*, *31*(2), 249–258. doi:10.1111/jar.12387

Lidia, B., Federica, G., & Maria, V. E. (2016). The Patient-Centered Medicine as the Theoretical Framework for Patient Engagement. In G. Graffigna (Ed.), *Promoting Patient Engagement and Participation for Effective Healthcare Reform* (pp. 25–39). Hershey, PA: IGI Global. doi:10.4018/978-1-4666-9992-2.ch002

Lieber, A. (2017). Understanding Atypical Depression: Symptoms & Treatment. Psycom. Retrieved from https://www.psycom.net

Lightfoot, E., & Kalomo, E. N. (2010). The interplay of population aging and HIV/AIDS on social development in Southern Africa: The case of Namibia. *Social Development Issues*, *32*(1), 1–15.

Li, L. F., Chan, R. L. Y., Lu, L., Shen, J., Zhang, L., Wu, W. K. K., ... Cho, C. H. (2014). Cigarette smoking and gastrointestinal diseases: The causal relationship and underlying molecular mechanisms [Review]. *International Journal of Molecular Medicine*, *34*(2), 372–380. doi:10.3892/ijmm.2014.1786 PMID:24859303

Lindner, L. M. E., Rathmann, W., & Rosenbauer, J. (2018). Inequalities in glycaemic control, hypoglycaemia and diabetic ketoacidosis according to socio-economic status and area-level deprivation in Type 1 diabetes mellitus: A systematic review. *Diabetic Medicine*, *35*(1), 12–32. doi:10.1111/dme.13519

Lindsey, E., Hirschfeld, M., Tlou, S., & Ncube, M. (2003). Home-based care in Botswana: Experiences of older women and young girls. *Health Care for Women International*, *24*(6), 486–501. doi:10.1080/07399330390199384 PMID:12851169

Littrell, M., Murphy, L., Kumwenda, M., & Macintyre, K. (2012). Gogo Care and protection of vulnerable children in rural Malawi: Changing responsibilities, capacity to provide, and implications for well-being in the era of HIV and AIDS. *Journal of Cross-Cultural Gerontology*, *27*(4), 335–355. doi:10.100710823-012-9174-1 PMID:22869344

Love, L., & McDowelle, D. (2018). Developing a Comprehensive Wellness Program for Medical Students. In C. Smith (Ed.), *Exploring the Pressures of Medical Education From a Mental Health and Wellness Perspective* (pp. 190–208). Hershey, PA: IGI Global. doi:10.4018/978-1-5225-2811-1.ch008

Lovell, K. L. (2017). Development and Evaluation of Neuroscience Computer-Based Modules for Medical Students: Instructional Design Principles and Effectiveness. In J. Stefaniak (Ed.), *Advancing Medical Education Through Strategic Instructional Design* (pp. 262–276). Hershey, PA: IGI Global. doi:10.4018/978-1-5225-2098-6.ch013

Lubin, R., & Hamlin, M. D. (2018). Medical Student Burnout: A Social Cognitive Learning Perspective on Medical Student Mental Health and Wellness. In C. Smith (Ed.), *Exploring the Pressures of Medical Education From a Mental Health and Wellness Perspective* (pp. 92–121). Hershey, PA: IGI Global. doi:10.4018/978-1-5225-2811-1.ch004

Luk, C. Y. (2018). Moving Towards Universal Health Coverage: Challenges for the Present and Future in China. In B. Fong, A. Ng, & P. Yuen (Eds.), *Sustainable Health and Long-Term Care Solutions for an Aging Population* (pp. 19–45). Hershey, PA: IGI Global. doi:10.4018/978-1-5225-2633-9.ch002

Lundgren, J. D., Babiker, A. G., Gordin, F., Emery, S., & Grund, B. (2015). INSIGHT Start Study Group. Initiation of antiretroviral therapy in early asymptomatic HIV infection. *The New England Journal of Medicine, 373*(9), 795–807. doi:10.1056/NEJMoa1506816 PMID:26192873

Lyons-Ruth, K., Wolfe, R., & Lyubchik, A. (2000). Depression and parenting of young children: Making the case for early preventative mental health services. *Harvard Review of Psychiatry, 8*(3), 148–153. doi:10.1080/hrp_8.3.148 PMID:10973939

Maartens, G., Celum, C., & Lewin, S. R. (2014). HIV infection: Epidemiology, pathogenesis, treatment and prevention. *Lancet, 384*(9939), 258–271. doi:10.1016/S0140-6736(14)60164-1 PMID:24907868

MacArthur, C., Knox, E. G., & Lancashire, R. J. (2001, January). Effects at age nine of maternal smoking in pregnancy: Experimental and observational findings. *BJOG, 108*(1), 67–73. doi:10.1111/j.1471-0528.2001.00006.x PMID:11213007

Madhavan, S., Schatz, E., Gomes-Olive, F. X., & Collinson, W. (2017). Social positioning of older persons in rural South Africa. *Change or Stability or Journal of South African Studies, 43*(6), 1293–1307. doi:10.1080/03057070.2017.1365522 PMID:30686854

Mahat, M., & Pettigrew, A. (2017). The Regulatory Environment of Non-Profit Higher Education and Research Institutions and Its Implications for Managerial Strategy: The Case of Medical Education and Research. In L. West & A. Worthington (Eds.), *Handbook of Research on Emerging Business Models and Managerial Strategies in the Nonprofit Sector* (pp. 336–351). Hershey, PA: IGI Global. doi:10.4018/978-1-5225-2537-0.ch017

Maia, A. C., Braga Ade, A., Brouwers, A., Nardi, A. E., & Oliveira e Silva, A. C. (2012). Prevalence of psychiatric disorders in patients with diabetes types 1 and 2. *Comprehensive Psychiatry, 53*(8), 1169–1173. doi:10.1016/j.comppsych.2012.03.011

Maitra, I. K., & Bandhyopadhyaay, S. K. (2017). Adaptive Edge Detection Method towards Features Extraction from Diverse Medical Imaging Technologies. In S. Bhattacharyya, S. De, I. Pan, & P. Dutta (Eds.), *Intelligent Multidimensional Data Clustering and Analysis* (pp. 159–192). Hershey, PA: IGI Global. doi:10.4018/978-1-5225-1776-4.ch007

Malawi Malaria Indicator Survey. (2017). MMIS document: Ministry of health. National Malaria Control Program. Retrieved from https://dhsprogram.com/pubs/pdf/mis28/pdf

Mangu, V. P. (2017). Mobile Health Care: A Technology View. In C. Bhatt & S. Peddoju (Eds.), *Cloud Computing Systems and Applications in Healthcare* (pp. 1–18). Hershey, PA: IGI Global. doi:10.4018/978-1-5225-1002-4.ch001

Manirabona, A., Fourati, L. C., & Boudjit, S. (2017). Investigation on Healthcare Monitoring Systems: Innovative Services and Applications. *International Journal of E-Health and Medical Communications*, *8*(1), 1–18. doi:10.4018/IJEHMC.2017010101

Mannai, M. M., & Karâa, W. B. (2016). Biomedical Image Processing Overview. In W. Karâa & N. Dey (Eds.), *Biomedical Image Analysis and Mining Techniques for Improved Health Outcomes* (pp. 1–12). Hershey, PA: IGI Global. doi:10.4018/978-1-4666-8811-7.ch001

Mannucci, E., Rotella, F., Ricca, V., Moretti, S., Placidi, G. F., & Rotella, C. M. (2005). Eating disorders in patients with type 1 diabetes: A meta-analysis. *Journal of Endocrinological Investigation*, *28*(7), 417–419. doi:10.1007/BF03347221

Manzoor, A. (2016). RFID in Health Care-Building Smart Hospitals for Quality Healthcare. *International Journal of User-Driven Healthcare*, *6*(2), 21–45. doi:10.4018/IJUDH.2016070102

Margoob, A. M., & Ahmad, S. A. (2006). Community prevalence of adult post traumatic stress disorder in south Asia: Experience from Kashmir. *Jammu Kashmir Practitioner*, *13*(1), S18–S25.

Margoob, A. M., Firdosi, M. M., Ali, Z., Hussain, A., Mushtaq, H., Khan, A. Y., & ... Muzamil, M. (2006). Treatment seeking post-traumatic stress disorder patient population - Experience from Kashmir. *Jammu and Kashmir Practitioner*, *13*(1), S57–S60.

Margoob, M. A., Beg, A. A., & Dutta, K. S. (1993). Depressive disorders in kashmir; A changing Socio Demographic and Clinical Profile of patients over the past two decades. *JK Practitioner*, 22–24.

Mariotti, A. (2015). The effects of chronic stress on health: New insights into the molecular mechanisms of brain-body communication. *Future Science OA*, *1*(3), FSO23. doi:10.4155/fso.15.21

Marston, M., Michael, D., Wringe, A., Isingo, R., Clark, B. D., Jonas, A., ... Urassa, M. (2012). The impact of antiretroviral therapy on adult mortality in rural Tanzania. *Tropical Medicine & International Health*, *17*(8), 58–65. doi:10.1111/j.1365-3156.2011.02924.x PMID:22943380

Martin, B. (2018). What are the risk factors for depression? Psych Central. Retrieved from https://www.com

Marufu, C. T., Ahankari, A., Coleman, T., & Lewis, S. (2015). Maternal smoking and the risk of still birth: Systematic review and meta-analysis. *BMC Public Health*, *15*(239), 1–15. doi:10.118612889-015-1552-5 PMID:25885887

Marwan, M., Kartit, A., & Ouahmane, H. (2018). A Framework to Secure Medical Image Storage in Cloud Computing Environment. *Journal of Electronic Commerce in Organizations*, *16*(1), 1–16. doi:10.4018/JECO.2018010101

Mascolini, M. (2010). HIV raises heart disease risk 60% in people over 49. In *Proceedings of the XVIII International AIDS Conference*. Academic Press.

Masoud, M. P., Nejad, M. K., Darebaghi, H., Chavoshi, M., & Farahani, M. (2018). The Decision Support System and Conventional Method of Telephone Triage by Nurses in Emergency Medical Services: A Comparative Investigation. *International Journal of E-Business Research, 14*(1), 77–88. doi:10.4018/IJEBR.2018010105

Mazigo, H. D., Obasy, E., Mauka, W., Manyiri, P., Zinga, M., Kweka, E. J., & Henkelbach, J. (2010). Knowledge, attitude and practices about malaria and its control in rural North West Tanzania. *Malaria Research and Treatment, 10*, 1–9. doi:10.4061/2010/794261 PubMed

McCrae, R. R., & Costa, P. T. (2008). The five-factor theory of personality. In O. P. John, R. W. Robins, & L. A. Pervin (Eds.), *Handbook of personality: Theory and research* (Vol. 3, pp. 159–181). New York, NY: Guilford Press.

McDonald, W. G., Martin, M., & Salzberg, L. D. (2018). From Medical Student to Medical Resident: Graduate Medical Education and Mental Health in the United States. In C. Smith (Ed.), *Exploring the Pressures of Medical Education From a Mental Health and Wellness Perspective* (pp. 145–169). Hershey, PA: IGI Global. doi:10.4018/978-1-5225-2811-1.ch006

Médecins Sans Frontières. (2012). *Undetectable-how viral load monitoring can improve HIV treatment in developing countries*. Geneva: Médecins Sans Frontières.

Medhekar, A. (2017). The Role of Social Media for Knowledge Dissemination in Medical Tourism: A Case of India. In R. Chugh (Ed.), *Harnessing Social Media as a Knowledge Management Tool* (pp. 25–54). Hershey, PA: IGI Global. doi:10.4018/978-1-5225-0495-5.ch002

Medhekar, A., & Haq, F. (2018). Urbanization and New Jobs Creation in Healthcare Services in India: Challenges and Opportunities. In U. Benna & I. Benna (Eds.), *Urbanization and Its Impact on Socio-Economic Growth in Developing Regions* (pp. 198–218). Hershey, PA: IGI Global. doi:10.4018/978-1-5225-2659-9.ch010

Mehta, G., Dutta, M. K., & Kim, P. S. (2016). An Efficient and Lossless Cryptosystem for Security in Tele-Ophthalmology Applications Using Chaotic Theory. *International Journal of E-Health and Medical Communications, 7*(4), 28–47. doi:10.4018/IJEHMC.2016100102

Mehta, P. (2017). Framework of Indian Healthcare System and its Challenges: An Insight. In V. Bryan & J. Bird (Eds.), *Healthcare Community Synergism between Patients, Practitioners, and Researchers* (pp. 247–271). Hershey, PA: IGI Global. doi:10.4018/978-1-5225-0640-9.ch011

Mendenhall, E., & Norris, S. A. (2015). When HIV is ordinary and diabetes new: Remaking suffering in a South African township. *Global Public Health: An International Journal for Research, Policy and Practice, 10*(4), 449–462. doi:10.1080/17441692.2014.998698 PMID:25643001

Mercy Corps. (2011). *Youth Entrepreneurship in Kashmir: challenges and opportunities. Kashmir*. Mercy Corp.

Metelmann, B., & Metelmann, C. (2016). M-Health in Prehospital Emergency Medicine: Experiences from the EU funded Project LiveCity. In A. Moumtzoglou (Ed.), *M-Health Innovations for Patient-Centered Care* (pp. 197–212). Hershey, PA: IGI Global. doi:10.4018/978-1-4666-9861-1.ch010

Meyers, T., Moulrie, H., Naidoo, K., Cotton, M., Eley, B., & ... (2007). Challenges to pediatric HIV care and treatment in South Africa. *The Journal of Infectious Diseases*, *196*(3), 474–481. doi:10.1086/521116 PMID:18181697

Mhaka-Mutepfa, M., Mpofu, E., & Cumming, R. (2014). Impact of protective factors on resilience of grandparent carers fostering orphans and non-orphans in Zimbabwe. *Journal of Aging and Health*, *27*(3), 454–479. doi:10.1177/0898264314551333 PMID:25260649

Middleton, L., Nicolson, G., & O'Neil, V. (2012). *Juta's nursing psychology: Applying psychological concepts to nursing practice*. Johannesburg: Juta.

Middleton, L., & Uys, L. (2014). *Mental Health Nursing: A South African Perspective* (6th ed.). Cape Town: Juta&Co.Ltd.

Miglioretti, M., Mariani, F., & Vecchio, L. (2016). Could Patient Engagement Promote a Health System Free From Malpractice Litigation Risk? In G. Graffigna (Ed.), *Promoting Patient Engagement and Participation for Effective Healthcare Reform* (pp. 240–264). Hershey, PA: IGI Global. doi:10.4018/978-1-4666-9992-2.ch012

Milburn, N. G., Stein, J. A., Lopez, S. A., Hilberg, A. M., Veprinsky, A., Arnold, E. M., ... Comulada, W. S. (2019). Trauma, family factors and the mental health of homeless adolescents. *Journal of Child & Adolescent Trauma*, *12*(1), 37–47. doi:10.100740653-017-0157-9

Millea, J.P., Brodie, J.J. (2002). Tension type headache. *American Family Physician*, *66*(5), 797-803.

Miller, C., Gruskin, S., Subramanian, S., Rajaraman, D., & Heymann, J. (2006). Orphan care in Botswana's working households: Growing responsibilities in the absence of adequate support. *American Journal of Public Health*, *96*(8), 1429–1435. doi:10.2105/AJPH.2005.072280 PMID:16809585

Miller-Cribbs, J. E., Wen, F., Coon, K. A., Jelley, M. J., Foulks-Rodriguez, K., & Stearns, J. (2016). Adverse childhood experiences and inequalities in adult health care access. *International Public Health Journal*, *8*(2), 257–270.

Miller, K. E., & Rasmussen, A. (2010). War exposure, daily stressors, and mental health in conflict and post-conflict settings: Bridging the divide between trauma-focused and psychosocial frameworks. *Social Science & Medicine*, *70*(1), 7–16. doi:10.1016/j.socscimed.2009.09.029 PMID:19854552

Mi, M. (2017). Informal Learning in Medical Education. In J. Stefaniak (Ed.), *Advancing Medical Education Through Strategic Instructional Design* (pp. 225–244). Hershey, PA: IGI Global. doi:10.4018/978-1-5225-2098-6.ch011

Ministry of Health and Social Services (MoHSS). (1995). *Integrated health care delivery: The challenge of implementation. A situational analysis and practical implementation guide*. Windhoek, Namibia: Government of the Republic of Namibia.

Ministry of Health and Social Services (MoHSS). (2006). *Progress Report on the Third Medium Term Plan on HIV/AIDS 2004–2006*. Windhoek: Directorate of Special Programmes, MOHSS.

Ministry of Health and Social Services (MoHSS). (2010a). *PHC Guidelines for Namibia*. Windhoek: Government of Republic of Namibia.

Ministry of Health and Social Services (MoHSS). (2010b). *National Community Based Care*. Windhoek: Government of Republic of Namibia.

Ministry of Health and Social Services (MoHSS). (2010c). *National Health Policy Framework 2010–2020*. Windhoek: Government of Republic of Namibia.

Ministry of Health and Social Services (MoHSS). (2013). *Namibia demographic and health services*. Windhoek: Government of Republic of Namibia.

Ministry of Health and Social Services. (2008). *National Policy on Community Based Health Care*. Windhoek: Directorate of Primary Care Services.

Ministry of Health and Social Services. (2010). *National policy for mental health*. Windhoek, Namibia.

Misra, S. C., & Bisui, S. (2016). Feasibility of Large Scale Implementation of Personalized Medicine in the Current Scenario. *International Journal of E-Health and Medical Communications*, *7*(2), 30–49. doi:10.4018/IJEHMC.2016040103

Misra, S. C., Bisui, S., & Fantazy, K. (2016). Identifying Critical Changes in Adoption of Personalized Medicine (PM) in Healthcare Management. *International Journal of E-Health and Medical Communications*, *7*(3), 1–15. doi:10.4018/IJEHMC.2016070101

Mohammadian, M., Hatzinakos, D., Spachos, P., & Jentzsh, R. (2016). An Intelligent and Secure Framework for Wireless Information Technology in Healthcare for User and Data Classification in Hospitals. In V. Wang (Ed.), *Handbook of Research on Advancing Health Education through Technology* (pp. 452–479). Hershey, PA: IGI Global. doi:10.4018/978-1-4666-9494-1.ch019

Mohan, D., Mander, H., Singh, N., Philipose, P., & Bose, T. (2018). Unending trauma: The heavy toll of ongoing violence on mental health in Kashmir. In Blood, censored: When Kashmiris Become the 'Enemy.' Yoda Press.

Mokeddem, S., & Atmani, B. (2016). Assessment of Clinical Decision Support Systems for Predicting Coronary Heart Disease. *International Journal of Operations Research and Information Systems*, *7*(3), 57–73. doi:10.4018/IJORIS.2016070104

Mokrzycka, A., & Kowalska-Bobko, I. (2016). Public Health Legislation and Patient's Rights: Health2020 Strategy, European Perspective. In A. Rosiek & K. Leksowski (Eds.), *Organizational Culture and Ethics in Modern Medicine* (pp. 298–322). Hershey, PA: IGI Global. doi:10.4018/978-1-4666-9658-7.ch013

Moon, J. D., & Galea, M. P. (2016). Overview of Clinical Decision Support Systems in Healthcare. In J. Moon & M. Galea (Eds.), *Improving Health Management through Clinical Decision Support Systems* (pp. 1–27). Hershey, PA: IGI Global. doi:10.4018/978-1-4666-9432-3.ch001

Moore, A. R. (2007-2008). Older poor parents who lost an adult child to AIDS in Togo, West Africa: A Qualitative study. *Omega*, *56*(3), 289–304. doi:10.2190/OM.56.3.e PMID:18300652

Moore, B., & Woodcock, S. (2017). Resilience, bullying, and mental health: Factors associated with improved outcomes. *Psychology in the Schools*, *54*(7), 689–702. doi:10.1002/pits.22028

Morojele, N. K., Brook, J. S., & Brook, D. W. (2016). Tobacco and Alcohol Use Among Adolescents in South Africa: Shared and Unshared Risks. *Journal of Child and Adolescent Mental Health*, *28*(2), 139–152. doi:10.2989/17280583.2016.1200586 PMID:27562001

Mosadeghrad, A. M., & Woldemichael, A. (2017). Application of Quality Management in Promoting Patient Safety and Preventing Medical Errors. In M. Riga (Ed.), *Impact of Medical Errors and Malpractice on Health Economics, Quality, and Patient Safety* (pp. 91–112). Hershey, PA: IGI Global. doi:10.4018/978-1-5225-2337-6.ch004

Moumtzoglou, A. (2017). Digital Medicine: The Quality Standpoint. In A. Moumtzoglou (Ed.), *Design, Development, and Integration of Reliable Electronic Healthcare Platforms* (pp. 179–195). Hershey, PA: IGI Global. doi:10.4018/978-1-5225-1724-5.ch011

Moumtzoglou, A., & Pouliakis, A. (2018). Population Health Management and the Science of Individuality. *International Journal of Reliable and Quality E-Healthcare*, *7*(2), 1–26. doi:10.4018/IJRQEH.2018040101

Mouradian, C., Naboulsi, D., Yangui, S., Glitho, R. H., Morrow, M. J., & Polakos, P. A. (2017). A comprehensive survey on fog computing: State-of-the-art and research challenges. IEEE Communications Surveys & Tutorials, 20(1), 416-464. Retrieved from https://ieeexplore.ieee.org/abstract/document/8100873/authors#authors

Mouri, M. I., & Badireddy, M. (2019). *Hyperglycemia*. StatPearls Publishing. Retrieved from https://www.ncbi.nlm.nih.gov/books/NBK430900/

Mpofu, C. (2016). International Medical Experiences Outbound New Zealand: An Economic and Medical Workforce Strategy. In D. Velliaris & D. Coleman-George (Eds.), *Handbook of Research on Study Abroad Programs and Outbound Mobility* (pp. 446–469). Hershey, PA: IGI Global. doi:10.4018/978-1-5225-0169-5.ch018

MSF. (n.d.). Kashmir Mental Health Survey-2015.

Muga, G. O., & Onyango-Ouma, W. (2009). Changing household composition and food security among the elderly caretakers in rural Western Kenya. *Journal of Cross-Cultural Gerontology*, *24*(3), 259–272. doi:10.100710823-008-9090-6 PMID:19137419

Mukhtar, W. F., & Abuelyaman, E. S. (2017). Opportunities and Challenges of Big Data in Healthcare. In N. Wickramasinghe (Ed.), *Handbook of Research on Healthcare Administration and Management* (pp. 47–58). Hershey, PA: IGI Global. doi:10.4018/978-1-5225-0920-2.ch004

Mullaly, J. W., Hall, K., & Goldstein, R. (2009, November/December). Efficacy of BF in the Treatment of Migraine and Tension Type Headaches. *Pain Physician*, *12*(1), 1005–1011. PMID:19935987

Munugala, S., Brar, G. K., Syed, A., Mohammad, A., & Halgamuge, M. N. (2018). The Much Needed Security and Data Reforms of Cloud Computing in Medical Data Storage. In M. Lytras & P. Papadopoulou (Eds.), *Applying Big Data Analytics in Bioinformatics and Medicine* (pp. 99–113). Hershey, PA: IGI Global. doi:10.4018/978-1-5225-2607-0.ch005

Musoke, D., Karani, G., Ssempebwa, J. C., Etajak, S., Guwatudde, D., & Musoke, B. M. (2015). Knowledge and practices on malaria prevention in two rural communities in Wakiss District, Ugandan. *African Health Sciences*, *15*(2), 401–412. doi:10.4314/ahs.v15i2.13 PubMed

Mychasiuk, R., Muhammad, A., Carroll, C., & Kolb, B. (2013). Does prenatal nicotine exposure alter the brain's response to nicotine in adolescence? A neuroanatomical analysis. *The European Journal of Neuroscience*, *38*(4), 2491–2503. doi:10.1111/ejn.12245 PMID:23679187

Naikaku.EN. (2018). *Knowledge, attitudes and practices of medical doctors on pharmacotherapy for smoking cessation in Khomas region, Namibia. Master in Public Health*. Windhoek: University of Namibia.

Namibia Population-Based HIV Impact Assessment (NAMPHIA). (2018). Summary Sheet: Preliminary Findings.

Namibia Tobacco Control Policies. (2006). Retrieved from https://www.tobaccocontrollaws.org/legislation/fakctsheet/policy_status/namibia

Narasimhamurthy, A. (2016). An Overview of Machine Learning in Medical Image Analysis: Trends in Health Informatics. In N. Dey & A. Ashour (Eds.), *Classification and Clustering in Biomedical Signal Processing* (pp. 23–45). Hershey, PA: IGI Global. doi:10.4018/978-1-5225-0140-4.ch002

National Institute for Health & Clinical Excellence. (2011). COMMON MENTAL HEALTH DISORDERS: The nice guideline on identification and pathways to care. The British Psychological Society & The Royal College of Psychiatrists. Leicester. United Kingdom. Retrieved from: https://www.ncbi.nlm.nih.gov/books/NBK92266/pdf/Bookshelf_NBK92266.pdf

Nemade, R., Staats Reiss, N. S., & Dombeck, M. (2015a). Current understanding of major depression: Biopsychosocial model. *MentalHelp.net*. Retrieved from https://www.mentalhelp.net

Nemade, R., Staats Reiss, N., & Dombeck, M. (2015b). *Sociology of depression: Effects of culture*. Retrieved from https://www.mentalhelp.net/

New Era Newspaper. (2015). Call for more alcoholism rehab Centres. Etrieved from https://neweralive.na/posts/calls-alcoholism-rehab-centres

Newcomb-Fernandez, J. (2003). Cancer in the HIV-infected population. *Research Initiative, Treatment Action*, *9*(1), 5–13. PMID:14971360

Ngara, R. (2017). Multiple Voices, Multiple Paths: Towards Dialogue between Western and Indigenous Medical Knowledge Systems. In P. Ngulube (Ed.), *Handbook of Research on Theoretical Perspectives on Indigenous Knowledge Systems in Developing Countries* (pp. 332–358). Hershey, PA: IGI Global. doi:10.4018/978-1-5225-0833-5.ch015

Nicolau, J., Simó, R., Sanchís, P., Ayala, L., Fortuny, R., Zubillaga, I., & Masmiquel, L. (2015). Eating disorders are frequent among Type 2 diabetic patients and are associated with worse metabolic and psychological outcomes: Results from a cross-sectional study in primary and secondary care settings. *Acta Diabetologica*, *52*(6), 1037–1044. doi:10.100700592-015-0742-z

Nigeria Federal Ministry of Health, Nigeria (2014). FMoHN and NMEP document: National Malaria Elimination Programme (NMEP, Nigeria) and the National Malaria Strategic Plan, 2014-2020.

Nigerian Centre for Diseases. (2016). NCDC document on Malaria: Protecting the health of Nigerians.

Njororai, F., &Njororai, W. W. S. (2012). Older adult caregivers to people with HIV/AIDS in sub-Saharan Africa: A review of literature and policy implications for change. *International Journal of Health Promotion and Education*. iFirst.

Nolen-Hoeksema, S. (2001). Gender differences in depression. *Current Directions in Psychological Science*.

Nouwen, A., Nefs, G., Caramlau, I., Connock, M., Winkley, K., Lloyd, C. E., ... Pouwer, F.European Depression in Diabetes Research Consortium. (2011). Prevalence of depression in individuals with impaired glucose metabolism or undiagnosed diabetes: A systematic review and meta-analysis of the European Depression in Diabetes (EDID) Research Consortium. *Diabetes Care*, *34*(3), 752–762. doi:10.2337/dc10-1414

Nurius, P. S., Green, S., Logan-Greene, P., Longhi, D., & Song, C. (2016). Stress pathways to health inequalities: Embedding ACEs within social and behavioral contexts. *International Public Health Journal*, *8*(2), 241–256.

Nyavor, K., Kweku, M., Agbemafle, I., Takramah, W., Norman, I., Tarkang, E., & Binka, F. (2017). Assessing the ownership, usage and knowledge of Insecticide Treated Nets (ITNs) in Malaria Prevention in the Hohoe-Municipality, Ghana. *The Pan African Medical Journal*, *28*, 67. doi:10.11604/pamj.2017.28.67.9934

O'Connor, Y., & Heavin, C. (2018). Defining and Characterising the Landscape of eHealth. In M. Khosrow-Pour, D.B.A. (Ed.), Encyclopedia of Information Science and Technology, Fourth Edition (pp. 5864-5875). Hershey, PA: IGI Global. doi:10.4018/978-1-5225-2255-3.ch510

O'Connor, C., Finkbiner, C., & Watson, L. (2012). *Adverse childhood experiences in Wisconsin: Findings from the 2010 behavioral risk factor survey*. Madison, WI: Wisconsin Children's Trust Fund and Child Abuse Prevention Fund of Children's Hospital and Health System.

Ochonogor, W. C., & Okite-Amughoro, F. A. (2018). Building an Effective Digital Library in a University Teaching Hospital (UTH) in Nigeria. In A. Tella & T. Kwanya (Eds.), *Handbook of Research on Managing Intellectual Property in Digital Libraries* (pp. 184–204). Hershey, PA: IGI Global. doi:10.4018/978-1-5225-3093-0.ch010

Ogunmefun, C., Gilbert, L., & Schatz, E. (2011). Older female caregivers and HIV/AIDS-related secondary stigma in rural South Africa. *Journal of Cross-Cultural Gerontology. Journal of Cross-Cultural Gerontology*, *27*(1), 85–102. doi:10.100710823-010-9129-3 PMID:20957421

Ojikutu, B., Higgins-Biddle, M., Greeson, D., Phelps, B. R., Amzel, A., Okechukwu, E., ... Hirschhorn, L. R. (2014). The association between quality of HIV care, loss to follow-up and mortality in pediatric and adolescent patients receiving antiretroviral therapy in Nigeria. *PLoS One*, *9*(7), e100039. doi:10.1371/journal.pone.0100039 PMID:25075742

Okafor, F. U., & Oko-Ose, J. N. (2012). Prevalence of malaria infections among children aged 6 months -11 years in a tertiary institution in Benin City, Nigeria. *Global Advanced Research Journal of Medicine and Medical Sciences*, *1*(10), 273–279.

Okafor, I. P., Ezekwe, C., Oluwole, E. O., & Onogbogi, O. O. (2019). A community based study on the knowledge, perception and prevention among Nigerian women. *Journal of Family Medicine and Primary Health Care*, *8*(40), 1359–1364.

Okwa, O. O. (2019). Nipping the malaria vectors in the bud: Focus on Nigeria: In Malaria. In-Tech Publishers. doi:10.5772.83554

Okwa, O. O., Bello, B. A., & Olundegun, S. A. (2011). Social Aspects of Malaria among Students in Two Tertiary Institutions in Lagos, Nigeria. Sierra Leone Journal Biomedical Research, 3(2), 97- 103. Retrieved from **Error! Hyperlink reference not valid.**www.sljbr.com

Okwa, O. O., Soremekun, B. M., Adeseko, O., & Raheem, A. M. (2012b). Artisans and traders knowledge, attitude and practices of malaria in selected areas of Lagos, Nigeria. Global Advanced Research Journal of Medicine and Medical Sciences, 1(3), 68-74. Retrieved from http://garj.org/garjmms/index.htm

Okwa, O. O., Akinmolayan, F. I., Carter, V., & Hurd, H. (2009). Transmission dynamics of malaria in four selected ecological zones of Nigeria in the rainy season. *Annals of African Medicine*, *8*(1), 1–9. Retrieved from http://www.ajol.info

Okwa, O. O., & Ibidapo, C. A. (2010). Malaria situation, perception of cause and treatment in a Nigerian University. *Journal of Medicine and Medical Sciences*, *1*(6), 213–222.

Okwa, O. O., Sanyaolu, L. O., & Olatokunbo, A. F. (2012a). Malaria and working performance of academic staff in a Nigerian University. *Research Journal of Biology*, *2*(5), 151–156.

Okwa, O. O., & Savage, A. (2018). Oviposition and breeding water sites preferences of mosquitoes within Ojo Area, Lagos State, Nigeria. *Biomedical Journal of Scientific and Technical Research*, *7*(5), 1–7. doi:10.26717/BJSTR.07.001565

Oladimeji, K. E., Tsoka-Gwegweni, J. M., Ojewole, E., & Yunga, S. T. (2019). Knowledge of malaria prevention among pregnant and non-pregnant mothers of children aged under 5 years in Ibadan, South West Nigeria. *Malaria Journal*, *18*(92), 92. doi:10.1186/s12936-019-2706-1 PubMed

Olaniran, B. A. (2016). ICT Use and Multidisciplinary Healthcare Teams in the Age of e-Health. *International Journal of Reliable and Quality E-Healthcare*, *5*(1), 18–31. doi:10.4018/IJRQEH.2016010102

Olaniran, B. A. (2016). ICTs, E-health, and Multidisciplinary Healthcare Teams: Promises and Challenges. *International Journal of Privacy and Health Information Management*, *4*(2), 62–75. doi:10.4018/IJPHIM.2016070105

Olivares, S. L., Cruz, A. G., Cabrera, M. V., Regalado, A. I., & García, J. E. (2017). An Assessment Study of Quality Model for Medical Schools in Mexico. In S. Mukerji & P. Tripathi (Eds.), *Handbook of Research on Administration, Policy, and Leadership in Higher Education* (pp. 404–439). Hershey, PA: IGI Global. doi:10.4018/978-1-5225-0672-0.ch016

Omidoyin, E. O., Opeke, R. O., & Osagbemi, G. K. (2016). Utilization Pattern and Privacy Issues in the use of Health Records for Research Practice by Doctors: Selected Nigerian Teaching Hospitals as Case Study. *International Journal of Privacy and Health Information Management*, *4*(1), 1–11. doi:10.4018/IJPHIM.2016010101

Omoruyi, E. A., & Omidele, F. (2018). Resident Physician and Medical Academic Faculty Burnout: A Review of Current Literature. In C. Smith (Ed.), *Exploring the Pressures of Medical Education From a Mental Health and Wellness Perspective* (pp. 171–189). Hershey, PA: IGI Global. doi:10.4018/978-1-5225-2811-1.ch007

Onah, I. E., Adesina, F. P., Uweh, P. O., & Anumba, J. U. (2017). Challenges of malaria elimination in Nigeria (A Review). *International Journal of Infectious Diseases and Therapy*, *2*(4), 79–85. doi:10.11648/j.ijidt.20170204.14

openPr. (2018). Antiviral drugs market: New investments expected to boost the demand with rising awareness regarding vast benefits to drive market. Retrieved from https://www.openpr.com/news/990905/Antiviral-Drugs-Market-New-Investments-Expected-to-boost-the-Demand-with-Rising-Awareness-Regarding-Vast-Benefits-to-Drive-Market.html

Ordinioha, B. (2012). The use and misuse of mass distributed free insecticide treated nets in a semi urban community in Rivers State, Nigeria. *Annals of African Medicine*, *11*(3), 163–168. doi:10.4103/1596-3519.96879 PubMed

Osop, H., & Sahama, T. (2016). Data-Driven and Practice-Based Evidence: Design and Development of Efficient and Effective Clinical Decision Support System. In J. Moon & M. Galea (Eds.), *Improving Health Management through Clinical Decision Support Systems* (pp. 295–328). Hershey, PA: IGI Global. doi:10.4018/978-1-4666-9432-3.ch014

Ossowski, R., & Izdebski, P. (2016). Ethical Aspects of Talking to a Patient. In A. Rosiek & K. Leksowski (Eds.), *Organizational Culture and Ethics in Modern Medicine* (pp. 203–235). Hershey, PA: IGI Global. doi:10.4018/978-1-4666-9658-7.ch009

Owusu, D. A., Cremer, A. L., Brown, C. A., & Grosbusch, M. (2018). Knowledge, attitudes and practices regarding malaria in people living with HIV in rural and urban Ghana. *Acta Tropica*, *181*, 16–20. doi:10.1016/j.actatropica.2018.01.016 PubMed

Oyedeji, O. A., Elemile, P. O., Adepoju, A. A., & Oyedeji, G. A. (2009). An evaluation of the use of ITNs among children presenting with malaria at a Nigerian health facility. *International Journal of Medical and Medical Sciences*, *1*(11), 501–504.

Ozougwu, J. C., Obimba, K., Belonwu, C. D., & Unakalamba, C. B. (2013). The pathogenesis and pathophysiology of type 1 and type 2 diabetes mellitus. *Journal of Physiology and Pathophysiology*, *4*(4), 46–57. doi:10.5897/JPAP2013.0001

Palattiyil, G., & Chakrabarti, M. (2008). Coping strategies of families in HIV/AIDS care: Some exploratory data from two developmental contexts. *AIDS Care*, *20*(7), 881–885. doi:10.1080/09540120701767166 PMID:18608058

Palidofsky, M., & Stolbach, B. C. (2012). Dramatic healing: The evolution of a trauma-informed musical theatre program for incarcerated girls. *Journal of Child & Adolescent Trauma*, *5*(3), 239–256. doi:10.1080/19361521.2012.697102

Pandian, P. S. (2016). An Overview of Telemedicine Technologies for Healthcare Applications. *International Journal of Biomedical and Clinical Engineering*, *5*(2), 29–52. doi:10.4018/IJBCE.2016070103

Pan, X. R., Yang, W. Y., Li, G. W., & Liu, J. (1997). Prevalence of diabetes and its risk factors in China, 1994. National Diabetes Prevention and Control Cooperative Group. *Diabetes Care*, *20*(11), 1664–1669. doi:10.2337/diacare.20.11.1664

Papadopoulou, P., Lytras, M., & Marouli, C. (2018). Bioinformatics as Applied to Medicine: Challenges Faced Moving from Big Data to Smart Data to Wise Data. In M. Lytras & P. Papadopoulou (Eds.), *Applying Big Data Analytics in Bioinformatics and Medicine* (pp. 1–25). Hershey, PA: IGI Global. doi:10.4018/978-1-5225-2607-0.ch001

Paraskou, A., & George, B. P. (2018). An Overview of Reproductive Tourism. In *Legal and Economic Considerations Surrounding Reproductive Tourism: Emerging Research and Opportunities* (pp. 1–17). Hershey, PA: IGI Global. doi:10.4018/978-1-5225-2694-0.ch001

Parekh, R. (2017). Seasonal Affective Disorder (SAD). American Psychiatric Association. Retrieved from https://www.psychiatry.org

Parkhill, M. R., & Pickett, S. M. (2016). Difficulties in emotion regulation as a mediator of the relationship between child sexual abuse victimization and sexual aggression perpetration in male college students. *Journal of Child Sexual Abuse*, *25*(6), 674–685. doi:10.1080/10538712.2016.1205161

Park, S., & Moon, J. (2016). Strategic Approach towards Clinical Information Security. In J. Moon & M. Galea (Eds.), *Improving Health Management through Clinical Decision Support Systems* (pp. 329–359). Hershey, PA: IGI Global. doi:10.4018/978-1-4666-9432-3.ch015

Patel, L., Knijn, T., Gorman-Smith, D., Hochfeld, T., Isserow, M., Garthe, R., & Kgaohola, I. (2017). *Families, the child support grant, and child well-being outcomes*. Johannesburg: Centre for Social Development in Africa.

Penckofer, S., Ferrans, C. E., Velsor-Friedrich, B., & Savoy, S. (2007). The psychological impact of living with diabetes: Women's day-to-day experiences. *The Diabetes Educator*, *33*(4), 680–690. doi:10.1177/0145721707304079

Pereira, D., Castro, A., Gomes, P., Areias, J. C., Reis, Z. S., Coimbra, M. T., & Cruz-Correia, R. (2016). Digital Auscultation: Challenges and Perspectives. In M. Cruz-Cunha, I. Miranda, R. Martinho, & R. Rijo (Eds.), *Encyclopedia of E-Health and Telemedicine* (pp. 910–927). Hershey, PA: IGI Global. doi:10.4018/978-1-4666-9978-6.ch070

Perkins, K. A., Conklin, C. A., & Levine, M. D. (2008). *Cognitive-behavioural therapy for smoking cessation:A practical guidebook to the most effective treatments*. New York, NY: Routledge.

Peters, R. A., & Cruz, M. (2016). The States as Generators of Incremental Change in American Health Care Policy: 1935 to 1965. In R. Gholipour & K. Rouzbehani (Eds.), *Social, Economic, and Political Perspectives on Public Health Policy-Making* (pp. 86–114). Hershey, PA: IGI Global. doi:10.4018/978-1-4666-9944-1.ch005

Phuritsabam, B., & Devi, A. B. (2017). Information Seeking Behavior of Medical Scientists at Jawaharlal Nehru Institute of Medical Science: A Study. In S. Ram (Ed.), *Library and Information Services for Bioinformatics Education and Research* (pp. 177–187). Hershey, PA: IGI Global. doi:10.4018/978-1-5225-1871-6.ch010

Pieczka, B. (2018). Management of Risk and Adverse Events in Medical Entities. In A. Rosiek-Kryszewska & K. Leksowski (Eds.), *Healthcare Administration for Patient Safety and Engagement* (pp. 31–46). Hershey, PA: IGI Global. doi:10.4018/978-1-5225-3946-9.ch003

Pinzone, M. R., Fiorica, F., Di Rosa, M., Malaguarnera, G., Malaguarnera, L., Cacopardo, B., & … . (2012). Non-AIDS-defining cancers among HIV-infected people. *European Review for Medical and Pharmacological Sciences*, *16*(10), 1377–1388. PMID:23104654

Plagerson, S., Patel, V., Harpham, T., Kielmann, K., & Mathee, A. (2011). Does money matter for mental health? Evidence from the child support grants in Johannesburg. *Global Public Health: An International Journal for Research, Policy and Practice*, *6*(7), 760–776. doi:10.1080/17441692.2010.516267 PMID:20938853

PMI. (2019). MOP document: CDC, USAID & United State Presidents Malaria initiative FY 2018 and FY 2019. Retrieved from https://www.pmi.gov/docs/default-source/default-document-library/malaria-operational-plan

Poduval, J. (2016). Curriculum Development. In *Optimizing Medicine Residency Training Programs* (pp. 45–102). Hershey, PA: IGI Global. doi:10.4018/978-1-4666-9527-6.ch003

Poduval, J. (2016). Ethics and Professionalism. In *Optimizing Medicine Residency Training Programs* (pp. 103–133). Hershey, PA: IGI Global. doi:10.4018/978-1-4666-9527-6.ch004

Poduval, J. (2016). Management Skills and Leadership. In *Optimizing Medicine Residency Training Programs* (pp. 182–205). Hershey, PA: IGI Global. doi:10.4018/978-1-4666-9527-6.ch008

Poduval, J. (2016). Medicine Residency Training. In *Optimizing Medicine Residency Training Programs* (pp. 1–27). Hershey, PA: IGI Global. doi:10.4018/978-1-4666-9527-6.ch001

Poduval, J. (2016). Personal Issues. In *Optimizing Medicine Residency Training Programs* (pp. 206–221). Hershey, PA: IGI Global. doi:10.4018/978-1-4666-9527-6.ch009

Poduval, J. (2017). Medical Errors: Impact on Health Care Quality. In M. Riga (Ed.), *Impact of Medical Errors and Malpractice on Health Economics, Quality, and Patient Safety* (pp. 33–60). Hershey, PA: IGI Global. doi:10.4018/978-1-5225-2337-6.ch002

Pogosyan, M. (2017). How culture affects depression. *Psychology today*. Retrieved from https://www.psychologytoday.com/

Politis, D., Stagiopoulos, P., Aidona, S., Kyriafinis, G., & Constantinidis, I. (2018). Autonomous Learning and Skill Accreditation: A Paradigm for Medical Studies. In A. Kumar (Ed.), *Optimizing Student Engagement in Online Learning Environments* (pp. 266–296). Hershey, PA: IGI Global. doi:10.4018/978-1-5225-3634-5.ch012

Pollack, C. E., Chideya, S., Cubbin, C., Williams, B., Dekker, M., & Braveman, P. (2007). Should health studies measure wealth? A systematic review. *American Journal of Preventive Medicine*, *33*(3), 250–264. doi:10.1016/j.amepre.2007.04.033

Pollock, J. D., Koustova, E., Hoffman, A., Shurtleff, D., & Volkow, N. D. (2009). Treatments for nicotine addiction should be a top priority. *Lancet*, *374*(9689), 513–514. doi:10.1016/S0140-6736(09)60352-4 PMID:19394686

Polonsky, W. H., & Henry, R. R. (2016). Poor medication adherence in type 2 diabetes: Recognizing the scope of the problem and its key contributors. *Patient Preference and Adherence*, *10*, 1299–1307. doi:10.2147/PPA.S106821

Pomares-Quimbaya, A., Gonzalez, R. A., Quintero, S., Muñoz, O. M., Bohórquez, W. R., García, O. M., & Londoño, D. (2016). A Review of Existing Applications and Techniques for Narrative Text Analysis in Electronic Medical Records. In M. Cruz-Cunha, I. Miranda, R. Martinho, & R. Rijo (Eds.), *Encyclopedia of E-Health and Telemedicine* (pp. 796–811). Hershey, PA: IGI Global. doi:10.4018/978-1-4666-9978-6.ch062

Pomares-Quimbaya, A., González, R. A., Sierra, A., Daza, J. C., Muñoz, O., García, A., ... Bohórquez, W. R. (2017). ICT for Enabling the Quality Evaluation of Health Care Services: A Case Study in a General Hospital. In A. Moumtzoglou (Ed.), *Design, Development, and Integration of Reliable Electronic Healthcare Platforms* (pp. 196–210). Hershey, PA: IGI Global. doi:10.4018/978-1-5225-1724-5.ch012

Pouliakis, A., Margari, N., Karakitsou, E., Archondakis, S., & Karakitsos, P. (2018). Emerging Technologies Serving Cytopathology: Big Data, the Cloud, and Mobile Computing. In I. El Naqa (Ed.), *Emerging Developments and Practices in Oncology* (pp. 114–152). Hershey, PA: IGI Global. doi:10.4018/978-1-5225-3085-5.ch005

Powell, R. A., Honey, P. L., & Symbaluk, D. G. (2016). *Introduction to learning and behavior* (5th ed.). Belmont, CA: Wadsworth Publishing Company.

Power, R. A., Lecky-Thompson, L., Fisher, H. L., Cohen-Woods, S., Hosang, G. M., Uher, R., ... McGuffin, P. (2013). The interaction between child maltreatment, adult stressful life events and the 5-HTTLPR in major depression. *Journal of Psychiatric Research*, *47*(8), 1032–1035. doi:10.1016/j.jpsychires.2013.03.017

Price, G. (2017). *Is India Getting Serious About Dialogue in Kashmir?* Chatham House.

Psychiatric Mental Health. (n.d.). Retrieved from https://www.ncbi.nlm.nih.gov

Punthakee, Z., Goldenberg, R., & Katz, P. (2018). Definition, classification and diagnosis of diabetes, prediabetes and metabolic syndrome. *Canadian Journal of Diabetes*, *42*, S10–S15. doi:10.1016/j.jcjd.2017.10.003

Purse, M. (2019). Types of bipolar episodes according to DSM-5. *Verywellmind*. Retrieved from https://www.verywellmind.com

Queirós, A., Silva, A. G., Ferreira, A., Caravau, H., Cerqueira, M., & Rocha, N. P. (2016). Assessing Mobile Applications Considered Medical Devices. In M. Cruz-Cunha, I. Miranda, R. Martinho, & R. Rijo (Eds.), *Encyclopedia of E-Health and Telemedicine* (pp. 111–127). Hershey, PA: IGI Global. doi:10.4018/978-1-4666-9978-6.ch010

Quraishi, H. (2004). *Kashmir- The Untold Story*. India: Penguin Books.

Racicka, E., & Bryńska, A. (2015). Eating disorders in children and adolescents with Type 1 and Type 2 Diabetes: Prevalence, risk factors, warning signs. *Psychiatria Polska*, *49*(5), 1017–1024. doi:10.12740/PP/39536

Raffaeli, L., Spinsante, S., & Gambi, E. (2016). Integrated Smart TV-Based Personal e-Health System. *International Journal of E-Health and Medical Communications*, *7*(1), 48–64. doi:10.4018/IJEHMC.2016010103

Rai, A., Kothari, R., & Singh, D. P. (2017). Assessment of Available Technologies for Hospital Waste Management: A Need for Society. In R. Singh, A. Singh, & V. Srivastava (Eds.), *Environmental Issues Surrounding Human Overpopulation* (pp. 172–188). Hershey, PA: IGI Global. doi:10.4018/978-1-5225-1683-5.ch010

Ramamoorthy, S., & Sivasubramaniam, R. (2018). Image Processing Including Medical Liver Imaging: Medical Image Processing from Big Data Perspective, Ultrasound Liver Images, Challenges. In M. Lytras & P. Papadopoulou (Eds.), *Applying Big Data Analytics in Bioinformatics and Medicine* (pp. 380–392). Hershey, PA: IGI Global. doi:10.4018/978-1-5225-2607-0.ch016

Ramkisson, S., Pillay, B. J., & Sibanda, W. (2017). Social support and coping in adults with type 2 diabetes. *African Journal of Primary Health Care & Family Medicine*, *9*(1), e1–e8. doi:10.4102/phcfm.v9i1.1405

Rastogi, R., Chaturvedi, D. K., Satya, S., Arora, N., & Chauhan, S. (2018a). An optimized biofeedback therapy for chronic TTH between electromyography and galvanic skin resistance biofeedback on audio, visual and audio visual modes on various medical symptoms. In *Proceedings of the national Conference on 3rd MDNCPDR-2018*. Academic Press.

Rastogi, R., Chaturvedi, D. K., Satya, S., Arora, N., Singhal, P., & Gulati, M. (2018f). Statistical Resultant Analysis of Spiritual & Psychosomatic Stress Survey on Various Human Personality Indicators. In *Proceedings of ICCI 2018*. Academic Press. doi:10.1007/978-981-13-8222-2_25

Rastogi, R., Chaturvedi, D. K., Satya, S., Arora, N., Yadav, V., Chauhan, S., & Sharma, P. (2018c). SF-36 Scores Analysis for EMG and GSR Therapy on Audio, Visual and Audio Visual Modes for Chronic TTH. In Proceedings of the ICCIDA-2018. Academic Press.

Rather, F. (2013). Armed conflict in j&k and its impact on society: A case study of Kashmir valley. *International journal of Scientific and Research Publications*, *3*(2).

Rathor, G. P., & Gupta, S. K. (2017). Improving Multimodality Image Fusion through Integrate AFL and Wavelet Transform. In V. Tiwari, B. Tiwari, R. Thakur, & S. Gupta (Eds.), *Pattern and Data Analysis in Healthcare Settings* (pp. 143–157). Hershey, PA: IGI Global. doi:10.4018/978-1-5225-0536-5.ch008

Rawat, D. B., & Bhattacharya, S. (2016). Wireless Body Area Network for Healthcare Applications. In N. Meghanathan (Ed.), *Advanced Methods for Complex Network Analysis* (pp. 343–358). Hershey, PA: IGI Global. doi:10.4018/978-1-4666-9964-9.ch014

Rea, P. M. (2016). Advances in Anatomical and Medical Visualisation. In M. Pinheiro & D. Simões (Eds.), *Handbook of Research on Engaging Digital Natives in Higher Education Settings* (pp. 244–264). Hershey, PA: IGI Global. doi:10.4018/978-1-5225-0039-1.ch011

Rechenberg, K., Whittemore, R., & Grey, M. (2017). Anxiety in youth with type 1 diabetes. *Journal of Pediatric Nursing*, *32*, 64–71. doi:10.1016/j.pedn.2016.08.007

Reddy, P., Zuma, K., Shisana, O., Jonas, K., & Sewpaul, R. (2015). Prevalence of tobacco use among adults in South Africa: Results from the first South African National Health and Nutrition Examination Survey. *SAMJ: South African Medical Journal.*, *105*(8), 648. doi:10.7196/SAMJnew.7932 PMID:26449697

Redford, J. (Producer). (2015, September 21). *ACES primer* [Video file]. Retrieved from https://vimeo.com/139998006

Regehr, C. (2018). *Stress, trauma, and decision-making for social workers*. New York, NY: Columbia University Press. doi:10.7312/rege18012

Reinert, K., Campbell, J., Bandeen-Roche, K., Lee, J., & Szanton, S. (2016). The role of religious involvement in the relationship between early trauma and health outcomes among adult survivors. *Journal of Child & Adolescent Trauma*, *9*(3), 231–241. doi:10.100740653-015-0067-7

Retrieved fromhttp://www.unaids.org/en/regionscountries/countries/namibia

Rexhepi, H., & Persson, A. (2017). Challenges to Implementing IT Support for Evidence Based Practice Among Nurses and Assistant Nurses: A Qualitative Study. *Journal of Electronic Commerce in Organizations*, *15*(2), 61–76. doi:10.4018/JECO.2017040105

Reychav, I., & Azuri, J. (2016). Including Elderly Patients in Decision Making via Electronic Health Literacy. In M. Cruz-Cunha, I. Miranda, R. Martinho, & R. Rijo (Eds.), *Encyclopedia of E-Health and Telemedicine* (pp. 241–249). Hershey, PA: IGI Global. doi:10.4018/978-1-4666-9978-6.ch020

Richards, D., & Caldwell, P. H. (2016). Gamification to Improve Adherence to Clinical Treatment Advice: Improving Adherence to Clinical Treatment. In D. Novák, B. Tulu, & H. Brendryen (Eds.), *Handbook of Research on Holistic Perspectives in Gamification for Clinical Practice* (pp. 47–77). Hershey, PA: IGI Global. doi:10.4018/978-1-4666-9522-1.ch004

Rissman, B. (2016). Medical Conditions Associated with NLD. In B. Rissman (Ed.), *Medical and Educational Perspectives on Nonverbal Learning Disability in Children and Young Adults* (pp. 27–66). Hershey, PA: IGI Global. doi:10.4018/978-1-4666-9539-9.ch002

Robinson, L., Smith, M., Shubin, J., & Segal, J. (2019). Depression in Men. *HelpGuide*. Retrieved from https://www.helpguide.org

Rodin, G., Olmsted, M. P., Rydall, A. C., Maharaj, S. I., Colton, P. A., Jones, J. M., & Daneman, D. (2002). Eating disorders in young women with Type 1 diabetes mellitus. *Journal of Psychosomatic Research*, *53*(4), 943–949. doi:10.1016/S0022-3999(02)00305-7

Rodríguez Calvín, J. L., Zapatero Gaviria, A., & Martín Ríos, M. D. (2015). Prevalence of depression in type 2 diabetes mellitus. *Revista Clínica Española*, *215*(3), 156–164. doi:10.1016/j.rceng.2014.12.001

Roncaglia, I. (2014). Coping Styles: A Better Understanding of Stress and Anxiety in Individuals With Autism Spectrum Conditions Through Sport and Exercise Models. *Psychological Thought*, *7*(2), 134–143. doi:10.5964/psyct.v7i2.115

Roper, N. A., Bilous, R. W., Kelly, W. F., Unwin, N. C., & Connolly, V. M. (2001). Excess mortality in a population with diabetes and the impact of material deprivation: Longitudinal, population based study. *BMJ (Clinical Research Ed.)*, *322*(7299), 1389–1393. doi:10.1136/bmj.322.7299.1389

Rosiek, A. (2018). The Assessment of Actions of the Environment and the Impact of Preventive Medicine for Public Health in Poland. In A. Rosiek-Kryszewska & K. Leksowski (Eds.), *Healthcare Administration for Patient Safety and Engagement* (pp. 106–119). Hershey, PA: IGI Global. doi:10.4018/978-1-5225-3946-9.ch006

Rosiek, A., Leksowski, K., Goch, A., Rosiek-Kryszewska, A., & Leksowski, Ł. (2016). Medical Treatment and Difficult Ethical Decisions in Interdisciplinary Hospital Teams. In A. Rosiek & K. Leksowski (Eds.), *Organizational Culture and Ethics in Modern Medicine* (pp. 121–153). Hershey, PA: IGI Global. doi:10.4018/978-1-4666-9658-7.ch006

Rosiek, A., & Rosiek-Kryszewska, A. (2018). Managed Healthcare: Doctor Life Satisfaction and Its Impact on the Process of Communicating With the Patient. In A. Rosiek-Kryszewska & K. Leksowski (Eds.), *Healthcare Administration for Patient Safety and Engagement* (pp. 244–261). Hershey, PA: IGI Global. doi:10.4018/978-1-5225-3946-9.ch013

Rosiek-Kryszewska, A., Leksowski, Ł., Rosiek, A., Leksowski, K., & Goch, A. (2016). Clinical Communication in the Aspect of Development of New Technologies and E-Health in the Doctor-Patient Relationship. In A. Rosiek & K. Leksowski (Eds.), *Organizational Culture and Ethics in Modern Medicine* (pp. 18–51). Hershey, PA: IGI Global. doi:10.4018/978-1-4666-9658-7.ch002

Rosiek-Kryszewska, A., & Rosiek, A. (2018). The Impact of Management and Leadership Roles in Building Competitive Healthcare Units. In A. Rosiek-Kryszewska & K. Leksowski (Eds.), *Healthcare Administration for Patient Safety and Engagement* (pp. 13–30). Hershey, PA: IGI Global. doi:10.4018/978-1-5225-3946-9.ch002

Rosiek-Kryszewska, A., & Rosiek, A. (2018). The Involvement of the Patient and his Perspective Evaluation of the Quality of Healthcare. In A. Rosiek-Kryszewska & K. Leksowski (Eds.), *Healthcare Administration for Patient Safety and Engagement* (pp. 121–144). Hershey, PA: IGI Global. doi:10.4018/978-1-5225-3946-9.ch007

Roşu, S. M., Păvăloiu, I. B., Dragoi, G., Apostol, C. G., & Munteanu, D. (2016). Telemedicine Based on LMDS in the Urban/Metropolitan Area: A Romanian Case Study. In M. Cruz-Cunha, I. Miranda, R. Martinho, & R. Rijo (Eds.), *Encyclopedia of E-Health and Telemedicine* (pp. 96–109). Hershey, PA: IGI Global. doi:10.4018/978-1-4666-9978-6.ch009

Rouzbehani, K. (2017). Health Policy Implementation: Moving Beyond Its Barriers in United States. In N. Wickramasinghe (Ed.), *Handbook of Research on Healthcare Administration and Management* (pp. 541–552). Hershey, PA: IGI Global. doi:10.4018/978-1-5225-0920-2.ch032

Rubin, A. (1999). Biofeedback and binocular vision. *Journal of Behavioral Optometry*, *3*(4), 95–98.

Ruiz, I. M., Cohen, D. S., & Marco, Á. M. (2016). ISO/IEEE11073 Family of Standards: Trends and Applications on E-Health Monitoring. In M. Cruz-Cunha, I. Miranda, R. Martinho, & R. Rijo (Eds.), *Encyclopedia of E-Health and Telemedicine* (pp. 646–660). Hershey, PA: IGI Global. doi:10.4018/978-1-4666-9978-6.ch050

Rush, A. J., Fava, M., Wisniewski, S. R., Lavori, P. W., Trivedi, M. H., Sackeim, H. A., ... Niederehe, G.STAR*D Investigators Group. (2004). Sequenced treatment alternatives to relieve depression (STAR*D): Rationale and design. *Controlled Clinical Trials*, *25*(1), 119–142. doi:10.1016/S0197-2456(03)00112-0 PMID:15061154

Sacco, W. P., & Yanover, T. (2006). Diabetes and depression: The role of social support and medical symptoms. *Journal of Behavioral Medicine*, *29*(6), 523–531. doi:10.100710865-006-9072-5

Sack, W., Him, C., & Dickason, D. (1999). Twelve year follow up study of khmer youths who suffered massive war trauma as children. *Journal of the American Academy of Child and Adolescent Psychiatry*, *38*(9), 1173–1179. doi:10.1097/00004583-199909000-00023 PMID:10504817

Saini, H., Rastogi, R., Chaturvedi, D. K., Satya, S., Arora, N., Gupta, M., & Verma, H. (2019c). An Optimized Biofeedback EMG and GSR Biofeedback Therapy for Chronic TTH on SF-36 Scores of Different MMBD Modes on Various Medical Symptoms. In Hybrid Machine Intelligence for Medical Image Analysis (Ch. 8). Springer Nature. doi:10.1007/978-981-13-8930-6_8

Salinero-Fort, M. A., Gómez-Campelo, P., San Andrés-Rebollo, F. J., Cárdenas-Valladolid, J., Abánades-Herranz, J. C., Carrillo de Santa Pau, E., ... De Burgos-Lunar, C. (2018). Prevalence of depression in patients with type 2 diabetes mellitus in Spain (the DIADEMA Study): Results from the MADIABETES cohort. *BMJ Open*, *8*(9), e020768. doi:10.1136/bmjopen-2017-020768

Salomon, J. A. (2014) Disability-Adjusted Life Years (DALY). In Encyclopedia of Health Economics Science Direct (pp. 200-203). Academic Press. doi:10.1016/B978-0-12-375678-7.00511-3

Sam, S. (2017). Mobile Phones and Expanding Human Capabilities in Plural Health Systems. In K. Moahi, K. Bwalya, & P. Sebina (Eds.), *Health Information Systems and the Advancement of Medical Practice in Developing Countries* (pp. 93–114). Hershey, PA: IGI Global. doi:10.4018/978-1-5225-2262-1.ch006

Sankaranarayanan, S., & Ganesan, S. (2016). Applications of Intelligent Agents in Health Sector-A Review. *International Journal of E-Health and Medical Communications*, *7*(1), 1–30. doi:10.4018/IJEHMC.2016010101

Santos-Trigo, M., Suaste, E., & Figuerola, P. (2018). Technology Design and Routes for Tool Appropriation in Medical Practices. In M. Khosrow-Pour, D.B.A. (Ed.), Encyclopedia of Information Science and Technology, Fourth Edition (pp. 3794-3804). Hershey, PA: IGI Global. doi:10.4018/978-1-5225-2255-3.ch329

Sarivougioukas, J., Vagelatos, A., Parsopoulos, K. E., & Lagaris, I. E. (2018). Home UbiHealth. In M. Khosrow-Pour, D.B.A. (Ed.), Encyclopedia of Information Science and Technology, Fourth Edition (pp. 7765-7774). Hershey, PA: IGI Global. doi:10.4018/978-1-5225-2255-3.ch675

Sarkar, B. K. (2017). Big Data and Healthcare Data: A Survey. *International Journal of Knowledge-Based Organizations*, *7*(4), 50–77. doi:10.4018/IJKBO.2017100104

Sarwar, N., Gao, P., Seshasai, S. R., Gobin, R., Kaptoge, S., Di Angelantonio, E., ... Danesh, J. (2010). Diabetes mellitus, fasting blood glucose concentration, and risk of vascular disease: A collaborative meta-analysis of 102 prospective studies. Emerging Risk Factors Collaboration. *Lancet*, *375*(9733), 2215–2222. doi:10.1016/S0140-6736(10)60484-9

Satya, S., Arora, N., Trivedi, P., Singh, A., Sharma, A., Singh, A., Rastogi, R., Chaturvedi, D.K. (2019a). Intelligent Analysis for Personality Detection on Various Indicators by Clinical Reliable Psychological TTH and Stress Surveys. In *Proceedings of CIPR 2019*. Academic Press.

Satya, S., Rastogi, R., Chaturvedi, D. K., Arora, N., Singh, P., & Vyas, P. (2018e). Statistical Analysis for Effect of Positive Thinking on Stress Management and Creative Problem Solving for Adolescents. In *Proceedings of the 12th INDIA-Com* (pp. 245-251). Academic Press.

Saxena, K., & Banodha, U. (2017). An Essence of the SOA on Healthcare. In R. Bhadoria, N. Chaudhari, G. Tomar, & S. Singh (Eds.), *Exploring Enterprise Service Bus in the Service-Oriented Architecture Paradigm* (pp. 283–304). Hershey, PA: IGI Global. doi:10.4018/978-1-5225-2157-0.ch018

Schatz, E., & Ogunmefun, C. (2007). Caring and Contributing: The role of older women in rural South Africa multi-generational households in the HIV/AIDS era. *World Development*, *35*(8), 1390–1403. doi:10.1016/j.worlddev.2007.04.004

Scheffer, M., van de Leemput, I. A., van Nes, E. H., Gijzel, S. M. W., Romero, L. M., & Bolhuis, J. E., … Martin, C. M. (2018). Quantifying resilience of humans and other animals. In *Proceedings of the National Academy of Sciences of the United States of America* (pp. 11883–11890). Academic Press. 10.1073/pnas.1810630115

Schimelpfening, N. (2019). Common types of depression. *VeryWellMind*. Retrieved from https://www.verywellmind.com/common-types-of-depression-1067313

Schimelpfening, N. (2019). Is depression different in males and females? Understanding the subtle differences. *VeryWellMind*. Retrieved from https://www.verywellmind.com/common-types-of-depression-1067313

Schmeida, M., & McNeal, R. (2016). Consulting Online Healthcare Information: E-Caregivers as Knowledgeable Decision Makers. *International Journal of Computers in Clinical Practice*, *1*(1), 42–52. doi:10.4018/IJCCP.2016010104

Schneiderman, N., Ironson, G., & Siegel, S. D. (2005). Stress and health: Psychological, behavioral, and biological determinants. *Annual Review of Clinical Psychology*, *1*(1), 607–628. doi:10.1146/annurev.clinpsy.1.102803.144141

Schroeder, E., & Nichola, T. (2006). The adoption of HIV/AIDS orphans and food security in rural Ingwavuma, South Africa. *International Journal of Technology Management & Sustainable Development*, *5*(2), 173–187. doi:10.1386/ijtm.5.2.173_1

Scott, E. (2019). 17 Highly Effective Stress Relievers. Very Well Mind. Retrieved from https://www.verywellmind.com/tips-to-reduce-stress-3145195#citation-5

Scott, A., Chambers, D., Goyder, E., & O'Cathain, A. (2017). Socioeconomic inequalities in mortality, morbidity and diabetes management for adults with type 1 diabetes: A systematic review. *PLoS One*, *12*(5), e0177210. doi:10.1371/journal.pone.0177210

Scott, D. S., & Lundeen, T. F. (2004). Myofascial pain involving the masticatory muscles: An experimental model. *Pain*, *8*(2), 207–215. doi:10.1016/0304-3959(88)90008-5 PMID:7402684

Secrest, A. M., Costacou, T., Gutelius, B., Miller, R. G., Songer, T. J., & Orchard, T. J. (2011). Associations between socioeconomic status and major complications in type 1 diabetes: The Pittsburgh epidemiology of diabetes complication (EDC) Study. *Annals of Epidemiology*, *21*(5), 374–381. doi:10.1016/j.annepidem.2011.02.007

Segal, E. A., Gerdes, K. E., & Steiner, S. (2019). *An introduction to the profession of social work* (6th ed.). Boston, MA: Cengage Learning.

Semenkovich, K., Brown, M. E., Svrakic, D. M., & Lustman, P. J. (2015). Depression in type 2 diabetes mellitus: Prevalence, impact, and treatment. *Drugs*, *75*(6), 577–587. doi:10.100740265-015-0347-4

Sen, K., & Ghosh, K. (2018). Incorporating Global Medical Knowledge to Solve Healthcare Problems: A Framework for a Crowdsourcing System. *International Journal of Healthcare Information Systems and Informatics*, *13*(1), 1–14. doi:10.4018/IJHISI.2018010101

Seshasai, S. R., Kaptoge, S., & Thompson, A.Emerging Risk Factors Collaboration. (2011). Diabetes mellitus, fasting glucose, and risk of cause-specific death. *The New England Journal of Medicine*, *364*(9), 829–841. doi:10.1056/NEJMoa1008862

Shah, A. V. (1982). Integration of mental health. *Indian Journal of Psychiatry*, *24*, 3–7. PMID:21965877

Shakdher, A., & Pandey, K. (2017). REDAlert+: Medical/Fire Emergency and Warning System using Android Devices. *International Journal of E-Health and Medical Communications*, *8*(1), 37–51. doi:10.4018/IJEHMC.2017010103

Sharma, S., Rastogi, R., Chaturvedi, D. K., Bansal, A., & Agrawal, A. (2018g). Audio visual EMG & GSR Biofeedback analysis for effect of spiritual techniques on human behavior and psychic challenges. In *Proceedings of the 12th INDIACom* (pp. 252-258). Academic Press.

Shekarian, E., Abdul-Rashid, S. H., & Olugu, E. U. (2017). An Integrated Fuzzy VIKOR Method for Performance Management in Healthcare. In M. Tavana, K. Szabat, & K. Puranam (Eds.), *Organizational Productivity and Performance Measurements Using Predictive Modeling and Analytics* (pp. 40–61). Hershey, PA: IGI Global. doi:10.4018/978-1-5225-0654-6.ch003

Sherman, A. (2016). Learned helplessness and depression: Dysfunction interrupted. *PsychCentral*. Retrieved from https://www.blogs.psychcentral.com

Shern, D. L., Blanch, A. K., & Steverman, S. M. (2016). Toxic stress, behavioral health, and the next major era in public health. *The American Journal of Orthopsychiatry*, *86*(2), 109–123. doi:10.1037/ort0000120

Shifiona, N. N., Poggenpoel, M., & Myburgh, C. P. H. (2006). Life stories of depressed adult women in peri-urban Namibia. *Curationis, 29*(2), 5–11. doi:10.4102/curationis.v29i2.1063 PMID:16910128

Shi, J., Erdem, E., & Liu, H. (2016). Expanding Role of Telephone Systems in Healthcare: Developments and Opportunities. In A. Dwivedi (Ed.), *Reshaping Medical Practice and Care with Health Information Systems* (pp. 87–131). Hershey, PA: IGI Global. doi:10.4018/978-1-4666-9870-3.ch004

Shijina, V., & John, S. J. (2017). Multiple Relations and its Application in Medical Diagnosis. *International Journal of Fuzzy System Applications, 6*(4), 47–62. doi:10.4018/IJFSA.2017100104

Shipley, N., & Chakraborty, J. (2018). Big Data and mHealth: Increasing the Usability of Healthcare Through the Customization of Pinterest – Literary Perspective. In J. Machado, A. Abelha, M. Santos, & F. Portela (Eds.), *Next-Generation Mobile and Pervasive Healthcare Solutions* (pp. 46–66). Hershey, PA: IGI Global. doi:10.4018/978-1-5225-2851-7.ch004

Shoib, S., Maqbool, D., Bashir, H., Qayoom, G., & Arif, T. (2012). Psychiatric morbidity and the socio-demographic determinants of patients attempting suicide in Kashmir Valley: A cross-sectional study. *International Journal of Health Sciences and Research, 2*(7), 45–53.

Shrivastava, S. R., Shrivastava, P. S., & Ramasamy, J. (2013). Role of self-care in management of diabetes mellitus. *Journal of Diabetes and Metabolic Disorders, 12*(1), 14. doi:10.1186/2251-6581-12-14

Siddiqi, K. (2019). Tobacco Use in Sub-Saharan Africa: The Risks and Challenges. *Nicotine & Tobacco Research: Official Journal of the Society for Research on Nicotine and Tobacco, 21*(8), 1–4. doi:10.1093/ntr/ntz086 PMID:31112602

Siebers, A. (2016). Does culture influence our response to depression? *Perspective*. Retrieved from https://www.genre.com/knowledge/blog/

Silove, D., Liddell, B., Rees, S., Chey, T., Nickerson, A., Tam, N., ... Steel, Z. (2014). Effects of recurrent violence on post-traumatic stress disorder and severe distress in conflict-affected Timor-Leste: A 6-year longitudinal study. *The Lancet. Global Health, 2*(5), 293–300. doi:10.1016/S2214-109X(14)70196-2 PMID:25103168

Silva, L. C. C. D., Araújo, A. J. D., Queiroz, Â. M. D. D., Sales, M. D. P. U., & Castellano, M. V. C. D. O. (2016). Smoking control: challenges and achievements. *Journal Brasilileiro de Pneumologia. 42*(4), 290-298. doi:10.1590/S1806-37562016000000145

Simon, V., Ho, D. D., & Abdool, K. Q. (2006). HIV/AIDS epidemiology, pathogenesis, prevention and treatment. *Lancet, 368*(9534), 489–504. doi:10.1016/S0140-6736(06)69157-5 PMID:16890836

Singh, A., Rastogi, R., Chaturvedi, D. K., Satya, S., Arora, N., Sharma, A., & Singh, A. (2019d). Intelligent Personality Analysis on Indicators inIoT-MMBD Enabled Environment. In Multimedia Big Data Computing for IoT Applications: Concepts, Paradigms, and Solutions (Ch. 7). Springer Nature. doi:10.1007/978-981-13-8759-3_7

Singh, A., & Dutta, M. K. (2017). A Reversible Data Hiding Scheme for Efficient Management of Tele-Ophthalmological Data. *International Journal of E-Health and Medical Communications*, *8*(3), 38–54. doi:10.4018/IJEHMC.2017070103

Singhal, P., Rastogi, R., Chaturvedi, D. K., Satya, S., Arora, N., Gupta, M., … Gulati, M. (2019b). Statistical Analysis of Exponential and Polynomial Models of EMG & GSR Biofeedback for Correlation between Subjects Medications Movement & Medication Scores. *IJITEE*, *8*(6S), 625-635. Retrieved from https://www.ijitee.org/download/volume-8-issue-6S/

Singh, H., Raju, M. S., Dubey, V., Kurrey, R., Bansal, S., & Malik, M. (2014). A study of sociodemographic clinical and glycemic control factors associated with co-morbid depression in type 2 diabetes mellitus. *Industrial Psychiatry Journal*, *23*(2), 134–142. doi:10.4103/0972-6748.151687

Singh, R., Musa, J., Singh, S., & Ukatu, V. E. (2014). Knowledge, attitudes and practices of malaria in Aleiro, Kebbi State, Northern Nigeria. *Journal of Family Medicine and Primary Care*, *3*(1), 39–44. doi:10.4103/2249-4863.130271 PubMed

Siu, A. L. (2015). Behavioral and Pharmacotherapy Interventions for Tobacco Smoking Cessation in Adults, Including Pregnant Women: U.S. Preventive Services Task Force Recommendation Statement. *Annals of Internal Medicine*, *2015*(163), 622–634. doi:10.7326/M15-2023 PMID:26389730

Sivaji, A., Radjo, H. K., Amin, M., & Abu Hashim, M. A. (2016). Design of a Hospital Interactive Wayfinding System: Designing for Malaysian Users. In N. Mohamed, T. Mantoro, M. Ayu, & M. Mahmud (Eds.), *Critical Socio-Technical Issues Surrounding Mobile Computing* (pp. 88–123). Hershey, PA: IGI Global. doi:10.4018/978-1-4666-9438-5.ch005

Skourti, P. K., & Pavlakis, A. (2017). The Second Victim Phenomenon: The Way Out. In M. Riga (Ed.), *Impact of Medical Errors and Malpractice on Health Economics, Quality, and Patient Safety* (pp. 197–222). Hershey, PA: IGI Global. doi:10.4018/978-1-5225-2337-6.ch008

Skovdal, M., Mwasiaji, W., Webale, A., & Tomkins, A. (2011). Building orphan competent communities: Experiences from a community-based capital cash transfer initiative in Kenya. *Health Policy and Planning*, *16*(3), 233–241. doi:10.1093/heapol/czq039 PMID:20805235

Small, R., Lumley, J., & Yelland, J. (2003). Cross-cultural experiences of maternal depression: Associations and contributing factors for Vietnamese, Turkish and Fillipino Immigrant women in Victoria, Australia. *Ethnicity & Health*, *8*(3), 189–206. doi:10.1080/1355785032000136416 PMID:14577995

Smith, M., Robinson, L., & Segal, J. (2019). *Coping with Depression: Tips for overcoming depression one step at a time. HelpGuide.org* Retrieved from https://www.helpguide.org/

Smith, C. R. (2018). Medical Students' Quest Towards the Long White Coat: Impact on Mental Health and Well-Being. In C. Smith (Ed.), *Exploring the Pressures of Medical Education From a Mental Health and Wellness Perspective* (pp. 1–42). Hershey, PA: IGI Global. doi:10.4018/978-1-5225-2811-1.ch001

Smith, K. J., Béland, M., Clyde, M., Gariépy, G., Page, V., Badawi, G., ... Schmitz, N. (2013). Association of diabetes with anxiety: A systematic review and meta-analysis. *Journal of Psychosomatic Research*, *74*(2), 89–99. doi:10.1016/j.jpsychores.2012.11.013

Smith, S. I., & Dandignac, M. (2018). Perfectionism: Addressing Lofty Expectations in Medical School. In C. Smith (Ed.), *Exploring the Pressures of Medical Education From a Mental Health and Wellness Perspective* (pp. 68–91). Hershey, PA: IGI Global. doi:10.4018/978-1-5225-2811-1.ch003

Snoek, F. J., Bremmer, M. A., & Hermanns, N. (2015). Constructs of depression and distress in diabetes: Time for an appraisal. *The Lancet. Diabetes & Endocrinology*, *3*(6), 450–460. doi:10.1016/S2213-8587(15)00135-7

Sobrinho, Á. A., Dias da Silva, L., Perkusich, A., Cunha, P., Pinheiro, M. E., & Melo de Medeiros, L. (2016). Towards Medical Systems to Aid the Detection and Treatment of Chronic Diseases. In D. Fotiadis (Ed.), *Handbook of Research on Trends in the Diagnosis and Treatment of Chronic Conditions* (pp. 50–69). Hershey, PA: IGI Global. doi:10.4018/978-1-4666-8828-5.ch003

Social Impact Assessment and Policy Analysis Corporation (SIAPAC). (2002). *Situational analysis of orphan children in Namibia.* Windhoek, Namibia: Ministry of Health and Social Services.

Soczywko, J., & Rutkowska, D. (2018). The Patient/Provider Relationship in Emergency Medicine: Organization, Communication, and Understanding. In A. Rosiek-Kryszewska & K. Leksowski (Eds.), *Healthcare Administration for Patient Safety and Engagement* (pp. 74–105). Hershey, PA: IGI Global. doi:10.4018/978-1-5225-3946-9.ch005

Sołtysik-Piorunkiewicz, A., Furmankiewicz, M., & Ziuziański, P. (2016). Web Healthcare Applications in Poland: Trends, Standards, Barriers and Possibilities of Implementation and Usage of E-Health Systems. In I. Deliyannis, P. Kostagiolas, & C. Banou (Eds.), *Experimental Multimedia Systems for Interactivity and Strategic Innovation* (pp. 258–283). Hershey, PA: IGI Global. doi:10.4018/978-1-4666-8659-5.ch013

Soni, P. (2018). Implications of HIPAA and Subsequent Regulations on Information Technology. In M. Gupta, R. Sharman, J. Walp, & P. Mulgund (Eds.), *Information Technology Risk Management and Compliance in Modern Organizations* (pp. 71–98). Hershey, PA: IGI Global. doi:10.4018/978-1-5225-2604-9.ch004

Soomro, A. (2019, August 17). Fear and uncertainty around Kashmir's future. *Lancet*, *394*(10198), 542. doi:10.1016/S0140-6736(19)31939-7 PMID:31423985

South African Depression and Anxiety Group (SADAG). (2006). *Depression in black South Africans.* Retrieved from https://www.sadag.com

Sperry, D. M., & Widom, C. S. (2013). Child abuse and neglect, social support, and psychopathology in adulthood: A prospective investigation. *Child Abuse & Neglect*, *37*(6), 415–425. doi:10.1016/j.chiabu.2013.02.006

Spinelli, R., & Benevolo, C. (2016). From Healthcare Services to E-Health Applications: A Delivery System-Based Taxonomy. In A. Dwivedi (Ed.), *Reshaping Medical Practice and Care with Health Information Systems* (pp. 205–245). Hershey, PA: IGI Global. doi:10.4018/978-1-4666-9870-3.ch007

Srivastava, A., & Aggarwal, A. K. (2018). Medical Image Fusion in Spatial and Transform Domain: A Comparative Analysis. In M. Anwar, A. Khosla, & R. Kapoor (Eds.), *Handbook of Research on Advanced Concepts in Real-Time Image and Video Processing* (pp. 281–300). Hershey, PA: IGI Global. doi:10.4018/978-1-5225-2848-7.ch011

Srivastava, S. K., & Roy, S. N. (2018). Recommendation System: A Potential Tool for Achieving Pervasive Health Care. In J. Machado, A. Abelha, M. Santos, & F. Portela (Eds.), *Next-Generation Mobile and Pervasive Healthcare Solutions* (pp. 111–127). Hershey, PA: IGI Global. doi:10.4018/978-1-5225-2851-7.ch008

Ssengonzi, R. (2007). The plight of older persons as caregivers to people infected/affected by HIV/AIDS: Evidence from Uganda. *Journal of Cross-Cultural Gerontology*, *22*(4), 339–353. doi:10.100710823-007-9043-5 PMID:17694427

Ssewamala, F. M., Neilands, T. B., Waldfogel, J., & Ismayilova, L. (2012). The impact of a comprehensive microfinance intervention on depression levels of AIDS-orphaned children in Uganda. *The Journal of Adolescent Health*, *50*(4), 346–352. doi:10.1016/j.jadohealth.2011.08.008 PMID:22443837

SSQ financial solution. (2013). Reference document: Stress management. Paris. France. Retrieved from https://ssq.ca/sites/default/files/archives/ac/Chroniques_sante/Stress_management_-reference_document-.pdf

Stancu, A. (2016). Correlations and Patterns of Food and Health Consumer Expenditure. In A. Jean-Vasile (Ed.), *Food Science, Production, and Engineering in Contemporary Economies* (pp. 44–101). Hershey, PA: IGI Global. doi:10.4018/978-1-5225-0341-5.ch003

Stanimirovic, D. (2017). Digitalization of Death Certification Model: Transformation Issues and Implementation Concerns. In S. Saeed, Y. Bamarouf, T. Ramayah, & S. Iqbal (Eds.), *Design Solutions for User-Centric Information Systems* (pp. 22–43). Hershey, PA: IGI Global. doi:10.4018/978-1-5225-1944-7.ch002

Starace, F., Ammassari, A., Trotta, M. P., Murri, R., De Longis, P., Izzo, C., ... Antinori, A. (2002). Depression is a risk factor for suboptimal adherence to highly active antiretroviral therapy. *JAIDS Journal of Acquired Immune Deficiency Syndromes*, *31*(3), 136–139. doi:10.1097/00126334-200212153-00010 PMID:12562037

Staveteig, S., Croft, T. N., Kampa, K. T., & Head, S. K. (2017). Reaching the 'first 90': Gaps in coverage of HIV testing among people living with HIV in 16 African countries. *PLoS One*, *12*(10), e0186316. doi:10.1371/journal.pone.0186316 PMID:29023510

Stavros, A., Vavoulidis, E., & Nasioutziki, M. (2016). The Use of Mobile Health Applications for Quality Control and Accreditational Purposes in a Cytopathology Laboratory. In A. Moumtzoglou (Ed.), *M-Health Innovations for Patient-Centered Care* (pp. 262–283). Hershey, PA: IGI Global. doi:10.4018/978-1-4666-9861-1.ch013

Stead, L. F., Perera, R., Bullen, C., Mant, D., & Lancaster, T. (2008). *Nicotine replacement therapy for smoking cessation (Review)*. Oxford, UK: John Wiley & Sons; doi:10.1002/14651858

Steel, Z., Chey, T., Silove, D., Marnane, C., Bryant, R.A., & van Ommeren, M. (2009). Association of torture and other potentially traumatic events with mental health outcomes among populations exposed to mass conflict and displacements: A systematic review and meta-analysis. *American Medical Association*, *302*(5), 537-549.

Stetson, B., Minges, K. E., & Richardson, C. R. (2017). New directions for diabetes prevention and management in behavioral medicine. *Journal of Behavioral Medicine*, *40*(1), 127–144. doi:10.100710865-016-9802-2

Stevens, L. M., Lynm, C., & Golub, R. M. (2012). HIV infection: The basics. *Journal of the American Medical Association*, *308*(4), 419. doi:10.1001/jama.2012.4079 PMID:22820800

Stoa, E. M., Meling, S., Nyhus, L. K., Stromstad, G., Mangerud, K. M., Helgerud, J., ... Storen, O. (2017). High-intensity aerobic interval training improves aerobic fitness and HbA1c among persons diagnosed with type 2 diabetes. *European Journal of Applied Physiology*, *117*(3), 455–467. doi:10.100700421-017-3540-1

Stolar, M. W. (2010). Defining and achieving treatment success in patients with type 2 diabetes mellitus. *Mayo Clinic Proceedings*, *85*(12 Suppl.), S50–S59. doi:10.4065/mcp.2010.0471

Stoll, D. J. (2015). *Running head: A biopsychosocial analysis of smoking*.

Strom, J. L., & Egede, L. E. (2012). The impact of social support on outcomes in adult patients with type 2 diabetes: A systematic review. *Current Diabetes Reports*, *12*(6), 769–781. doi:10.100711892-012-0317-0

Substance Abuse and Mental Health Services Administration. (2014). Trauma-Informed Care in Behavioral Health Services. Treatment Improvement Protocol (TIP) Series 57. Rockville, MD: Author.

Sukkird, V., & Shirahada, K. (2018). E-Health Service Model for Asian Developing Countries: A Case of Emergency Medical Service for Elderly People in Thailand. In M. Khosrow-Pour (Ed.), *Optimizing Current Practices in E-Services and Mobile Applications* (pp. 214–232). Hershey, PA: IGI Global. doi:10.4018/978-1-5225-5026-6.ch011

Sumari, D., Dillip, A., Ndume, V., Mugasa, J. P., & Gwakisa, P. S. (2016). Knowledge, attitudes and practices on malaria in relation to its transmission among primary school children in Bagamoyo district, Tanzania. *MalariaWorld Journal*, *7*(2), 1–7.

Summerfield, D. (2000). War and mental health: A brief overview. *British Medical Journal*, *321*(7255), 232–235. doi:10.1136/bmj.321.7255.232 PMID:10903662

Sustainable Development starts with safe, healthy and well educated children. (2013). UNICEF.

Suthar, A. B., Lawn, S. D., Del Amo, J., Getahun, H., Dye, C., Sculier, D., ... & Granich, R. M. (2012). Antiretroviral therapy for prevention of HIV-associated tuberculosis in developing countries: A systematic review and meta-analysis. *PLoS Medicine*, *9*. doi:10.1371/journal.pmed.1001270

Syed, H. R., Zachrisson, H. D., Dalgard, O. S., Dalen, I., & Ahlberg, N. (2008). Concordance between Hopkins Symptom Checklist (HSCL-10) and Pakistan Anxiety and Depression Questionnaire. *BMC Psychiatry*, *8*(59). PMID:18647394

Sygit, B., & Wąsik, D. (2016). Patients' Rights and Medical Personnel Duties in the Field of Hospital Care. In A. Rosiek & K. Leksowski (Eds.), *Organizational Culture and Ethics in Modern Medicine* (pp. 282–297). Hershey, PA: IGI Global. doi:10.4018/978-1-4666-9658-7.ch012

Sygit, B., & Wąsik, D. (2016). The Idea of Human Rights in Conditions of Hospital Treatment. In A. Rosiek & K. Leksowski (Eds.), *Organizational Culture and Ethics in Modern Medicine* (pp. 236–254). Hershey, PA: IGI Global. doi:10.4018/978-1-4666-9658-7.ch010

Tabish, A. (2004). Mental Health: Science and sensibility. In *The Future of Health* (1st ed., pp. 179–207). New Delhi: Paras Medical publishers.

Tabish, A. (2005). Mental Health: Neglected for far too long. *JK Practitioner*, *12*(1), 38–42.

Talbot, T. B. (2017). Making Lifelike Medical Games in the Age of Virtual Reality: An Update on "Playing Games with Biology" from 2013. In B. Dubbels (Ed.), *Transforming Gaming and Computer Simulation Technologies across Industries* (pp. 103–119). Hershey, PA: IGI Global. doi:10.4018/978-1-5225-1817-4.ch006

Tambo, E. (2019). World Malaria Day, April 25th 2019: Zero malaria starts with me. Bio Med Central. Retrieved from http://blogs.biomedcentral.com/onhealth/2019/04/25/zero-malaria-starts-with-me-practice

Tam, J., & van Walbeek, C. (2013). Tobacco control in namibia: The importance of government capacity, Media coverage and industry interference. *Tobacco Control*, *23*. doi:10.1136/tobaccocontrol-2012-050725 PMID:23788605

Tamposis, I., Pouliakis, A., Fezoulidis, I., & Karakitsos, P. (2016). Mobile Platforms Supporting Health Professionals: Need, Technical Requirements, and Applications. In A. Moumtzoglou (Ed.), *M-Health Innovations for Patient-Centered Care* (pp. 91–114). Hershey, PA: IGI Global. doi:10.4018/978-1-4666-9861-1.ch005

Tang, T. S., Brown, M. B., Funnell, M. M., & Anderson, R. M. (2008). Social support, quality of life, and self-care behaviors among African Americans with type 2 diabetes. *The Diabetes Educator*, *34*(2), 266–276. doi:10.1177/0145721708315680

Tan, M. L., Manski-Nankervis, J. A., Thuraisingam, S., Jenkins, A., O'Neal, D., & Furler, J. (2018). Socioeconomic status and time in glucose target range in people with type 2 diabetes: A baseline analysis of the GP-OSMOTIC study. *BMC Endocrine Disorders*, *18*(1), 47. doi:10.118612902-018-0279-6

Tassie, A. K. (2015). Vicarious resilience from attachment trauma: Reflections of long-term therapy with marginalized young people. *Journal of Social Work Practice*, *29*(2), 191–204. doi:10.1080/02650533.2014.933406

Taylor, R. (2018). Explaining intentions to seek mental health services among black Canadians. Retrieved from https://www.scholar.uwindsor.ca/

Teicher, M. H., Samson, J. A., Polcari, A., & McGreenery, C. E. (2006). Sticks, stones, and hurtful words: Relative effects of various forms of childhood maltreatment. *The American Journal of Psychiatry*, *163*(6), 993–1000. doi:10.1176/ajp.2006.163.6.993

Thapa, S. B., Martinez, P., & Clausen, T. (2014). Depression and its correlates in South Africa and Ghana among people aged 50 and above: Findings from the WHO study on Global AGEing and adult health. *Journal of Psychiatry*, *17*(6). PMID:25914902

The Body Pro. (2016). Virological response without routine viral load monitoring in children: Results from the ARROW Trial. Retrieved from https://www.thebodypro.com/content/78528/virological-response-without-routine-viral-load-mo.html

The Royal Australian College of General Practitioners. (2011). S*upporting smoking cessation: A guide for health professionals*. Retrieved from https://www.racgp.org.au/download/documents/Guidelines/smoking-cessation.pdf

The World Health Organization. (2003). Department of mental health and substance Dependence.

Thomas, M. 2018. Over half a million children in India are smoking cigarettes everyday. Retrieved from https://qz.com/india/1232112/indias-cigarette-smoking-epidemic-includes-over-600000-addicted-children/

Tiago, M. T., Tiago, F., Amaral, F. E., & Silva, S. (2016). Healthy 3.0: Healthcare Digital Dimensions. In A. Dwivedi (Ed.), *Reshaping Medical Practice and Care with Health Information Systems* (pp. 287–322). Hershey, PA: IGI Global. doi:10.4018/978-1-4666-9870-3.ch010

Tiv, M., Viel, J. F., Mauny, F., Eschwège, E., Weill, A., Fournier, C., ... Penfornis, A. (2012). Medication adherence in type 2 diabetes: The ENTRED study 2007, a French Population-Based Study. *PLoS One*, *7*(3), e32412. doi:10.1371/journal.pone.0032412

Tobacco Product Control Act. (2010). Republic of Namibia. Government printer. Retrieved from https://www.tobaccocontrollaws.org/files/live/Namibia/Namibia%20-%20Tobacco%20Products%20Control%20-%20national.pdf

Tomoda, A., Suzuki, H., Rabi, K., Sheu, Y. S., Polcari, A., & Teicher, M. H. (2009). Reduced prefrontal cortical gray matter volume in young adults exposed to harsh corporal punishment. *NeuroImage*, *47*, T66–T71. doi:10.1016/j.neuroimage.2009.03.005

Townsend, M. C. (1996). *Psychiatric-mental health nursing: Concepts of care*. Philadelphia, PA: F. A. Davis.

Trading Economics. (2019).Namibian unemployment rate. Retrieved from: https://tradingeconomics.com/namibia/youth-unemployment-rate

Trento, M., Passera, P., Tomalino, M., Bajardi, M., Pomero, F., Allione, A., ... Porta, M. (2001). Group visits improve metabolic control in type 2 diabetes: A 2-year follow-up. *Diabetes Care*, *24*(6), 995–1000. doi:10.2337/diacare.24.6.995

Trief, P. M., Grant, W., Elbert, K., & Weinstock, R. S. (1998). Family environment, glycemic control, and the psychosocial adaptation of adults with diabetes. *Diabetes Care*, *21*(2), 241–245. doi:10.2337/diacare.21.2.241

Trinh, T. T., Montague, B. T., Flanigan, T. P., & Gerard, H. M. (2011). HIV suppression among patients on treatment in Vietnam: A review of HIV viral load testing in a public urban clinic in Ho Chi Minh City. *AIDS Research and Treatment*. doi:10.1155/2011/230953 PMID:21490776

Tripathy, B. (2016). Application of Rough Set Based Models in Medical Diagnosis. In S. Dash & B. Subudhi (Eds.), *Handbook of Research on Computational Intelligence Applications in Bioinformatics* (pp. 144–168). Hershey, PA: IGI Global. doi:10.4018/978-1-5225-0427-6.ch008

Truschel, J. (2019). PMDD: Premenstrual Dysphoric Disorder Symptoms, Causes, Treatment. Psycom.net. Retrieved from https://www.psycom.net

Turcu, C. E., & Turcu, C. O. (2017). Social Internet of Things in Healthcare: From Things to Social Things in Internet of Things. In C. Reis & M. Maximiano (Eds.), *Internet of Things and Advanced Application in Healthcare* (pp. 266–295). Hershey, PA: IGI Global. doi:10.4018/978-1-5225-1820-4.ch010

U.S Department of Health and Human Services. (1999) Mental health: A Report of the surgeon general. Rockville, MD: U.S. Department of Health and Human Services; Substance Abuse and Mental health services Administration, enter for mental Health Services, National institute of Health, National institute of mental health.

Umwangange, M. L., Chironda, G., & Mukeshimana, M. (2018). Knowledge, Attitude and Practice towards malaria prevention among school children aged 5 -14 years in sub-Saharan Africa - A review of literature. *Rwanda Journal of Medicine and Health Sciences*, *1*(1), 22–30. doi:10.4314/rjmhs.v1i1.4

UNAIDS. (2012). *Global report: UNAIDS report on the global AIDS epidemic*. Geneva: UNAIDS.

UNAIDS. (2015). *How AIDS changed everything*. Retrieved from https://www.unaids.org/sites/default/files/media_asset/MDG6Report_en.pdf

UNAIDS. (2017). State of the AIDS epidemic: UNAIDS data 2017. Retrieved from www.unaids.org/sites/default/files/media_asset/20170720_Data_book_2017_en.pdf

UNICEF. (2011). *Children and HIV & AIDS in Namibia*. Windhoek: UNICEF.

UNICEF. (2016). Seventh Stocktaking Report on Children & AIDS, 2016.

UNICEF. (2018). Malaria: Malaria mortality as a cause of death in children under five. Child Health. *Database*.

United Nations Programme on HIV/AIDS (UNAIDS). (2014).

United States Agency for International Development (UNAIDS). (2008). *Third annual report on orphans and vulnerable children in developing countries*. Washington, DC: USAID. Retrieved from www.healthpolicyinitiative.com/Publications/Documents/1346

Unwin, D. W., Sanzogni, L., & Sandhu, K. (2017). Developing and Measuring the Business Case for Health Information Technology. In K. Moahi, K. Bwalya, & P. Sebina (Eds.), *Health Information Systems and the Advancement of Medical Practice in Developing Countries* (pp. 262–290). Hershey, PA: IGI Global. doi:10.4018/978-1-5225-2262-1.ch015

Urooj, S., & Singh, S. P. (2016). Wavelet Transform-Based Soft Computational Techniques and Applications in Medical Imaging. In P. Saxena, D. Singh, & M. Pant (Eds.), *Problem Solving and Uncertainty Modeling through Optimization and Soft Computing Applications* (pp. 339–363). Hershey, PA: IGI Global. doi:10.4018/978-1-4666-9885-7.ch016

US Department of Health and Human Services. (2010). *How tobacco smoke causes disease: What It means to you. Atlanta: US Department of Health and Human Services, Centers for Disease Control and Prevention, National Center for Chronic Disease Prevention and Health Promotion, Office on Smoking and Health, 2010*. Retrieved from: https://www.ncbi.nlm.nih.gov/books/NBK53017/pdf/Bookshelf_NBK53017.pdf

Uys, L., & Middleton, L. (2014). *Mental health nursing: A South African perspective* (6th ed.). Johannesburg: Juta.

van der Heijden, M.M., van Dooren, F.E., Pop, V.J., &Pouwer, F. (2013). Effects of exercise training on quality of life, symptoms of depression, symptoms of anxiety and emotional well-being in type 2 diabetes mellitus: a systematic review. *Diabetologia*, *56*(6), 1210-1225.

van der Kolk, B. (2014). *The body keeps the score: Brain, mind, and body in the healing of trauma*. New York, NY: Penguin Books.

van der Sterren, A., Greenhalgh, E. M., Knoche, D., & Winstanley, M. H. (2019). 8.13 Policies for advancing tobacco control programs among Aboriginal and Torres Strait Islander peoples. In M.M. Scollo & M.H. Winstanley (Eds.), *Tobacco in Australia: Facts and issues*. Melbourne: Cancer Council Victoria. Retrieved from https://www.tobaccoinaustralia.org.au/chapter-8-aptsi/8-13-policy-recommendations-for-advancing-tobacco-

Van Dyck, D., De Greef, K., Deforche, B., Ruige, J., Tudor-Locke, C. E., Kaufman, J. M., ... Bourdeaudhuii, I. (2011). Mediators of physical activity change in a behavioral modification program for type 2 diabetes patients. *The International Journal of Behavioral Nutrition and Physical Activity*, *8*(1), 105. doi:10.1186/1479-5868-8-105

Vasant, P. (2018). A General Medical Diagnosis System Formed by Artificial Neural Networks and Swarm Intelligence Techniques. In U. Kose, G. Guraksin, & O. Deperlioglu (Eds.), *Nature-Inspired Intelligent Techniques for Solving Biomedical Engineering Problems* (pp. 130–145). Hershey, PA: IGI Global. doi:10.4018/978-1-5225-4769-3.ch006

Victor, A. A., Jim, A. W., Uusiku, P., Abdisalan, M. N., Robert, W. S., & Peter, M. A. (2012). Spatial modelling of healthcare utilisation for treatment of fever in Namibia. *International Journal of Health Geography, 11 (6), 1 -13.* https://doi.org/10.1186/1476-072X-11-6.

Voorthuis, A., Bhandari, R., Out, D., Veen, R., Bakermans-Kranenburg, M., & IJzendoorn, M. (2014). Childhood maltreatment experiences and child abuse potential: Temperamental sensitivity as moderator? *Journal of Family Violence*, *29*(7), 749–756. doi:10.100710896-014-9624-3

Vreeman, R. C., Wiehe, S. E., Pearce, E. C., & Winstone, N. M. (2008). A systematic review of pediatric adherence to antiretroviral therapy in low and middle-income countries. *The Pediatric Infectious Disease Journal*, *27*(8), 686–691. doi:10.1097/INF.0b013e31816dd325 PMID:18574439

Waegemann, C. P. (2016). mHealth: History, Analysis, and Implementation. In A. Moumtzoglou (Ed.), M-Health Innovations for Patient-Centered Care (pp. 1-19). Hershey, PA: IGI Global. doi:10.4018/978-1-4666-9861-1.ch001

Walker, R. J., Gebregziabher, M., Martin-Harris, B., & Egede, L. E. (2015). Quantifying direct effects of social determinants of health on glycemic control in adults with type 2 diabetes. *Diabetes Technology & Therapeutics*, *17*(2), 80–87. doi:10.1089/dia.2014.0166

Wang, M. P., Ho, S. Y., & Lam, T. H. (2011). Parental smoking, exposure to second-hand smoke at home, and smoking initiation among young children. *Nicotine & Tobacco Research: Official Journal of the Society for Research on Nicotine and Tobacco*, *13*(9), 827–832. doi:10.1093/ntr/ntr083 PMID:21525153

Wani, Z. A., & Margoob, M. A. (2006). Family study of Adult PTSD patients in south Asia: Experiences from Kashmir. *JK Practitioner*, 61–64.

Watfa, M. K., Majeed, H., & Salahuddin, T. (2016). Computer Based E-Healthcare Clinical Systems: A Comprehensive Survey. *International Journal of Privacy and Health Information Management*, *4*(1), 50–69. doi:10.4018/IJPHIM.2016010104

Webb, D., Cluver, L., & Luo, C. (2018). Evolution or extinction? Pediatric and adolescent HIV responses in the Agenda 2030 era. *Journal of the International AIDS Society*, *21*(S1), 1–3. doi:10.1002/jia2.25071 PMID:29485744

Weinberg, J. L., & Kovarik, C. L. (2010). The WHO clinical staging system for HIV/AIDS. *The Virtual Mentor*, *12*(3), 202–206. PMID:23140869

Weinberg, M., & Gil, S. (2016). Trauma as an objective or subjective experience: The association between types of traumatic events, personality traits, subjective experience of the event, and posttraumatic symptoms. *Journal of Loss and Trauma*, *21*(2), 137–146. doi:10.1080/15325024.2015.1011986

Weiten, W. (2017). *Psychology: Themes and variations* (10th ed.). Boston, MA: Cengage Learning.

Wenk-Sormaz, H. (2005). Meditation can reduce habitual responding. *Advances in Mind-Body*, *3*(4), 34–39.

Westaway, M. S., Seager, J. R., Rheeder, P., & Van Zyl, D. G. (2005). The effects of social support on health, well-being and management of diabetes mellitus: A black South African perspective. *Ethnicity & Health*, *10*(1), 73–89. doi:10.1080/1355785052000323047

West, R. (2017). Tobacco smoking: Health impact, prevalence, correlates and interventions. *Psychology & Health*, *32*(8), 1018–1036. doi:10.1080/08870446.2017.1325890 PMID:28553727

WHO. (2010). *Antiretroviral therapy for HIV infection in adults and adolescents: recommendations for a public health approach (2010 revision)*. Geneva: WHO.

WHO. (2013). Global Action Plan for the prevention and control of noncommunicable diseases 2013-2020. Retrieved from https://www.who.int/nmh/events/ncd_action_plan/en/

WHO. (2018). Global health observatory data. NCD mortality and morbidity. Retrieved from https://www.who.int/gho/ncd/mortality_morbidity/en/

WHO. (2018). Primary health care in Western Pacific. Retrieved from https://www.who.int/westernpacific/health-topics/primary-health-care

Wietholter, J. P., Coetzee, R., Nardella, B., Kincaid, S. E., & Slain, D. (2016). International Healthcare Experiences: Caring While Learning and Learning While Caring. In D. Velliaris & D. Coleman-George (Eds.), *Handbook of Research on Study Abroad Programs and Outbound Mobility* (pp. 470–496). Hershey, PA: IGI Global. doi:10.4018/978-1-5225-0169-5.ch019

Wikipedia. (n.d.). History of Kashmir online. from https://en.wikipedia.org/wiki/History_of_Kashmir

Wisting, L., Reas, D. L., Bang, L., Skrivarhaug, T., Dahl-Jorgensen, K., & Ro, O. (2017). Eating patterns in adolescents with type 1 diabetes: Associations with metabolic control, insulin omission, and eating disorder pathology. *Appetite*, *114*, 226–231. doi:10.1016/j.appet.2017.03.035

Witzke, K., & Specht, O. (2017). M-Health Telemedicine and Telepresence in Oral and Maxillofacial Surgery: An Innovative Prehospital Healthcare Concept in Structurally Weak Areas. *International Journal of Reliable and Quality E-Healthcare*, *6*(4), 37–48. doi:10.4018/IJRQEH.2017100105

Wójcik, A., & Chojnacki, M. (2016). Behavior and Ethical Problems in the Functioning of the Operating Theater (Case Study). In A. Rosiek & K. Leksowski (Eds.), *Organizational Culture and Ethics in Modern Medicine* (pp. 154–179). Hershey, PA: IGI Global. doi:10.4018/978-1-4666-9658-7.ch007

Wolk, K., & Marasek, K. P. (2016). Translation of Medical Texts using Neural Networks. *International Journal of Reliable and Quality E-Healthcare*, *5*(4), 51–66. doi:10.4018/IJRQEH.2016100104

Wong, A. K., & Lo, M. F. (2018). Using Pervasive Computing for Sustainable Healthcare in an Aging Population. In B. Fong, A. Ng, & P. Yuen (Eds.), *Sustainable Health and Long-Term Care Solutions for an Aging Population* (pp. 187–202). Hershey, PA: IGI Global. doi:10.4018/978-1-5225-2633-9.ch010

World Federation for Mental Health. (2015).

World Health Organization (WHO). (2014). Worlds AIDS Day: Business Unusual: Time to end the AIDS epidemic.

World Health Organization (WHO). (2017a). *Depression and other common mental disorders: Global health estimates.* Geneva: World Health Organization. Retrieved from https://apps.who.int/iris/bitstream/handle/10665/254610/WHO-MSD-MER-2017.2-eng.pdf?sequence=1

World Health Organization (WHO). (2017b). *Depression: Let's talk [News release].* Retrieved from https://www.who.int/

World Health Organization (WHO). (2017c). *Depression: Largest cause of disability worldwide.* Retrieved from https://www.voanews.com/a/who-depression-statistics/3737024.html

World Health Organization (WHO). (2018). *Suicide*. Retrieved from https://www.who.int/news-room/fact-sheets/detail/suicid

World Health Organization (WHO). (2019). *Suicide Data.* Retrieved from https://www.who.int/

World Health Organization. (2001). *Encouraging people to stop smoking*. Department of Mental Health and Substance Dependence. Retrieved from https://www.who.int/mental_health/evidence/stop_smoking_whomsdmdp01_4.pdf

World Health Organization. (2001d). strengthening mental health promotion. Geneva, World Health Organization (fact sheet no. 220).

World Health Organization. (2011). *Wolrd report on disability*. Geneva. USA. Retrived from https://www.who.int/disabilities/worldreport/2011/en/

World Health Organization. (2016). World Malaria Report 2016. Retrieved from https://www.who.int/malaria/publications/world-malaria-report-2016/report/en/

World Health Organization. (2017). World Malaria Report 2017. Retrieved from https://www.who.int/malaria/publications/world-malaria-report-2017/en/

World Health Organization. (2018) World Malaria Report 2018. Retrieved from https://www.who.int/malaria/publications/world-malaria-report-2018/en/

World Health Organization. (2019). Bulletin on the African Health Report. *The Health of the People*, *§§§*, 97.

Wu, B. (2018). Situational depression or clinical depression. *Medical News Today*. Retrieved from https://www.medicalnewstoday.com

Wu, G., Hu, Z., & Zheng, J. (2019). Role Stress, Job Burnout, and Job Performance in Construction Project Managers: The Moderating Role of Career Calling. *International Journal of Environmental Research and Public Health*, *16*(13), 2394. doi:10.3390/ijerph16132394

Wu, G., Wu, Y., Li, H., & Dan, C. (2018). Job Burnout, Work-Family Conflict and Project Performance for Construction Professionals: The Moderating Role of Organizational Support. *International Journal of Environmental Research and Public Health*, *15*(12), 2869. doi:10.3390/ijerph15122869

Wu, S. F., Young, L. S., Yeh, F. C., Jian, Y. M., Cheng, K. C., & Lee, M. C. (2013). Correlations among social support, depression, and anxiety in patients with type-2 diabetes. *The Journal of Nursing Research*, *21*(2), 129–138. doi:10.1097/jnr.0b013e3182921fe1

Wu, W., Martin, B. C., & Ni, C. (2017). A Systematic Review of Competency-Based Education Effort in the Health Professions: Seeking Order Out of Chaos. In K. Rasmussen, P. Northrup, & R. Colson (Eds.), *Handbook of Research on Competency-Based Education in University Settings* (pp. 352–378). Hershey, PA: IGI Global. doi:10.4018/978-1-5225-0932-5.ch018

Yadav, S., Ekbal, A., Saha, S., Pathak, P. S., & Bhattacharyya, P. (2017). Patient Data De-Identification: A Conditional Random-Field-Based Supervised Approach. In S. Saha, A. Mandal, A. Narasimhamurthy, S. V, & S. Sangam (Eds.), Handbook of Research on Applied Cybernetics and Systems Science (pp. 234-253). Hershey, PA: IGI Global. doi:10.4018/978-1-5225-2498-4.ch011

Yadav, N., Aliasgari, M., & Poellabauer, C. (2016). Mobile Healthcare in an Increasingly Connected Developing World. *International Journal of Privacy and Health Information Management*, *4*(2), 76–97. doi:10.4018/IJPHIM.2016070106

Yadav, V., Rastogi, R., Chaturvedi, D. K., Satya, S., Arora, N., Yadav, V., ... Chauhan, S. (2018j). Statistical Analysis of EMG & GSR Biofeedback Efficacy on Different Modes for Chronic TTH on Various Indicators. *Int. J. Advanced Intelligence Paradigms*, *13*(1), 251–275. doi:10.1504/IJAIP.2019.10021825

Yalewayler, T., Ashmelash, D., Anibachew, S., Eschetie, S., Addisu, A., & Zelek, A. J. (2019). The Prevalence of Malaria among pregnant women in Ethiopia: A systematic review and data analysis. *Journal of Parasitology Research*. doi:10.1155/2019/8390091

Yang, J., Su, S., Zhao, H., Wang, D., Wang, J., Zhang, F., & Zhao, Y. (2016). Prevalence and mortality of cancer among HIV-infected inpatients in Beijing, China. *BMC Infectious Diseases*, *16*(1), 82. doi:10.118612879-016-1416-3 PMID:26883427

Yaswi, A., & Haque, A. (2008). Prevalence of PTSD symptoms and Depression and level of coping among the victims of the Kashmir conflict. *Journal of Loss and Trauma*, *13*(5), 471–480. doi:10.1080/15325020802171441

Young, V., Eiser, C., Johnson, B., Brierley, S., Epton, T., Elliott, J., & Heller, S. (2013). Eating problems in adolescents with Type 1 diabetes: A systematic review with meta-analysis. *Diabetic Medicine*, *30*(2), 189–198. doi:10.1111/j.1464-5491.2012.03771.x

Yu, B., Wijesekera, D., & Costa, P. C. (2017). Informed Consent in Electronic Medical Record Systems. In I. Management Association (Ed.), Healthcare Ethics and Training: Concepts, Methodologies, Tools, and Applications (pp. 1029-1049). Hershey, PA: IGI Global. doi:10.4018/978-1-5225-2237-9.ch049

Yu, B., Wijesekera, D., & Costa, P. C. (2017). Informed Consent in Healthcare: A Study Case of Genetic Services. In A. Moumtzoglou (Ed.), *Design, Development, and Integration of Reliable Electronic Healthcare Platforms* (pp. 211–242). Hershey, PA: IGI Global. doi:10.4018/978-1-5225-1724-5.ch013

Yu, M., Li, J., & Wang, W. (2017). Creative Life Experience among Students in Medical Education. In C. Zhou (Ed.), *Handbook of Research on Creative Problem-Solving Skill Development in Higher Education* (pp. 158–184). Hershey, PA: IGI Global. doi:10.4018/978-1-5225-0643-0.ch008

Zagarins, S. E., Allen, N. A., Garb, J. L., & Welch, G. (2012). Improvement in glycemic control following a diabetes education intervention is associated with change in diabetes distress but not change in depressive symptoms. *Journal of Behavioral Medicine*, *35*(3), 299–304. doi:10.100710865-011-9359-z

Zahid M. (2017). Judicial Independence and Accountability of Judiciary in Pakistan. *International Journal of Research in Social Sciences*, *7*(12).

Zanella, A., Bui, N., Castellani, A., Vangelista, L., & Zorzi, M. (2004). Internet of things for smart cities. *IEEE Internet Things J.*, *1*(1), 22–32. doi:10.1109/JIOT.2014.2306328

Zanoveli, J. M., de Morais, H., Dias, I. C. da S., Schreiber, A. K., de Souza, C. P., & Cunha, J. M. (2016). Depression associated with diabetes: From pathophysiology to treatment. *Current Diabetes Reviews*, *12*(3), 165–178. doi:10.2174/1573399811666150515125349

Zare, M., Narayan, M., Lasway, A., Kitsantas, P., Wojtusiak, J., & Oetjen, C. A. (2018). Influence of Adverse Childhood Experiences on anxiety and depression in children aged 6 to 11 years. *Pediatric Nursing*, *44*(6), 267–274.

Zarour, K. (2017). Towards a Telehomecare in Algeria: Case of Diabetes Measurement and Remote Monitoring. *International Journal of E-Health and Medical Communications*, *8*(4), 61–80. doi:10.4018/IJEHMC.2017100104

Zastrow, C., & Kirst-Ashman, K. K. (2015). *Empowerment series: Understanding human behavior and the social environment* (10th ed.). Boston, MA: Cengage Learning.

Zavyalova, Y. V., Korzun, D. G., Meigal, A. Y., & Borodin, A. V. (2017). Towards the Development of Smart Spaces-Based Socio-Cyber-Medicine Systems. *International Journal of Embedded and Real-Time Communication Systems*, *8*(1), 45–63. doi:10.4018/IJERTCS.2017010104

Zeinali, A. A. (2018). Word Formation Study in Developing Naming Guidelines in the Translation of English Medical Terms Into Persian. In M. Khosrow-Pour, D.B.A. (Ed.), Encyclopedia of Information Science and Technology, Fourth Edition (pp. 5136-5147). Hershey, PA: IGI Global. doi:10.4018/978-1-5225-2255-3.ch446

Zerrudo, M. R. (2016). Theater of disaster, folk stories as vehicles for healing and survival. *Teaching Artist Journal, 14*(3), 161–170. doi:10.1080/15411796.2016.1209073

Zhang, W., Xu, H., Zhao, S., Yin, S., Wang, X., Guo, J., ... Tian, D. (2015). Prevalence and influencing factors of co-morbid depression in patients with type 2 diabetes mellitus: A General Hospital based study. *Diabetology & Metabolic Syndrome, 7*(1), 60. doi:10.118613098-015-0053-0

Zhao, F. F., Suhonen, R., Katajisto, J., & Leino-Kilpi, H. (2018). The association of diabetes-related self-care activities with perceived stress, anxiety, and fatigue: A cross-sectional study. *Patient Preference and Adherence, 12*, 1677–1686. doi:10.2147/PPA.S169826

Ziminski, T. B., Demurjian, S. A., Sanzi, E., & Agresta, T. (2016). Toward Integrating Healthcare Data and Systems: A Study of Architectural Alternatives. In T. Iyamu & A. Tatnall (Eds.), *Maximizing Healthcare Delivery and Management through Technology Integration* (pp. 270–304). Hershey, PA: IGI Global. doi:10.4018/978-1-4666-9446-0.ch016

Ziminski, T. B., Demurjian, S. A., Sanzi, E., Baihan, M., & Agresta, T. (2016). An Architectural Solution for Health Information Exchange. *International Journal of User-Driven Healthcare, 6*(1), 65–103. doi:10.4018/IJUDH.2016010104

Zineldin, M., & Vasicheva, V. (2018). Reducing Medical Errors and Increasing Patient Safety: TRM and 5 Q's Approaches for Better Quality of Life. In *Technological Tools for Value-Based Sustainable Relationships in Health: Emerging Research and Opportunities* (pp. 87–115). Hershey, PA: IGI Global. doi:10.4018/978-1-5225-4091-5.ch005

Related References

To continue our tradition of advancing information science and technology research, we have compiled a list of recommended IGI Global readings. These references will provide additional information and guidance to further enrich your knowledge and assist you with your own research and future publications.

Abu Seman, S. A., & Ramayah, T. (2017). Are We Ready to App?: A Study on mHealth Apps, Its Future, and Trends in Malaysia Context. In J. Pelet (Ed.), *Mobile Platforms, Design, and Apps for Social Commerce* (pp. 69–83). Hershey, PA: IGI Global. doi:10.4018/978-1-5225-2469-4.ch005

Aggarwal, S., & Azad, V. (2017). A Hybrid System Based on FMM and MLP to Diagnose Heart Disease. In S. Bhattacharyya, S. De, I. Pan, & P. Dutta (Eds.), *Intelligent Multidimensional Data Clustering and Analysis* (pp. 293–325). Hershey, PA: IGI Global. doi:10.4018/978-1-5225-1776-4.ch011

Akaichi, J., & Mhadhbi, L. (2016). A Clinical Decision Support System: Ontology-Driven Approach for Effective Emergency Management. In J. Moon & M. Galea (Eds.), *Improving Health Management through Clinical Decision Support Systems* (pp. 270–294). Hershey, PA: IGI Global. doi:10.4018/978-1-4666-9432-3.ch013

Akerkar, R. (2016). Towards an Intelligent Integrated Approach for Clinical Decision Support. In A. Aggarwal (Ed.), *Managing Big Data Integration in the Public Sector* (pp. 187–205). Hershey, PA: IGI Global. doi:10.4018/978-1-4666-9649-5.ch011

Al-Busaidi, S. S. (2018). Interdisciplinary Relationships Between Medicine and Social Sciences. In M. Al-Suqri, A. Al-Kindi, S. AlKindi, & N. Saleem (Eds.), *Promoting Interdisciplinarity in Knowledge Generation and Problem Solving* (pp. 124–137). Hershey, PA: IGI Global. doi:10.4018/978-1-5225-3878-3.ch009

Al Kareh, T., & Thoumy, M. (2018). The Impact of Health Information Digitization on the Physiotherapist-Patient Relationship: A Pilot Study of the Lebanese Community. *International Journal of Healthcare Information Systems and Informatics, 13*(2), 29–53. doi:10.4018/IJHISI.2018040103

Alenzuela, R. (2017). Research, Leadership, and Resource-Sharing Initiatives: The Role of Local Library Consortia in Access to Medical Information. In S. Ram (Ed.), *Library and Information Services for Bioinformatics Education and Research* (pp. 199–211). Hershey, PA: IGI Global. doi:10.4018/978-1-5225-1871-6.ch012

Ameri, H., Alizadeh, S., & Noughabi, E. A. (2017). Application of Data Mining Techniques in Clinical Decision Making: A Literature Review and Classification. In E. Noughabi, B. Raahemi, A. Albadvi, & B. Far (Eds.), *Handbook of Research on Data Science for Effective Healthcare Practice and Administration* (pp. 257–295). Hershey, PA: IGI Global. doi:10.4018/978-1-5225-2515-8.ch012

Anand, S. (2017). Medical Image Enhancement Using Edge Information-Based Methods. In B. Singh (Ed.), *Computational Tools and Techniques for Biomedical Signal Processing* (pp. 123–148). Hershey, PA: IGI Global. doi:10.4018/978-1-5225-0660-7.ch006

Angjellari-Dajci, F., Sapienza, C., Lawless, W. F., & Kavanagh, K. (2016). Human Capital Accumulation in Medical Simulated Learning Environments: A Framework for Economic Evaluation. In M. Russ (Ed.), *Quantitative Multidisciplinary Approaches in Human Capital and Asset Management* (pp. 65–88). Hershey, PA: IGI Global. doi:10.4018/978-1-4666-9652-5.ch004

Anil, M., Ayyildiz-Tamis, D., Tasdemir, S., Sendemir-Urkmez, A., & Gulce-Iz, S. (2016). Bioinspired Materials and Biocompatibility. In M. Bououdina (Ed.), *Emerging Research on Bioinspired Materials Engineering* (pp. 294–322). Hershey, PA: IGI Global. doi:10.4018/978-1-4666-9811-6.ch011

Anton, J. L., Soriano, J. V., Martinez, M. I., & Garcia, F. B. (2018). Comprehensive E-Learning Appraisal System. In M. Khosrow-Pour, D.B.A. (Ed.), Encyclopedia of Information Science and Technology, Fourth Edition (pp. 5787-5799). Hershey, PA: IGI Global. doi:10.4018/978-1-5225-2255-3.ch503

Arabi, M. (2016). Redesigning the Organizational Structure to Reach Efficiency: The Case of Ministry of Health and Medical Education of Iran. In R. Gholipour & K. Rouzbehani (Eds.), *Social, Economic, and Political Perspectives on Public Health Policy-Making* (pp. 257–294). Hershey, PA: IGI Global. doi:10.4018/978-1-4666-9944-1.ch012

Assis-Hassid, S., Heart, T., Reychav, I., & Pliskin, J. S. (2016). Modelling Factors Affecting Patient-Doctor-Computer Communication in Primary Care. *International Journal of Reliable and Quality E-Healthcare, 5*(1), 1–17. doi:10.4018/IJRQEH.2016010101

Atzori, B., Hoffman, H. G., Vagnoli, L., Messeri, A., & Grotto, R. L. (2018). Virtual Reality as Distraction Technique for Pain Management in Children and Adolescents. In M. Khosrow-Pour, D.B.A. (Ed.), Encyclopedia of Information Science and Technology, Fourth Edition (pp. 5955-5965). Hershey, PA: IGI Global. doi:10.4018/978-1-5225-2255-3.ch518

Audibert, M., Mathonnat, J., Pélissier, A., & Huang, X. X. (2018). The Impact of the New Rural Cooperative Medical Scheme on Township Hospitals' Utilization and Income Structure in Weifang Prefecture, China. In I. Management Association (Ed.), Health Economics and Healthcare Reform: Breakthroughs in Research and Practice (pp. 109-121). Hershey, PA: IGI Global. doi:10.4018/978-1-5225-3168-5.ch007

Ayyachamy, S. (2016). Analysis and Comparison of Developed 2D Medical Image Database Design using Registration Scheme, Retrieval Scheme, and Bag-of-Visual-Words. In N. Dey & A. Ashour (Eds.), *Classification and Clustering in Biomedical Signal Processing* (pp. 149–168). Hershey, PA: IGI Global. doi:10.4018/978-1-5225-0140-4.ch007

Babalola, A. C. (2016). Literacy and Decision Making on Health Issues among Married Women in Southwest Nigeria. In V. Wang (Ed.), *Handbook of Research on Advancing Health Education through Technology* (pp. 191–212). Hershey, PA: IGI Global. doi:10.4018/978-1-4666-9494-1.ch009

Babu, A., & Ayyappan, S. (2017). A Methodological Evaluation of Crypto-Watermarking System for Medical Images. In C. Bhatt & S. Peddoju (Eds.), *Cloud Computing Systems and Applications in Healthcare* (pp. 189–217). Hershey, PA: IGI Global. doi:10.4018/978-1-5225-1002-4.ch010

Bakke, A. (2017). Ethos in E-Health: From Informational to Interactive Websites. In M. Folk & S. Apostel (Eds.), *Establishing and Evaluating Digital Ethos and Online Credibility* (pp. 85–103). Hershey, PA: IGI Global. doi:10.4018/978-1-5225-1072-7.ch005

Bali, S. (2018). Enhancing the Reach of Health Care Through Telemedicine: Status and New Possibilities in Developing Countries. In U. Pandey & V. Indrakanti (Eds.), *Open and Distance Learning Initiatives for Sustainable Development* (pp. 339–354). Hershey, PA: IGI Global. doi:10.4018/978-1-5225-2621-6.ch019

Barrett, T. E. (2018). Essentials for Education and Training for Tomorrow's Physicians. In C. Smith (Ed.), *Exploring the Pressures of Medical Education From a Mental Health and Wellness Perspective* (pp. 230–252). Hershey, PA: IGI Global. doi:10.4018/978-1-5225-2811-1.ch010

Barrett, T. J. (2016). Knowledge in Action: Fostering Health Education through Technology. In V. Wang (Ed.), *Handbook of Research on Advancing Health Education through Technology* (pp. 39–62). Hershey, PA: IGI Global. doi:10.4018/978-1-4666-9494-1.ch003

Berrahal, S., & Boudriga, N. (2017). The Risks of Wearable Technologies to Individuals and Organizations. In A. Marrington, D. Kerr, & J. Gammack (Eds.), *Managing Security Issues and the Hidden Dangers of Wearable Technologies* (pp. 18–46). Hershey, PA: IGI Global. doi:10.4018/978-1-5225-1016-1.ch002

Bhagat, A. P., & Atique, M. (2016). Medical Image Mining Using Fuzzy Connectedness Image Segmentation: Efficient Retrieval of Patients' Stored Images. In W. Karâa & N. Dey (Eds.), *Biomedical Image Analysis and Mining Techniques for Improved Health Outcomes* (pp. 184–209). Hershey, PA: IGI Global. doi:10.4018/978-1-4666-8811-7.ch009

Bhargava, P. (2018). Blended Learning: An Effective Application to Clinical Teaching. In S. Tang & C. Lim (Eds.), *Preparing the Next Generation of Teachers for 21st Century Education* (pp. 302–320). Hershey, PA: IGI Global. doi:10.4018/978-1-5225-4080-9.ch018

Binh, N. T., & Tuyet, V. T. (2016). The Combination of Adaptive Filters to Improve the Quality of Medical Images in New Wavelet Domain. In N. Dey & A. Ashour (Eds.), *Classification and Clustering in Biomedical Signal Processing* (pp. 46–76). Hershey, PA: IGI Global. doi:10.4018/978-1-5225-0140-4.ch003

Bird, J. L. (2017). Writing Healing Narratives. In V. Bryan & J. Bird (Eds.), *Healthcare Community Synergism between Patients, Practitioners, and Researchers* (pp. 1–28). Hershey, PA: IGI Global. doi:10.4018/978-1-5225-0640-9.ch001

Bottrighi, A., Leonardi, G., Piovesan, L., & Terenziani, P. (2016). Knowledge-Based Support to the Treatment of Exceptions in Computer Interpretable Clinical Guidelines. *International Journal of Knowledge-Based Organizations*, *6*(3), 1–27. doi:10.4018/IJKBO.2016070101

Bougoulias, K., Kouris, I., Prasinos, M., Giokas, K., & Koutsouris, D. (2017). Ob/Gyn EMR Software: A Solution for Obstetricians and Gynecologists. In A. Moumtzoglou (Ed.), *Design, Development, and Integration of Reliable Electronic Healthcare Platforms* (pp. 101–111). Hershey, PA: IGI Global. doi:10.4018/978-1-5225-1724-5.ch006

Bouslimi, R., Ayadi, M. G., & Akaichi, J. (2018). Medical Image Retrieval in Healthcare Social Networks. *International Journal of Healthcare Information Systems and Informatics, 13*(2), 13–28. doi:10.4018/IJHISI.2018040102

Bouzaabia, O., Bouzaabia, R., & Mejri, K. (2017). Role of Internet in the Development of Medical Tourism Service in Tunisia. In A. Capatina & E. Rancati (Eds.), *Key Challenges and Opportunities in Web Entrepreneurship* (pp. 211–241). Hershey, PA: IGI Global. doi:10.4018/978-1-5225-2466-3.ch009

Briz-Ponce, L., Juanes-Méndez, J. A., & García-Peñalvo, F. J. (2016). The Role of Gender in Technology Acceptance for Medical Education. In M. Cruz-Cunha, I. Miranda, R. Martinho, & R. Rijo (Eds.), *Encyclopedia of E-Health and Telemedicine* (pp. 1013–1027). Hershey, PA: IGI Global. doi:10.4018/978-1-4666-9978-6.ch079

Briz-Ponce, L., Juanes-Méndez, J. A., & García-Peñalvo, F. J. (2016). A Research Contribution to the Analysis of Mobile Devices in Higher Education from Medical Students' Point of View. In L. Briz-Ponce, J. Juanes-Méndez, & F. García-Peñalvo (Eds.), *Handbook of Research on Mobile Devices and Applications in Higher Education Settings* (pp. 196–221). Hershey, PA: IGI Global. doi:10.4018/978-1-5225-0256-2.ch009

Brown-Jackson, K. L. (2018). Telemedicine and Telehealth: Academics Engaging the Community in a Call to Action. In S. Burton (Ed.), *Engaged Scholarship and Civic Responsibility in Higher Education* (pp. 166–193). Hershey, PA: IGI Global. doi:10.4018/978-1-5225-3649-9.ch008

Bwalya, K. J. (2017). Next Wave of Tele-Medicine: Virtual Presence of Medical Personnel. In K. Moahi, K. Bwalya, & P. Sebina (Eds.), *Health Information Systems and the Advancement of Medical Practice in Developing Countries* (pp. 168–180). Hershey, PA: IGI Global. doi:10.4018/978-1-5225-2262-1.ch010

Carlton, E. L., Holsinger, J. W. Jr, & Anunobi, N. (2016). Physician Engagement with Health Information Technology: Implications for Practice and Professionalism. *International Journal of Computers in Clinical Practice, 1*(2), 51–73. doi:10.4018/IJCCP.2016070103

Castillo-Page, L., Eliason, J., Conrad, S. S., & Nivet, M. A. (2016). Diversity in Undergraduate Medical Education: An Examination of Organizational Culture and Climate in Medical Schools. In C. Scott & J. Sims (Eds.), *Developing Workforce Diversity Programs, Curriculum, and Degrees in Higher Education* (pp. 304–326). Hershey, PA: IGI Global. doi:10.4018/978-1-5225-0209-8.ch016

Cebeci, H. I., & Hiziroglu, A. (2016). Review of Business Intelligence and Intelligent Systems in Healthcare Domain. In N. Celebi (Ed.), *Intelligent Techniques for Data Analysis in Diverse Settings* (pp. 192–206). Hershey, PA: IGI Global. doi:10.4018/978-1-5225-0075-9.ch009

Celik, G. (2018). Determining Headache Diseases With Genetic Algorithm. In U. Kose, G. Guraksin, & O. Deperlioglu (Eds.), *Nature-Inspired Intelligent Techniques for Solving Biomedical Engineering Problems* (pp. 249–262). Hershey, PA: IGI Global. doi:10.4018/978-1-5225-4769-3.ch012

Chakraborty, C., Gupta, B., & Ghosh, S. K. (2016). Mobile Telemedicine Systems for Remote Patient's Chronic Wound Monitoring. In A. Moumtzoglou (Ed.), *M-Health Innovations for Patient-Centered Care* (pp. 213–239). Hershey, PA: IGI Global. doi:10.4018/978-1-4666-9861-1.ch011

Chakraborty, S., Chatterjee, S., Ashour, A. S., Mali, K., & Dey, N. (2018). Intelligent Computing in Medical Imaging: A Study. In N. Dey (Ed.), *Advancements in Applied Metaheuristic Computing* (pp. 143–163). Hershey, PA: IGI Global. doi:10.4018/978-1-5225-4151-6.ch006

Chavez, A., & Kovarik, C. (2017). Open Source Technology for Medical Practice in Developing Countries. In K. Moahi, K. Bwalya, & P. Sebina (Eds.), *Health Information Systems and the Advancement of Medical Practice in Developing Countries* (pp. 33–59). Hershey, PA: IGI Global. doi:10.4018/978-1-5225-2262-1.ch003

Chen, E. T. (2016). Examining the Influence of Information Technology on Modern Health Care. In P. Manolitzas, E. Grigoroudis, N. Matsatsinis, & D. Yannacopoulos (Eds.), *Effective Methods for Modern Healthcare Service Quality and Evaluation* (pp. 110–136). Hershey, PA: IGI Global. doi:10.4018/978-1-4666-9961-8.ch006

Chin, S. (2016). Surviving Sandy: Recovering Collections after a Natural Disaster. In E. Decker & J. Townes (Eds.), *Handbook of Research on Disaster Management and Contingency Planning in Modern Libraries* (pp. 366–388). Hershey, PA: IGI Global. doi:10.4018/978-1-4666-8624-3.ch016

Chojnacki, M., & Wójcik, A. (2016). Security and the Role of New Technologies and Innovation in Medical Ethics. In A. Rosiek & K. Leksowski (Eds.), *Organizational Culture and Ethics in Modern Medicine* (pp. 52–77). Hershey, PA: IGI Global. doi:10.4018/978-1-4666-9658-7.ch003

Cılız, N., Yıldırım, H., & Temizel, Ş. (2016). Structure Development for Effective Medical Waste and Hazardous Waste Management System. In U. Akkucuk (Ed.), *Handbook of Research on Waste Management Techniques for Sustainability* (pp. 303–327). Hershey, PA: IGI Global. doi:10.4018/978-1-4666-9723-2.ch016

Ciufudean, C. (2018). Innovative Formalism for Biological Data Analysis. In M. Khosrow-Pour, D.B.A. (Ed.), Encyclopedia of Information Science and Technology, Fourth Edition (pp. 1814-1824). Hershey, PA: IGI Global. doi:10.4018/978-1-5225-2255-3.ch158

Ciufudean, C., & Ciufudean, O. (2016). Tele-Monitoring for Medical Diagnosis Availability. In M. Cruz-Cunha, I. Miranda, R. Martinho, & R. Rijo (Eds.), *Encyclopedia of E-Health and Telemedicine* (pp. 401–411). Hershey, PA: IGI Global. doi:10.4018/978-1-4666-9978-6.ch032

Colaguori, R., & Danesi, M. (2017). Medical Semiotics: A Revisitation and an Exhortation. *International Journal of Semiotics and Visual Rhetoric*, *1*(1), 11–18. doi:10.4018/IJSVR.2017010102

Cole, A. W., & Salek, T. A. (2017). Adopting a Parasocial Connection to Overcome Professional Kakoethos in Online Health Information. In M. Folk & S. Apostel (Eds.), *Establishing and Evaluating Digital Ethos and Online Credibility* (pp. 104–120). Hershey, PA: IGI Global. doi:10.4018/978-1-5225-1072-7.ch006

Contreras, E. C., & Puente, G. J. (2016). How to Identify Rheumatic Diseases by General Physicians. In T. Gasmelseid (Ed.), *Advancing Pharmaceutical Processes and Tools for Improved Health Outcomes* (pp. 136–166). Hershey, PA: IGI Global. doi:10.4018/978-1-5225-0248-7.ch006

D'Andrea, A., Ferri, F., & Grifoni, P. (2016). RFID Technologies in Healthcare Setting: Applications and Future Perspectives. *International Journal of Computers in Clinical Practice*, *1*(1), 15–27. doi:10.4018/IJCCP.2016010102

Damianakis, A., Kallonis, P., Loudos, G., Tsatsos, D., & Tsoukalis, A. (2016). Exploiting 3D Medical Equipment Simulations to Support Biomedical Engineering Academic Courses: Design Methodology and Implementation in a Small Scale National Project. In B. Khan (Ed.), *Revolutionizing Modern Education through Meaningful E-Learning Implementation* (pp. 277–295). Hershey, PA: IGI Global. doi:10.4018/978-1-5225-0466-5.ch015

Demiroz, E. (2016). Principles of Instructional Design for E-Learning and Online Learning Practices: Implications for Medical Education. In V. Wang (Ed.), *Handbook of Research on Advancing Health Education through Technology* (pp. 419–451). Hershey, PA: IGI Global. doi:10.4018/978-1-4666-9494-1.ch018

Deperlioglu, O. (2018). Intelligent Techniques Inspired by Nature and Used in Biomedical Engineering. In U. Kose, G. Guraksin, & O. Deperlioglu (Eds.), *Nature-Inspired Intelligent Techniques for Solving Biomedical Engineering Problems* (pp. 51–77). Hershey, PA: IGI Global. doi:10.4018/978-1-5225-4769-3.ch003

Dey, N., & Ashour, A. S. (2018). Meta-Heuristic Algorithms in Medical Image Segmentation: A Review. In N. Dey (Ed.), *Advancements in Applied Metaheuristic Computing* (pp. 185–203). Hershey, PA: IGI Global. doi:10.4018/978-1-5225-4151-6.ch008

Dey, N., Ashour, A. S., & Althoupety, A. S. (2017). Thermal Imaging in Medical Science. In V. Santhi (Ed.), *Recent Advances in Applied Thermal Imaging for Industrial Applications* (pp. 87–117). Hershey, PA: IGI Global. doi:10.4018/978-1-5225-2423-6.ch004

Di Virgilio, F., Camillo, A. A., & Camillo, I. C. (2017). The Impact of Social Network on Italian Users' Behavioural Intention for the Choice of a Medical Tourist Destination. *International Journal of Tourism and Hospitality Management in the Digital Age*, *1*(1), 36–49. doi:10.4018/IJTHMDA.2017010103

Dias, C. M., Ribeiro, A. G., & Furtado, S. F. (2016). An Overview about the Use of Healthcare Applications on Mobile Devices. In M. Cruz-Cunha, I. Miranda, R. Martinho, & R. Rijo (Eds.), *Encyclopedia of E-Health and Telemedicine* (pp. 285–298). Hershey, PA: IGI Global. doi:10.4018/978-1-4666-9978-6.ch024

Dogra, A. K., & Dogra, P. (2017). The Medical Tourism Industry in the BRIC Nations: An Indian Analysis. In M. Dhiman (Ed.), *Opportunities and Challenges for Tourism and Hospitality in the BRIC Nations* (pp. 320–336). Hershey, PA: IGI Global. doi:10.4018/978-1-5225-0708-6.ch020

Drowos, J. L., & Wood, S. K. (2017). Preparing Future Physicians to Adapt to the Changing Health Care System: Promoting Humanism through Curricular Design. In V. Bryan & J. Bird (Eds.), *Healthcare Community Synergism between Patients, Practitioners, and Researchers* (pp. 106–125). Hershey, PA: IGI Global. doi:10.4018/978-1-5225-0640-9.ch006

Dulam, K. (2017). Medical Patents and Impact on Availability and Affordability of Essential Medicines in India. In R. Aggarwal & R. Kaur (Eds.), *Patent Law and Intellectual Property in the Medical Field* (pp. 41–57). Hershey, PA: IGI Global. doi:10.4018/978-1-5225-2414-4.ch003

Dutta, P. (2017). Decision Making in Medical Diagnosis via Distance Measures on Interval Valued Fuzzy Sets. *International Journal of System Dynamics Applications*, *6*(4), 63–83. doi:10.4018/IJSDA.2017100104

Edoh, T. O., Pawar, P. A., Brügge, B., & Teege, G. (2016). A Multidisciplinary Remote Healthcare Delivery System to Increase Health Care Access, Pathology Screening, and Treatment in Developing Countries: The Case of Benin. *International Journal of Healthcare Information Systems and Informatics*, *11*(4), 1–31. doi:10.4018/IJHISI.2016100101

El Guemhioui, K., & Demurjian, S. A. (2017). Semantic Reconciliation of Electronic Health Records Using Semantic Web Technologies. *International Journal of Information Technology and Web Engineering*, *12*(2), 26–48. doi:10.4018/IJITWE.2017040102

Ellouze, N., Rekhis, S., & Boudriga, N. (2016). Forensic Investigation of Digital Crimes in Healthcare Applications. In O. Isafiade & A. Bagula (Eds.), *Data Mining Trends and Applications in Criminal Science and Investigations* (pp. 169–210). Hershey, PA: IGI Global. doi:10.4018/978-1-5225-0463-4.ch007

Eneanya, A. N. (2016). Health Policy Implementation and Its Barriers: The Case Study of US Health System. In R. Gholipour & K. Rouzbehani (Eds.), *Social, Economic, and Political Perspectives on Public Health Policy-Making* (pp. 42–63). Hershey, PA: IGI Global. doi:10.4018/978-1-4666-9944-1.ch003

Entico, G. J. (2016). Knowledge Management and the Medical Health Librarians: A Perception Study. In J. Yap, M. Perez, M. Ayson, & G. Entico (Eds.), *Special Library Administration, Standardization and Technological Integration* (pp. 52–77). Hershey, PA: IGI Global. doi:10.4018/978-1-4666-9542-9.ch003

Ferradji, M. A., & Zidani, A. (2016). Collaborative Environment for Remote Clinical Reasoning Learning. *International Journal of E-Health and Medical Communications*, *7*(4), 62–81. doi:10.4018/IJEHMC.2016100104

Fisher, J. (2018). Sociological Perspectives on Improving Medical Diagnosis Emphasizing CAD. In M. Khosrow-Pour, D.B.A. (Ed.), Encyclopedia of Information Science and Technology, Fourth Edition (pp. 1017-1024). Hershey, PA: IGI Global. doi:10.4018/978-1-5225-2255-3.ch088

Flores, C. D., Respício, A., Coelho, H., Bez, M. R., & Fonseca, J. M. (2016). Simulation for Medical Training. In M. Cruz-Cunha, I. Miranda, R. Martinho, & R. Rijo (Eds.), *Encyclopedia of E-Health and Telemedicine* (pp. 827–842). Hershey, PA: IGI Global. doi:10.4018/978-1-4666-9978-6.ch064

Frank, E. M. (2018). Healthcare Education: Integrating Simulation Technologies. In V. Bryan, A. Musgrove, & J. Powers (Eds.), *Handbook of Research on Human Development in the Digital Age* (pp. 163–182). Hershey, PA: IGI Global. doi:10.4018/978-1-5225-2838-8.ch008

Garner, G. (2018). Foundations for Yoga Practice in Rehabilitation. In S. Telles & N. Singh (Eds.), *Research-Based Perspectives on the Psychophysiology of Yoga* (pp. 263–307). Hershey, PA: IGI Global. doi:10.4018/978-1-5225-2788-6.ch015

Gasmelseid, T. M. (2016). Improving Pharmaceutical Care through the Use of Intelligent Pharmacoinformatics. In T. Gasmelseid (Ed.), *Advancing Pharmaceutical Processes and Tools for Improved Health Outcomes* (pp. 167–188). Hershey, PA: IGI Global. doi:10.4018/978-1-5225-0248-7.ch007

Gavurová, B., Kováč, V., & Šoltés, M. (2018). Medical Equipment and Economic Determinants of Its Structure and Regulation in the Slovak Republic. In M. Khosrow-Pour, D.B.A. (Ed.), Encyclopedia of Information Science and Technology, Fourth Edition (pp. 5841-5852). Hershey, PA: IGI Global. doi:10.4018/978-1-5225-2255-3.ch508

Ge, X., Wang, Q., Huang, K., Law, V., & Thomas, D. C. (2017). Designing Simulated Learning Environments and Facilitating Authentic Learning Experiences in Medical Education. In J. Stefaniak (Ed.), *Advancing Medical Education Through Strategic Instructional Design* (pp. 77–100). Hershey, PA: IGI Global. doi:10.4018/978-1-5225-2098-6.ch004

Gewald, H., & Gewald, C. (2018). Inhibitors of Physicians' Use of Mandatory Hospital Information Systems (HIS). *International Journal of Healthcare Information Systems and Informatics, 13*(1), 29–44. doi:10.4018/IJHISI.2018010103

Ghosh, D., & Dinda, S. (2017). Health Infrastructure and Economic Development in India. In R. Das (Ed.), *Social, Health, and Environmental Infrastructures for Economic Growth* (pp. 99–119). Hershey, PA: IGI Global. doi:10.4018/978-1-5225-2364-2.ch006

Ghosh, K., & Sen, K. C. (2017). The Potential of Crowdsourcing in the Health Care Industry. In N. Wickramasinghe (Ed.), *Handbook of Research on Healthcare Administration and Management* (pp. 418–427). Hershey, PA: IGI Global. doi:10.4018/978-1-5225-0920-2.ch024

Ghrab, S., & Saad, I. (2016). Identifying Crucial Know-How and Knowing-That for Medical Decision Support. *International Journal of Decision Support System Technology, 8*(4), 14–33. doi:10.4018/IJDSST.2016100102

Giokas, K., Tsirmpas, C., Anastasiou, A., Iliopoulou, D., Costarides, V., & Koutsouris, D. (2016). Contemporary Heart Failure Treatment Based on Improved Knowledge and Personalized Care of Comorbidities. In D. Fotiadis (Ed.), *Handbook of Research on Trends in the Diagnosis and Treatment of Chronic Conditions* (pp. 301–314). Hershey, PA: IGI Global. doi:10.4018/978-1-4666-8828-5.ch014

Gopalan, V., Chan, E., & Ho, D. T. (2018). Deliberate Self-Harm and Suicide Ideology in Medical Students. In C. Smith (Ed.), *Exploring the Pressures of Medical Education From a Mental Health and Wellness Perspective* (pp. 122–143). Hershey, PA: IGI Global. doi:10.4018/978-1-5225-2811-1.ch005

Goswami, S., Dey, U., Roy, P., Ashour, A., & Dey, N. (2017). Medical Video Processing: Concept and Applications. In N. Dey, A. Ashour, & P. Patra (Eds.), *Feature Detectors and Motion Detection in Video Processing* (pp. 1–17). Hershey, PA: IGI Global. doi:10.4018/978-1-5225-1025-3.ch001

Goswami, S., Mahanta, K., Goswami, S., Jigdung, T., & Devi, T. P. (2018). Ageing and Cancer: The Epigenetic Basis, Alternative Treatment, and Care. In B. Prasad & S. Akbar (Eds.), *Handbook of Research on Geriatric Health, Treatment, and Care* (pp. 206–235). Hershey, PA: IGI Global. doi:10.4018/978-1-5225-3480-8.ch012

Gouva, M. I. (2017). The Psychological Impact of Medical Error on Patients, Family Members, and Health Professionals. In M. Riga (Ed.), *Impact of Medical Errors and Malpractice on Health Economics, Quality, and Patient Safety* (pp. 171–196). Hershey, PA: IGI Global. doi:10.4018/978-1-5225-2337-6.ch007

Gürcü, M., & Tengilimoğlu, D. (2017). Health Tourism-Based Destination Marketing. In A. Bayraktar & C. Uslay (Eds.), *Strategic Place Branding Methodologies and Theory for Tourist Attraction* (pp. 308–331). Hershey, PA: IGI Global. doi:10.4018/978-1-5225-0579-2.ch015

Gürsel, G. (2016). Mobility in Healthcare: M-Health. In A. Panagopoulos (Ed.), *Handbook of Research on Next Generation Mobile Communication Systems* (pp. 485–511). Hershey, PA: IGI Global. doi:10.4018/978-1-4666-8732-5.ch019

Gürsel, G. (2017). For Better Healthcare Mining Health Data. In S. Bhattacharyya, S. De, I. Pan, & P. Dutta (Eds.), *Intelligent Multidimensional Data Clustering and Analysis* (pp. 135–158). Hershey, PA: IGI Global. doi:10.4018/978-1-5225-1776-4.ch006

Guzman-Lugo, G., Lopez-Martinez, M., Lopez-Ramirez, B., & Avila-Vazquez, D. (2016). City-Driven Approach to Determine Health Services Based on Current User Location and Collaborative Information. *International Journal of Knowledge Society Research, 7*(1), 53–62. doi:10.4018/IJKSR.2016010104

Gyaase, P. O., Darko-Lartey, R., William, H., & Borkloe, F. (2017). Towards an Integrated Electronic Medical Records System for Quality Healthcare in Ghana: An Exploratory Factor Analysis. *International Journal of Computers in Clinical Practice, 2*(2), 38–55. doi:10.4018/IJCCP.2017070103

Handayani, P. W., Sandhyaduhita, P. I., Hidayanto, A. N., Pinem, A. A., Fajrina, H. R., Junus, K. M., ... Ayuningtyas, D. (2016). Integrated Hospital Information System Architecture Design in Indonesia. In T. Iyamu & A. Tatnall (Eds.), *Maximizing Healthcare Delivery and Management through Technology Integration* (pp. 207–236). Hershey, PA: IGI Global. doi:10.4018/978-1-4666-9446-0.ch013

Hanel, P. (2017). Is China Catching Up?: Health-Related Applications of Biotechnology. In T. Bas & J. Zhao (Eds.), *Comparative Approaches to Biotechnology Development and Use in Developed and Emerging Nations* (pp. 465–520). Hershey, PA: IGI Global. doi:10.4018/978-1-5225-1040-6.ch016

Harmsen, C. A., & Royle, R. N. (2016). St. Stephen's Hospital Hervey Bay: Study of Developing a Digital Hospital. In J. Moon & M. Galea (Eds.), *Improving Health Management through Clinical Decision Support Systems* (pp. 127–153). Hershey, PA: IGI Global. doi:10.4018/978-1-4666-9432-3.ch006

Harp, D., Shim, R. S., Johnson, J., Harp, J. A., Wilcox, W. C., & Wilcox, J. K. (2016). Race and Gender Inequalities in Medicine and Biomedical Research. In U. Thomas & J. Drake (Eds.), *Critical Research on Sexism and Racism in STEM Fields* (pp. 115–134). Hershey, PA: IGI Global. doi:10.4018/978-1-5225-0174-9.ch006

Hartman, A., & Brown, S. (2017). Synergism through Therapeutic Visual Arts. In V. Bryan & J. Bird (Eds.), *Healthcare Community Synergism between Patients, Practitioners, and Researchers* (pp. 29–48). Hershey, PA: IGI Global. doi:10.4018/978-1-5225-0640-9.ch002

Hazra, J., Chowdhury, A. R., & Dutta, P. (2016). Cluster Based Medical Image Registration Using Optimized Neural Network. In S. Bhattacharyya, P. Banerjee, D. Majumdar, & P. Dutta (Eds.), *Handbook of Research on Advanced Hybrid Intelligent Techniques and Applications* (pp. 551–581). Hershey, PA: IGI Global. doi:10.4018/978-1-4666-9474-3.ch018

Hung, S., Huang, W., Yen, D. C., Chang, S., & Lu, C. (2016). Effect of Information Service Competence and Contextual Factors on the Effectiveness of Strategic Information Systems Planning in Hospitals. *Journal of Global Information Management, 24*(1), 14–36. doi:10.4018/JGIM.2016010102

Iltchev, P., Śliwczyński, A., Szynkiewicz, P., & Marczak, M. (2016). Mobile Health Applications Assisting Patients with Chronic Diseases: Examples from Asthma Care. In A. Moumtzoglou (Ed.), *M-Health Innovations for Patient-Centered Care* (pp. 170–196). Hershey, PA: IGI Global. doi:10.4018/978-1-4666-9861-1.ch009

Iqbal, S., Ahmad, S., & Willis, I. (2017). Influencing Factors for Adopting Technology Enhanced Learning in the Medical Schools of Punjab, Pakistan. *International Journal of Information and Communication Technology Education, 13*(3), 27–39. doi:10.4018/IJICTE.2017070103

Jagan, J., Dalkiliç, Y., & Samui, P. (2016). Utilization of SVM, LSSVM and GP for Predicting the Medical Waste Generation. In G. Hua (Ed.), *Smart Cities as a Solution for Reducing Urban Waste and Pollution* (pp. 224–251). Hershey, PA: IGI Global. doi:10.4018/978-1-5225-0302-6.ch008

Jagiello, K., Sosnowska, A., Mikolajczyk, A., & Puzyn, T. (2017). Nanomaterials in Medical Devices: Regulations' Review and Future Perspectives. *Journal of Nanotoxicology and Nanomedicine, 2*(2), 1–11. doi:10.4018/JNN.2017070101

Jena, T. K. (2018). Skill Training Process in Medicine Through Distance Mode. In U. Pandey & V. Indrakanti (Eds.), *Optimizing Open and Distance Learning in Higher Education Institutions* (pp. 228–243). Hershey, PA: IGI Global. doi:10.4018/978-1-5225-2624-7.ch010

Jesus, Â., & Gomes, M. J. (2016). Web 2.0 Tools in Biomedical and Pharmaceutical Education: Updated Review and Commentary. In T. Gasmelseid (Ed.), *Advancing Pharmaceutical Processes and Tools for Improved Health Outcomes* (pp. 52–78). Hershey, PA: IGI Global. doi:10.4018/978-1-5225-0248-7.ch003

Joseph, V., & Miller, J. M. (2018). Medical Students' Perceived Stigma in Seeking Care: A Cultural Perspective. In C. Smith (Ed.), *Exploring the Pressures of Medical Education From a Mental Health and Wellness Perspective* (pp. 44–67). Hershey, PA: IGI Global. doi:10.4018/978-1-5225-2811-1.ch002

Joyce, B. L., & Swanberg, S. M. (2017). Using Backward Design for Competency-Based Undergraduate Medical Education. In J. Stefaniak (Ed.), *Advancing Medical Education Through Strategic Instructional Design* (pp. 53–76). Hershey, PA: IGI Global. doi:10.4018/978-1-5225-2098-6.ch003

Kaljo, K., & Jacques, L. (2018). Flipping the Medical School Classroom. In M. Khosrow-Pour, D.B.A. (Ed.), Encyclopedia of Information Science and Technology, Fourth Edition (pp. 5800-5809). Hershey, PA: IGI Global. doi:10.4018/978-1-5225-2255-3.ch504

Karon, R. (2016). Utilisation of Health Information Systems for Service Delivery in the Namibian Environment. In T. Iyamu & A. Tatnall (Eds.), *Maximizing Healthcare Delivery and Management through Technology Integration* (pp. 169–183). Hershey, PA: IGI Global. doi:10.4018/978-1-4666-9446-0.ch011

Kasina, H., Bahubalendruni, M. V., & Botcha, R. (2017). Robots in Medicine: Past, Present and Future. *International Journal of Manufacturing, Materials, and Mechanical Engineering*, *7*(4), 44–64. doi:10.4018/IJMMME.2017100104

Katehakis, D. G. (2018). Electronic Medical Record Implementation Challenges for the National Health System in Greece. *International Journal of Reliable and Quality E-Healthcare*, *7*(1), 16–30. doi:10.4018/IJRQEH.2018010102

Katz, A., & Shtub, A. (2016). Design and Build a Wizard of Oz (WOZ) Telemedicine Simulator Platform. In M. Cruz-Cunha, I. Miranda, R. Martinho, & R. Rijo (Eds.), *Encyclopedia of E-Health and Telemedicine* (pp. 128–141). Hershey, PA: IGI Global. doi:10.4018/978-1-4666-9978-6.ch011

Kaur, P. D., & Sharma, P. (2017). Success Dimensions of ICTs in Healthcare. In B. Singh (Ed.), *Computational Tools and Techniques for Biomedical Signal Processing* (pp. 149–173). Hershey, PA: IGI Global. doi:10.4018/978-1-5225-0660-7.ch007

Kaushik, P. (2018). Comorbidity of Medical and Psychiatric Disorders in Geriatric Population: Treatment and Care. In B. Prasad & S. Akbar (Eds.), *Handbook of Research on Geriatric Health, Treatment, and Care* (pp. 448–474). Hershey, PA: IGI Global. doi:10.4018/978-1-5225-3480-8.ch025

Khachane, M. Y. (2017). Organ-Based Medical Image Classification Using Support Vector Machine. *International Journal of Synthetic Emotions*, *8*(1), 18–30. doi:10.4018/IJSE.2017010102

Kirci, P. (2018). Intelligent Techniques for Analysis of Big Data About Healthcare and Medical Records. In N. Shah & M. Mittal (Eds.), *Handbook of Research on Promoting Business Process Improvement Through Inventory Control Techniques* (pp. 559–582). Hershey, PA: IGI Global. doi:10.4018/978-1-5225-3232-3.ch029

Kldiashvili, E. (2016). Cloud Computing as the Useful Resource for Application of the Medical Information System for Quality Assurance Purposes. *International Journal of Computers in Clinical Practice*, *1*(2), 1–23. doi:10.4018/IJCCP.2016070101

Kldiashvili, E. (2018). Cloud Approach for the Medical Information System: MIS on Cloud. In M. Khosrow-Pour (Ed.), *Incorporating Nature-Inspired Paradigms in Computational Applications* (pp. 238–261). Hershey, PA: IGI Global. doi:10.4018/978-1-5225-5020-4.ch008

Kldiashvili, E., Burduli, A., Ghortlishvili, G., & Sheklashvili, I. (2016). Georgian Experience in Telecytology. In M. Cruz-Cunha, I. Miranda, R. Martinho, & R. Rijo (Eds.), *Encyclopedia of E-Health and Telemedicine* (pp. 62–71). Hershey, PA: IGI Global. doi:10.4018/978-1-4666-9978-6.ch006

Ko, H., Mesicek, L., Choi, J., Choi, J., & Hwang, S. (2018). A Study on Secure Contents Strategies for Applications With DRM on Cloud Computing. *International Journal of Cloud Applications and Computing*, *8*(1), 143–153. doi:10.4018/IJCAC.2018010107

Komendziński, T., Dreszer-Drogorób, J., Mikołajewska, E., Mikołajewski, D., & Bałaj, B. (2016). Interdisciplinary Education for Research and Everyday Clinical Practice: Lessons Learned from InteRDoCTor Project. In A. Rosiek & K. Leksowski (Eds.), *Organizational Culture and Ethics in Modern Medicine* (pp. 78–110). Hershey, PA: IGI Global. doi:10.4018/978-1-4666-9658-7.ch004

Komendziński, T., Mikołajewska, E., & Mikołajewski, D. (2018). Cross-Cultural Decision-Making in Healthcare: Theory and Practical Application in Real Clinical Conditions. In A. Rosiek-Kryszewska & K. Leksowski (Eds.), *Healthcare Administration for Patient Safety and Engagement* (pp. 276–298). Hershey, PA: IGI Global. doi:10.4018/978-1-5225-3946-9.ch015

Konecny, L. T. (2018). Medical School Wellness Initiatives. In C. Smith (Ed.), *Exploring the Pressures of Medical Education From a Mental Health and Wellness Perspective* (pp. 209–228). Hershey, PA: IGI Global. doi:10.4018/978-1-5225-2811-1.ch009

Konieczna, A., & Słomkowski, P. (2016). Confrontation of Human Rights in Daily Clinical Situations. In A. Rosiek & K. Leksowski (Eds.), *Organizational Culture and Ethics in Modern Medicine* (pp. 255–281). Hershey, PA: IGI Global. doi:10.4018/978-1-4666-9658-7.ch011

Kromrei, H., Solomonson, W. L., & Juzych, M. S. (2017). Teaching Residents How to Teach. In J. Stefaniak (Ed.), *Advancing Medical Education Through Strategic Instructional Design* (pp. 164–185). Hershey, PA: IGI Global. doi:10.4018/978-1-5225-2098-6.ch008

Kulkarni, S., Savyanavar, A., Kulkarni, P., Stranieri, A., & Ghorpade, V. (2018). Framework for Integration of Medical Image and Text-Based Report Retrieval to Support Radiological Diagnosis. In M. Kolekar & V. Kumar (Eds.), *Biomedical Signal and Image Processing in Patient Care* (pp. 86–122). Hershey, PA: IGI Global. doi:10.4018/978-1-5225-2829-6.ch006

Kumar, A., & Sarkar, B. K. (2018). Performance Analysis of Nature-Inspired Algorithms-Based Bayesian Prediction Models for Medical Data Sets. In U. Singh, A. Tiwari, & R. Singh (Eds.), *Soft-Computing-Based Nonlinear Control Systems Design* (pp. 134–155). Hershey, PA: IGI Global. doi:10.4018/978-1-5225-3531-7.ch007

Kurtz, R. S. (2016). Fortitude: A Study of African Americans in Surgery in New York City. In U. Thomas & J. Drake (Eds.), *Critical Research on Sexism and Racism in STEM Fields* (pp. 153–169). Hershey, PA: IGI Global. doi:10.4018/978-1-5225-0174-9.ch009

Labbadi, W., & Akaichi, J. (2017). Efficient Algorithm for Answering Fuzzy Medical Requests in Pervasive Healthcare Information Systems. *International Journal of Healthcare Information Systems and Informatics, 12*(2), 46–64. doi:10.4018/IJHISI.2017040103

Lagumdzija, A., & Swing, V. K. (2017). Health, Digitalization, and Individual Empowerment. In F. Topor (Ed.), *Handbook of Research on Individualism and Identity in the Globalized Digital Age* (pp. 380–402). Hershey, PA: IGI Global. doi:10.4018/978-1-5225-0522-8.ch017

Lamey, T. W., & Davidson-Shivers, G. V. (2017). Instructional Strategies and Sequencing. In J. Stefaniak (Ed.), *Advancing Medical Education Through Strategic Instructional Design* (pp. 30–52). Hershey, PA: IGI Global. doi:10.4018/978-1-5225-2098-6.ch002

Leon, G. (2017). The Role of Forensic Medicine in Medical Errors. In M. Riga (Ed.), *Impact of Medical Errors and Malpractice on Health Economics, Quality, and Patient Safety* (pp. 144–170). Hershey, PA: IGI Global. doi:10.4018/978-1-5225-2337-6.ch006

Lidia, B., Federica, G., & Maria, V. E. (2016). The Patient-Centered Medicine as the Theoretical Framework for Patient Engagement. In G. Graffigna (Ed.), *Promoting Patient Engagement and Participation for Effective Healthcare Reform* (pp. 25–39). Hershey, PA: IGI Global. doi:10.4018/978-1-4666-9992-2.ch002

Love, L., & McDowelle, D. (2018). Developing a Comprehensive Wellness Program for Medical Students. In C. Smith (Ed.), *Exploring the Pressures of Medical Education From a Mental Health and Wellness Perspective* (pp. 190–208). Hershey, PA: IGI Global. doi:10.4018/978-1-5225-2811-1.ch008

Lovell, K. L. (2017). Development and Evaluation of Neuroscience Computer-Based Modules for Medical Students: Instructional Design Principles and Effectiveness. In J. Stefaniak (Ed.), *Advancing Medical Education Through Strategic Instructional Design* (pp. 262–276). Hershey, PA: IGI Global. doi:10.4018/978-1-5225-2098-6.ch013

Lubin, R., & Hamlin, M. D. (2018). Medical Student Burnout: A Social Cognitive Learning Perspective on Medical Student Mental Health and Wellness. In C. Smith (Ed.), *Exploring the Pressures of Medical Education From a Mental Health and Wellness Perspective* (pp. 92–121). Hershey, PA: IGI Global. doi:10.4018/978-1-5225-2811-1.ch004

Luk, C. Y. (2018). Moving Towards Universal Health Coverage: Challenges for the Present and Future in China. In B. Fong, A. Ng, & P. Yuen (Eds.), *Sustainable Health and Long-Term Care Solutions for an Aging Population* (pp. 19–45). Hershey, PA: IGI Global. doi:10.4018/978-1-5225-2633-9.ch002

Mahat, M., & Pettigrew, A. (2017). The Regulatory Environment of Non-Profit Higher Education and Research Institutions and Its Implications for Managerial Strategy: The Case of Medical Education and Research. In L. West & A. Worthington (Eds.), *Handbook of Research on Emerging Business Models and Managerial Strategies in the Nonprofit Sector* (pp. 336–351). Hershey, PA: IGI Global. doi:10.4018/978-1-5225-2537-0.ch017

Maitra, I. K., & Bandhyopadhyaay, S. K. (2017). Adaptive Edge Detection Method towards Features Extraction from Diverse Medical Imaging Technologies. In S. Bhattacharyya, S. De, I. Pan, & P. Dutta (Eds.), *Intelligent Multidimensional Data Clustering and Analysis* (pp. 159–192). Hershey, PA: IGI Global. doi:10.4018/978-1-5225-1776-4.ch007

Mangu, V. P. (2017). Mobile Health Care: A Technology View. In C. Bhatt & S. Peddoju (Eds.), *Cloud Computing Systems and Applications in Healthcare* (pp. 1–18). Hershey, PA: IGI Global. doi:10.4018/978-1-5225-1002-4.ch001

Manirabona, A., Fourati, L. C., & Boudjit, S. (2017). Investigation on Healthcare Monitoring Systems: Innovative Services and Applications. *International Journal of E-Health and Medical Communications*, *8*(1), 1–18. doi:10.4018/IJEHMC.2017010101

Mannai, M. M., & Karâa, W. B. (2016). Biomedical Image Processing Overview. In W. Karâa & N. Dey (Eds.), *Biomedical Image Analysis and Mining Techniques for Improved Health Outcomes* (pp. 1–12). Hershey, PA: IGI Global. doi:10.4018/978-1-4666-8811-7.ch001

Manzoor, A. (2016). RFID in Health Care-Building Smart Hospitals for Quality Healthcare. *International Journal of User-Driven Healthcare, 6*(2), 21–45. doi:10.4018/IJUDH.2016070102

Marwan, M., Kartit, A., & Ouahmane, H. (2018). A Framework to Secure Medical Image Storage in Cloud Computing Environment. *Journal of Electronic Commerce in Organizations, 16*(1), 1–16. doi:10.4018/JECO.2018010101

Masoud, M. P., Nejad, M. K., Darebaghi, H., Chavoshi, M., & Farahani, M. (2018). The Decision Support System and Conventional Method of Telephone Triage by Nurses in Emergency Medical Services: A Comparative Investigation. *International Journal of E-Business Research, 14*(1), 77–88. doi:10.4018/IJEBR.2018010105

McDonald, W. G., Martin, M., & Salzberg, L. D. (2018). From Medical Student to Medical Resident: Graduate Medical Education and Mental Health in the United States. In C. Smith (Ed.), *Exploring the Pressures of Medical Education From a Mental Health and Wellness Perspective* (pp. 145–169). Hershey, PA: IGI Global. doi:10.4018/978-1-5225-2811-1.ch006

Medhekar, A. (2017). The Role of Social Media for Knowledge Dissemination in Medical Tourism: A Case of India. In R. Chugh (Ed.), *Harnessing Social Media as a Knowledge Management Tool* (pp. 25–54). Hershey, PA: IGI Global. doi:10.4018/978-1-5225-0495-5.ch002

Medhekar, A., & Haq, F. (2018). Urbanization and New Jobs Creation in Healthcare Services in India: Challenges and Opportunities. In U. Benna & I. Benna (Eds.), *Urbanization and Its Impact on Socio-Economic Growth in Developing Regions* (pp. 198–218). Hershey, PA: IGI Global. doi:10.4018/978-1-5225-2659-9.ch010

Mehta, G., Dutta, M. K., & Kim, P. S. (2016). An Efficient and Lossless Cryptosystem for Security in Tele-Ophthalmology Applications Using Chaotic Theory. *International Journal of E-Health and Medical Communications, 7*(4), 28–47. doi:10.4018/IJEHMC.2016100102

Mehta, P. (2017). Framework of Indian Healthcare System and its Challenges: An Insight. In V. Bryan & J. Bird (Eds.), *Healthcare Community Synergism between Patients, Practitioners, and Researchers* (pp. 247–271). Hershey, PA: IGI Global. doi:10.4018/978-1-5225-0640-9.ch011

Metelmann, B., & Metelmann, C. (2016). M-Health in Prehospital Emergency Medicine: Experiences from the EU funded Project LiveCity. In A. Moumtzoglou (Ed.), *M-Health Innovations for Patient-Centered Care* (pp. 197–212). Hershey, PA: IGI Global. doi:10.4018/978-1-4666-9861-1.ch010

Mi, M. (2017). Informal Learning in Medical Education. In J. Stefaniak (Ed.), *Advancing Medical Education Through Strategic Instructional Design* (pp. 225–244). Hershey, PA: IGI Global. doi:10.4018/978-1-5225-2098-6.ch011

Miglioretti, M., Mariani, F., & Vecchio, L. (2016). Could Patient Engagement Promote a Health System Free From Malpractice Litigation Risk? In G. Graffigna (Ed.), *Promoting Patient Engagement and Participation for Effective Healthcare Reform* (pp. 240–264). Hershey, PA: IGI Global. doi:10.4018/978-1-4666-9992-2.ch012

Misra, S. C., & Bisui, S. (2016). Feasibility of Large Scale Implementation of Personalized Medicine in the Current Scenario. *International Journal of E-Health and Medical Communications*, *7*(2), 30–49. doi:10.4018/IJEHMC.2016040103

Misra, S. C., Bisui, S., & Fantazy, K. (2016). Identifying Critical Changes in Adoption of Personalized Medicine (PM) in Healthcare Management. *International Journal of E-Health and Medical Communications*, *7*(3), 1–15. doi:10.4018/IJEHMC.2016070101

Mohammadian, M., Hatzinakos, D., Spachos, P., & Jentzsh, R. (2016). An Intelligent and Secure Framework for Wireless Information Technology in Healthcare for User and Data Classification in Hospitals. In V. Wang (Ed.), *Handbook of Research on Advancing Health Education through Technology* (pp. 452–479). Hershey, PA: IGI Global. doi:10.4018/978-1-4666-9494-1.ch019

Mokeddem, S., & Atmani, B. (2016). Assessment of Clinical Decision Support Systems for Predicting Coronary Heart Disease. *International Journal of Operations Research and Information Systems*, *7*(3), 57–73. doi:10.4018/IJORIS.2016070104

Mokrzycka, A., & Kowalska-Bobko, I. (2016). Public Health Legislation and Patient's Rights: Health2020 Strategy, European Perspective. In A. Rosiek & K. Leksowski (Eds.), *Organizational Culture and Ethics in Modern Medicine* (pp. 298–322). Hershey, PA: IGI Global. doi:10.4018/978-1-4666-9658-7.ch013

Moon, J. D., & Galea, M. P. (2016). Overview of Clinical Decision Support Systems in Healthcare. In J. Moon & M. Galea (Eds.), *Improving Health Management through Clinical Decision Support Systems* (pp. 1–27). Hershey, PA: IGI Global. doi:10.4018/978-1-4666-9432-3.ch001

Mosadeghrad, A. M., & Woldemichael, A. (2017). Application of Quality Management in Promoting Patient Safety and Preventing Medical Errors. In M. Riga (Ed.), *Impact of Medical Errors and Malpractice on Health Economics, Quality, and Patient Safety* (pp. 91–112). Hershey, PA: IGI Global. doi:10.4018/978-1-5225-2337-6.ch004

Moumtzoglou, A. (2017). Digital Medicine: The Quality Standpoint. In A. Moumtzoglou (Ed.), *Design, Development, and Integration of Reliable Electronic Healthcare Platforms* (pp. 179–195). Hershey, PA: IGI Global. doi:10.4018/978-1-5225-1724-5.ch011

Moumtzoglou, A., & Pouliakis, A. (2018). Population Health Management and the Science of Individuality. *International Journal of Reliable and Quality E-Healthcare*, *7*(2), 1–26. doi:10.4018/IJRQEH.2018040101

Mpofu, C. (2016). International Medical Experiences Outbound New Zealand: An Economic and Medical Workforce Strategy. In D. Velliaris & D. Coleman-George (Eds.), *Handbook of Research on Study Abroad Programs and Outbound Mobility* (pp. 446–469). Hershey, PA: IGI Global. doi:10.4018/978-1-5225-0169-5.ch018

Mukhtar, W. F., & Abuelyaman, E. S. (2017). Opportunities and Challenges of Big Data in Healthcare. In N. Wickramasinghe (Ed.), *Handbook of Research on Healthcare Administration and Management* (pp. 47–58). Hershey, PA: IGI Global. doi:10.4018/978-1-5225-0920-2.ch004

Munugala, S., Brar, G. K., Syed, A., Mohammad, A., & Halgamuge, M. N. (2018). The Much Needed Security and Data Reforms of Cloud Computing in Medical Data Storage. In M. Lytras & P. Papadopoulou (Eds.), *Applying Big Data Analytics in Bioinformatics and Medicine* (pp. 99–113). Hershey, PA: IGI Global. doi:10.4018/978-1-5225-2607-0.ch005

Narasimhamurthy, A. (2016). An Overview of Machine Learning in Medical Image Analysis: Trends in Health Informatics. In N. Dey & A. Ashour (Eds.), *Classification and Clustering in Biomedical Signal Processing* (pp. 23–45). Hershey, PA: IGI Global. doi:10.4018/978-1-5225-0140-4.ch002

Ngara, R. (2017). Multiple Voices, Multiple Paths: Towards Dialogue between Western and Indigenous Medical Knowledge Systems. In P. Ngulube (Ed.), *Handbook of Research on Theoretical Perspectives on Indigenous Knowledge Systems in Developing Countries* (pp. 332–358). Hershey, PA: IGI Global. doi:10.4018/978-1-5225-0833-5.ch015

O'Connor, Y., & Heavin, C. (2018). Defining and Characterising the Landscape of eHealth. In M. Khosrow-Pour, D.B.A. (Ed.), Encyclopedia of Information Science and Technology, Fourth Edition (pp. 5864-5875). Hershey, PA: IGI Global. doi:10.4018/978-1-5225-2255-3.ch510

Ochonogor, W. C., & Okite-Amughoro, F. A. (2018). Building an Effective Digital Library in a University Teaching Hospital (UTH) in Nigeria. In A. Tella & T. Kwanya (Eds.), *Handbook of Research on Managing Intellectual Property in Digital Libraries* (pp. 184–204). Hershey, PA: IGI Global. doi:10.4018/978-1-5225-3093-0.ch010

Olaniran, B. A. (2016). ICTs, E-health, and Multidisciplinary Healthcare Teams: Promises and Challenges. *International Journal of Privacy and Health Information Management*, *4*(2), 62–75. doi:10.4018/IJPHIM.2016070105

Olaniran, B. A. (2016). ICT Use and Multidisciplinary Healthcare Teams in the Age of e-Health. *International Journal of Reliable and Quality E-Healthcare*, *5*(1), 18–31. doi:10.4018/IJRQEH.2016010102

Olivares, S. L., Cruz, A. G., Cabrera, M. V., Regalado, A. I., & García, J. E. (2017). An Assessment Study of Quality Model for Medical Schools in Mexico. In S. Mukerji & P. Tripathi (Eds.), *Handbook of Research on Administration, Policy, and Leadership in Higher Education* (pp. 404–439). Hershey, PA: IGI Global. doi:10.4018/978-1-5225-0672-0.ch016

Omidoyin, E. O., Opeke, R. O., & Osagbemi, G. K. (2016). Utilization Pattern and Privacy Issues in the use of Health Records for Research Practice by Doctors: Selected Nigerian Teaching Hospitals as Case Study. *International Journal of Privacy and Health Information Management*, *4*(1), 1–11. doi:10.4018/IJPHIM.2016010101

Omoruyi, E. A., & Omidele, F. (2018). Resident Physician and Medical Academic Faculty Burnout: A Review of Current Literature. In C. Smith (Ed.), *Exploring the Pressures of Medical Education From a Mental Health and Wellness Perspective* (pp. 171–189). Hershey, PA: IGI Global. doi:10.4018/978-1-5225-2811-1.ch007

Osop, H., & Sahama, T. (2016). Data-Driven and Practice-Based Evidence: Design and Development of Efficient and Effective Clinical Decision Support System. In J. Moon & M. Galea (Eds.), *Improving Health Management through Clinical Decision Support Systems* (pp. 295–328). Hershey, PA: IGI Global. doi:10.4018/978-1-4666-9432-3.ch014

Ossowski, R., & Izdebski, P. (2016). Ethical Aspects of Talking to a Patient. In A. Rosiek & K. Leksowski (Eds.), *Organizational Culture and Ethics in Modern Medicine* (pp. 203–235). Hershey, PA: IGI Global. doi:10.4018/978-1-4666-9658-7.ch009

Pandian, P. S. (2016). An Overview of Telemedicine Technologies for Healthcare Applications. *International Journal of Biomedical and Clinical Engineering*, *5*(2), 29–52. doi:10.4018/IJBCE.2016070103

Papadopoulou, P., Lytras, M., & Marouli, C. (2018). Bioinformatics as Applied to Medicine: Challenges Faced Moving from Big Data to Smart Data to Wise Data. In M. Lytras & P. Papadopoulou (Eds.), *Applying Big Data Analytics in Bioinformatics and Medicine* (pp. 1–25). Hershey, PA: IGI Global. doi:10.4018/978-1-5225-2607-0.ch001

Paraskou, A., & George, B. P. (2018). An Overview of Reproductive Tourism. In *Legal and Economic Considerations Surrounding Reproductive Tourism: Emerging Research and Opportunities* (pp. 1–17). Hershey, PA: IGI Global. doi:10.4018/978-1-5225-2694-0.ch001

Park, S., & Moon, J. (2016). Strategic Approach towards Clinical Information Security. In J. Moon & M. Galea (Eds.), *Improving Health Management through Clinical Decision Support Systems* (pp. 329–359). Hershey, PA: IGI Global. doi:10.4018/978-1-4666-9432-3.ch015

Pereira, D., Castro, A., Gomes, P., Areias, J. C., Reis, Z. S., Coimbra, M. T., & Cruz-Correia, R. (2016). Digital Auscultation: Challenges and Perspectives. In M. Cruz-Cunha, I. Miranda, R. Martinho, & R. Rijo (Eds.), *Encyclopedia of E-Health and Telemedicine* (pp. 910–927). Hershey, PA: IGI Global. doi:10.4018/978-1-4666-9978-6.ch070

Peters, R. A., & Cruz, M. (2016). The States as Generators of Incremental Change in American Health Care Policy: 1935 to 1965. In R. Gholipour & K. Rouzbehani (Eds.), *Social, Economic, and Political Perspectives on Public Health Policy-Making* (pp. 86–114). Hershey, PA: IGI Global. doi:10.4018/978-1-4666-9944-1.ch005

Phuritsabam, B., & Devi, A. B. (2017). Information Seeking Behavior of Medical Scientists at Jawaharlal Nehru Institute of Medical Science: A Study. In S. Ram (Ed.), *Library and Information Services for Bioinformatics Education and Research* (pp. 177–187). Hershey, PA: IGI Global. doi:10.4018/978-1-5225-1871-6.ch010

Pieczka, B. (2018). Management of Risk and Adverse Events in Medical Entities. In A. Rosiek-Kryszewska & K. Leksowski (Eds.), *Healthcare Administration for Patient Safety and Engagement* (pp. 31–46). Hershey, PA: IGI Global. doi:10.4018/978-1-5225-3946-9.ch003

Poduval, J. (2016). Curriculum Development. In *Optimizing Medicine Residency Training Programs* (pp. 45–102). Hershey, PA: IGI Global. doi:10.4018/978-1-4666-9527-6.ch003

Poduval, J. (2016). Ethics and Professionalism. In *Optimizing Medicine Residency Training Programs* (pp. 103–133). Hershey, PA: IGI Global. doi:10.4018/978-1-4666-9527-6.ch004

Poduval, J. (2016). Management Skills and Leadership. In *Optimizing Medicine Residency Training Programs* (pp. 182–205). Hershey, PA: IGI Global. doi:10.4018/978-1-4666-9527-6.ch008

Poduval, J. (2016). Medicine Residency Training. In *Optimizing Medicine Residency Training Programs* (pp. 1–27). Hershey, PA: IGI Global. doi:10.4018/978-1-4666-9527-6.ch001

Poduval, J. (2016). Personal Issues. In *Optimizing Medicine Residency Training Programs* (pp. 206–221). Hershey, PA: IGI Global. doi:10.4018/978-1-4666-9527-6.ch009

Poduval, J. (2017). Medical Errors: Impact on Health Care Quality. In M. Riga (Ed.), *Impact of Medical Errors and Malpractice on Health Economics, Quality, and Patient Safety* (pp. 33–60). Hershey, PA: IGI Global. doi:10.4018/978-1-5225-2337-6.ch002

Politis, D., Stagiopoulos, P., Aidona, S., Kyriafinis, G., & Constantinidis, I. (2018). Autonomous Learning and Skill Accreditation: A Paradigm for Medical Studies. In A. Kumar (Ed.), *Optimizing Student Engagement in Online Learning Environments* (pp. 266–296). Hershey, PA: IGI Global. doi:10.4018/978-1-5225-3634-5.ch012

Pomares-Quimbaya, A., Gonzalez, R. A., Quintero, S., Muñoz, O. M., Bohórquez, W. R., García, O. M., & Londoño, D. (2016). A Review of Existing Applications and Techniques for Narrative Text Analysis in Electronic Medical Records. In M. Cruz-Cunha, I. Miranda, R. Martinho, & R. Rijo (Eds.), *Encyclopedia of E-Health and Telemedicine* (pp. 796–811). Hershey, PA: IGI Global. doi:10.4018/978-1-4666-9978-6.ch062

Pomares-Quimbaya, A., González, R. A., Sierra, A., Daza, J. C., Muñoz, O., García, A., ... Bohórquez, W. R. (2017). ICT for Enabling the Quality Evaluation of Health Care Services: A Case Study in a General Hospital. In A. Moumtzoglou (Ed.), *Design, Development, and Integration of Reliable Electronic Healthcare Platforms* (pp. 196–210). Hershey, PA: IGI Global. doi:10.4018/978-1-5225-1724-5.ch012

Pouliakis, A., Margari, N., Karakitsou, E., Archondakis, S., & Karakitsos, P. (2018). Emerging Technologies Serving Cytopathology: Big Data, the Cloud, and Mobile Computing. In I. El Naqa (Ed.), *Emerging Developments and Practices in Oncology* (pp. 114–152). Hershey, PA: IGI Global. doi:10.4018/978-1-5225-3085-5.ch005

Queirós, A., Silva, A. G., Ferreira, A., Caravau, H., Cerqueira, M., & Rocha, N. P. (2016). Assessing Mobile Applications Considered Medical Devices. In M. Cruz-Cunha, I. Miranda, R. Martinho, & R. Rijo (Eds.), *Encyclopedia of E-Health and Telemedicine* (pp. 111–127). Hershey, PA: IGI Global. doi:10.4018/978-1-4666-9978-6.ch010

Raffaeli, L., Spinsante, S., & Gambi, E. (2016). Integrated Smart TV-Based Personal e-Health System. *International Journal of E-Health and Medical Communications*, *7*(1), 48–64. doi:10.4018/IJEHMC.2016010103

Rai, A., Kothari, R., & Singh, D. P. (2017). Assessment of Available Technologies for Hospital Waste Management: A Need for Society. In R. Singh, A. Singh, & V. Srivastava (Eds.), *Environmental Issues Surrounding Human Overpopulation* (pp. 172–188). Hershey, PA: IGI Global. doi:10.4018/978-1-5225-1683-5.ch010

Ramamoorthy, S., & Sivasubramaniam, R. (2018). Image Processing Including Medical Liver Imaging: Medical Image Processing from Big Data Perspective, Ultrasound Liver Images, Challenges. In M. Lytras & P. Papadopoulou (Eds.), *Applying Big Data Analytics in Bioinformatics and Medicine* (pp. 380–392). Hershey, PA: IGI Global. doi:10.4018/978-1-5225-2607-0.ch016

Rathor, G. P., & Gupta, S. K. (2017). Improving Multimodality Image Fusion through Integrate AFL and Wavelet Transform. In V. Tiwari, B. Tiwari, R. Thakur, & S. Gupta (Eds.), *Pattern and Data Analysis in Healthcare Settings* (pp. 143–157). Hershey, PA: IGI Global. doi:10.4018/978-1-5225-0536-5.ch008

Rawat, D. B., & Bhattacharya, S. (2016). Wireless Body Area Network for Healthcare Applications. In N. Meghanathan (Ed.), *Advanced Methods for Complex Network Analysis* (pp. 343–358). Hershey, PA: IGI Global. doi:10.4018/978-1-4666-9964-9.ch014

Rea, P. M. (2016). Advances in Anatomical and Medical Visualisation. In M. Pinheiro & D. Simões (Eds.), *Handbook of Research on Engaging Digital Natives in Higher Education Settings* (pp. 244–264). Hershey, PA: IGI Global. doi:10.4018/978-1-5225-0039-1.ch011

Rexhepi, H., & Persson, A. (2017). Challenges to Implementing IT Support for Evidence Based Practice Among Nurses and Assistant Nurses: A Qualitative Study. *Journal of Electronic Commerce in Organizations*, *15*(2), 61–76. doi:10.4018/JECO.2017040105

Reychav, I., & Azuri, J. (2016). Including Elderly Patients in Decision Making via Electronic Health Literacy. In M. Cruz-Cunha, I. Miranda, R. Martinho, & R. Rijo (Eds.), *Encyclopedia of E-Health and Telemedicine* (pp. 241–249). Hershey, PA: IGI Global. doi:10.4018/978-1-4666-9978-6.ch020

Richards, D., & Caldwell, P. H. (2016). Gamification to Improve Adherence to Clinical Treatment Advice: Improving Adherence to Clinical Treatment. In D. Novák, B. Tulu, & H. Brendryen (Eds.), *Handbook of Research on Holistic Perspectives in Gamification for Clinical Practice* (pp. 47–77). Hershey, PA: IGI Global. doi:10.4018/978-1-4666-9522-1.ch004

Rissman, B. (2016). Medical Conditions Associated with NLD. In B. Rissman (Ed.), *Medical and Educational Perspectives on Nonverbal Learning Disability in Children and Young Adults* (pp. 27–66). Hershey, PA: IGI Global. doi:10.4018/978-1-4666-9539-9.ch002

Rosiek, A. (2018). The Assessment of Actions of the Environment and the Impact of Preventive Medicine for Public Health in Poland. In A. Rosiek-Kryszewska & K. Leksowski (Eds.), *Healthcare Administration for Patient Safety and Engagement* (pp. 106–119). Hershey, PA: IGI Global. doi:10.4018/978-1-5225-3946-9.ch006

Rosiek, A., Leksowski, K., Goch, A., Rosiek-Kryszewska, A., & Leksowski, Ł. (2016). Medical Treatment and Difficult Ethical Decisions in Interdisciplinary Hospital Teams. In A. Rosiek & K. Leksowski (Eds.), *Organizational Culture and Ethics in Modern Medicine* (pp. 121–153). Hershey, PA: IGI Global. doi:10.4018/978-1-4666-9658-7.ch006

Rosiek, A., & Rosiek-Kryszewska, A. (2018). Managed Healthcare: Doctor Life Satisfaction and Its Impact on the Process of Communicating With the Patient. In A. Rosiek-Kryszewska & K. Leksowski (Eds.), *Healthcare Administration for Patient Safety and Engagement* (pp. 244–261). Hershey, PA: IGI Global. doi:10.4018/978-1-5225-3946-9.ch013

Rosiek-Kryszewska, A., Leksowski, Ł., Rosiek, A., Leksowski, K., & Goch, A. (2016). Clinical Communication in the Aspect of Development of New Technologies and E-Health in the Doctor-Patient Relationship. In A. Rosiek & K. Leksowski (Eds.), *Organizational Culture and Ethics in Modern Medicine* (pp. 18–51). Hershey, PA: IGI Global. doi:10.4018/978-1-4666-9658-7.ch002

Rosiek-Kryszewska, A., & Rosiek, A. (2018). The Involvement of the Patient and his Perspective Evaluation of the Quality of Healthcare. In A. Rosiek-Kryszewska & K. Leksowski (Eds.), *Healthcare Administration for Patient Safety and Engagement* (pp. 121–144). Hershey, PA: IGI Global. doi:10.4018/978-1-5225-3946-9.ch007

Rosiek-Kryszewska, A., & Rosiek, A. (2018). The Impact of Management and Leadership Roles in Building Competitive Healthcare Units. In A. Rosiek-Kryszewska & K. Leksowski (Eds.), *Healthcare Administration for Patient Safety and Engagement* (pp. 13–30). Hershey, PA: IGI Global. doi:10.4018/978-1-5225-3946-9.ch002

Roşu, S. M., Păvăloiu, I. B., Dragoi, G., Apostol, C. G., & Munteanu, D. (2016). Telemedicine Based on LMDS in the Urban/Metropolitan Area: A Romanian Case Study. In M. Cruz-Cunha, I. Miranda, R. Martinho, & R. Rijo (Eds.), *Encyclopedia of E-Health and Telemedicine* (pp. 96–109). Hershey, PA: IGI Global. doi:10.4018/978-1-4666-9978-6.ch009

Rouzbehani, K. (2017). Health Policy Implementation: Moving Beyond Its Barriers in United States. In N. Wickramasinghe (Ed.), *Handbook of Research on Healthcare Administration and Management* (pp. 541–552). Hershey, PA: IGI Global. doi:10.4018/978-1-5225-0920-2.ch032

Ruiz, I. M., Cohen, D. S., & Marco, Á. M. (2016). ISO/IEEE11073 Family of Standards: Trends and Applications on E-Health Monitoring. In M. Cruz-Cunha, I. Miranda, R. Martinho, & R. Rijo (Eds.), *Encyclopedia of E-Health and Telemedicine* (pp. 646–660). Hershey, PA: IGI Global. doi:10.4018/978-1-4666-9978-6.ch050

Sam, S. (2017). Mobile Phones and Expanding Human Capabilities in Plural Health Systems. In K. Moahi, K. Bwalya, & P. Sebina (Eds.), *Health Information Systems and the Advancement of Medical Practice in Developing Countries* (pp. 93–114). Hershey, PA: IGI Global. doi:10.4018/978-1-5225-2262-1.ch006

Sankaranarayanan, S., & Ganesan, S. (2016). Applications of Intelligent Agents in Health Sector-A Review. *International Journal of E-Health and Medical Communications*, *7*(1), 1–30. doi:10.4018/IJEHMC.2016010101

Santos-Trigo, M., Suaste, E., & Figuerola, P. (2018). Technology Design and Routes for Tool Appropriation in Medical Practices. In M. Khosrow-Pour, D.B.A. (Ed.), Encyclopedia of Information Science and Technology, Fourth Edition (pp. 3794-3804). Hershey, PA: IGI Global. doi:10.4018/978-1-5225-2255-3.ch329

Sarivougioukas, J., Vagelatos, A., Parsopoulos, K. E., & Lagaris, I. E. (2018). Home UbiHealth. In M. Khosrow-Pour, D.B.A. (Ed.), Encyclopedia of Information Science and Technology, Fourth Edition (pp. 7765-7774). Hershey, PA: IGI Global. doi:10.4018/978-1-5225-2255-3.ch675

Sarkar, B. K. (2017). Big Data and Healthcare Data: A Survey. *International Journal of Knowledge-Based Organizations*, *7*(4), 50–77. doi:10.4018/IJKBO.2017100104

Saxena, K., & Banodha, U. (2017). An Essence of the SOA on Healthcare. In R. Bhadoria, N. Chaudhari, G. Tomar, & S. Singh (Eds.), *Exploring Enterprise Service Bus in the Service-Oriented Architecture Paradigm* (pp. 283–304). Hershey, PA: IGI Global. doi:10.4018/978-1-5225-2157-0.ch018

Schmeida, M., & McNeal, R. (2016). Consulting Online Healthcare Information: E-Caregivers as Knowledgeable Decision Makers. *International Journal of Computers in Clinical Practice, 1*(1), 42–52. doi:10.4018/IJCCP.2016010104

Sen, K., & Ghosh, K. (2018). Incorporating Global Medical Knowledge to Solve Healthcare Problems: A Framework for a Crowdsourcing System. *International Journal of Healthcare Information Systems and Informatics, 13*(1), 1–14. doi:10.4018/IJHISI.2018010101

Shakdher, A., & Pandey, K. (2017). REDAlert+: Medical/Fire Emergency and Warning System using Android Devices. *International Journal of E-Health and Medical Communications, 8*(1), 37–51. doi:10.4018/IJEHMC.2017010103

Shekarian, E., Abdul-Rashid, S. H., & Olugu, E. U. (2017). An Integrated Fuzzy VIKOR Method for Performance Management in Healthcare. In M. Tavana, K. Szabat, & K. Puranam (Eds.), *Organizational Productivity and Performance Measurements Using Predictive Modeling and Analytics* (pp. 40–61). Hershey, PA: IGI Global. doi:10.4018/978-1-5225-0654-6.ch003

Shi, J., Erdem, E., & Liu, H. (2016). Expanding Role of Telephone Systems in Healthcare: Developments and Opportunities. In A. Dwivedi (Ed.), *Reshaping Medical Practice and Care with Health Information Systems* (pp. 87–131). Hershey, PA: IGI Global. doi:10.4018/978-1-4666-9870-3.ch004

Shijina, V., & John, S. J. (2017). Multiple Relations and its Application in Medical Diagnosis. *International Journal of Fuzzy System Applications, 6*(4), 47–62. doi:10.4018/IJFSA.2017100104

Shipley, N., & Chakraborty, J. (2018). Big Data and mHealth: Increasing the Usability of Healthcare Through the Customization of Pinterest – Literary Perspective. In J. Machado, A. Abelha, M. Santos, & F. Portela (Eds.), *Next-Generation Mobile and Pervasive Healthcare Solutions* (pp. 46–66). Hershey, PA: IGI Global. doi:10.4018/978-1-5225-2851-7.ch004

Singh, A., & Dutta, M. K. (2017). A Reversible Data Hiding Scheme for Efficient Management of Tele-Ophthalmological Data. *International Journal of E-Health and Medical Communications, 8*(3), 38–54. doi:10.4018/IJEHMC.2017070103

Sivaji, A., Radjo, H. K., Amin, M., & Abu Hashim, M. A. (2016). Design of a Hospital Interactive Wayfinding System: Designing for Malaysian Users. In N. Mohamed, T. Mantoro, M. Ayu, & M. Mahmud (Eds.), *Critical Socio-Technical Issues Surrounding Mobile Computing* (pp. 88–123). Hershey, PA: IGI Global. doi:10.4018/978-1-4666-9438-5.ch005

Skourti, P. K., & Pavlakis, A. (2017). The Second Victim Phenomenon: The Way Out. In M. Riga (Ed.), *Impact of Medical Errors and Malpractice on Health Economics, Quality, and Patient Safety* (pp. 197–222). Hershey, PA: IGI Global. doi:10.4018/978-1-5225-2337-6.ch008

Smith, C. R. (2018). Medical Students' Quest Towards the Long White Coat: Impact on Mental Health and Well-Being. In C. Smith (Ed.), *Exploring the Pressures of Medical Education From a Mental Health and Wellness Perspective* (pp. 1–42). Hershey, PA: IGI Global. doi:10.4018/978-1-5225-2811-1.ch001

Smith, S. I., & Dandignac, M. (2018). Perfectionism: Addressing Lofty Expectations in Medical School. In C. Smith (Ed.), *Exploring the Pressures of Medical Education From a Mental Health and Wellness Perspective* (pp. 68–91). Hershey, PA: IGI Global. doi:10.4018/978-1-5225-2811-1.ch003

Sobrinho, Á. A., Dias da Silva, L., Perkusich, A., Cunha, P., Pinheiro, M. E., & Melo de Medeiros, L. (2016). Towards Medical Systems to Aid the Detection and Treatment of Chronic Diseases. In D. Fotiadis (Ed.), *Handbook of Research on Trends in the Diagnosis and Treatment of Chronic Conditions* (pp. 50–69). Hershey, PA: IGI Global. doi:10.4018/978-1-4666-8828-5.ch003

Soczywko, J., & Rutkowska, D. (2018). The Patient/Provider Relationship in Emergency Medicine: Organization, Communication, and Understanding. In A. Rosiek-Kryszewska & K. Leksowski (Eds.), *Healthcare Administration for Patient Safety and Engagement* (pp. 74–105). Hershey, PA: IGI Global. doi:10.4018/978-1-5225-3946-9.ch005

Sołtysik-Piorunkiewicz, A., Furmankiewicz, M., & Ziuziański, P. (2016). Web Healthcare Applications in Poland: Trends, Standards, Barriers and Possibilities of Implementation and Usage of E-Health Systems. In I. Deliyannis, P. Kostagiolas, & C. Banou (Eds.), *Experimental Multimedia Systems for Interactivity and Strategic Innovation* (pp. 258–283). Hershey, PA: IGI Global. doi:10.4018/978-1-4666-8659-5.ch013

Soni, P. (2018). Implications of HIPAA and Subsequent Regulations on Information Technology. In M. Gupta, R. Sharman, J. Walp, & P. Mulgund (Eds.), *Information Technology Risk Management and Compliance in Modern Organizations* (pp. 71–98). Hershey, PA: IGI Global. doi:10.4018/978-1-5225-2604-9.ch004

Spinelli, R., & Benevolo, C. (2016). From Healthcare Services to E-Health Applications: A Delivery System-Based Taxonomy. In A. Dwivedi (Ed.), *Reshaping Medical Practice and Care with Health Information Systems* (pp. 205–245). Hershey, PA: IGI Global. doi:10.4018/978-1-4666-9870-3.ch007

Srivastava, A., & Aggarwal, A. K. (2018). Medical Image Fusion in Spatial and Transform Domain: A Comparative Analysis. In M. Anwar, A. Khosla, & R. Kapoor (Eds.), *Handbook of Research on Advanced Concepts in Real-Time Image and Video Processing* (pp. 281–300). Hershey, PA: IGI Global. doi:10.4018/978-1-5225-2848-7.ch011

Srivastava, S. K., & Roy, S. N. (2018). Recommendation System: A Potential Tool for Achieving Pervasive Health Care. In J. Machado, A. Abelha, M. Santos, & F. Portela (Eds.), *Next-Generation Mobile and Pervasive Healthcare Solutions* (pp. 111–127). Hershey, PA: IGI Global. doi:10.4018/978-1-5225-2851-7.ch008

Stancu, A. (2016). Correlations and Patterns of Food and Health Consumer Expenditure. In A. Jean-Vasile (Ed.), *Food Science, Production, and Engineering in Contemporary Economies* (pp. 44–101). Hershey, PA: IGI Global. doi:10.4018/978-1-5225-0341-5.ch003

Stanimirovic, D. (2017). Digitalization of Death Certification Model: Transformation Issues and Implementation Concerns. In S. Saeed, Y. Bamarouf, T. Ramayah, & S. Iqbal (Eds.), *Design Solutions for User-Centric Information Systems* (pp. 22–43). Hershey, PA: IGI Global. doi:10.4018/978-1-5225-1944-7.ch002

Stavros, A., Vavoulidis, E., & Nasioutziki, M. (2016). The Use of Mobile Health Applications for Quality Control and Accreditational Purposes in a Cytopathology Laboratory. In A. Moumtzoglou (Ed.), *M-Health Innovations for Patient-Centered Care* (pp. 262–283). Hershey, PA: IGI Global. doi:10.4018/978-1-4666-9861-1.ch013

Sukkird, V., & Shirahada, K. (2018). E-Health Service Model for Asian Developing Countries: A Case of Emergency Medical Service for Elderly People in Thailand. In M. Khosrow-Pour (Ed.), *Optimizing Current Practices in E-Services and Mobile Applications* (pp. 214–232). Hershey, PA: IGI Global. doi:10.4018/978-1-5225-5026-6.ch011

Sygit, B., & Wąsik, D. (2016). Patients' Rights and Medical Personnel Duties in the Field of Hospital Care. In A. Rosiek & K. Leksowski (Eds.), *Organizational Culture and Ethics in Modern Medicine* (pp. 282–297). Hershey, PA: IGI Global. doi:10.4018/978-1-4666-9658-7.ch012

Sygit, B., & Wąsik, D. (2016). The Idea of Human Rights in Conditions of Hospital Treatment. In A. Rosiek & K. Leksowski (Eds.), *Organizational Culture and Ethics in Modern Medicine* (pp. 236–254). Hershey, PA: IGI Global. doi:10.4018/978-1-4666-9658-7.ch010

Talbot, T. B. (2017). Making Lifelike Medical Games in the Age of Virtual Reality: An Update on "Playing Games with Biology" from 2013. In B. Dubbels (Ed.), *Transforming Gaming and Computer Simulation Technologies across Industries* (pp. 103–119). Hershey, PA: IGI Global. doi:10.4018/978-1-5225-1817-4.ch006

Tamposis, I., Pouliakis, A., Fezoulidis, I., & Karakitsos, P. (2016). Mobile Platforms Supporting Health Professionals: Need, Technical Requirements, and Applications. In A. Moumtzoglou (Ed.), *M-Health Innovations for Patient-Centered Care* (pp. 91–114). Hershey, PA: IGI Global. doi:10.4018/978-1-4666-9861-1.ch005

Tiago, M. T., Tiago, F., Amaral, F. E., & Silva, S. (2016). Healthy 3.0: Healthcare Digital Dimensions. In A. Dwivedi (Ed.), *Reshaping Medical Practice and Care with Health Information Systems* (pp. 287–322). Hershey, PA: IGI Global. doi:10.4018/978-1-4666-9870-3.ch010

Tripathy, B. (2016). Application of Rough Set Based Models in Medical Diagnosis. In S. Dash & B. Subudhi (Eds.), *Handbook of Research on Computational Intelligence Applications in Bioinformatics* (pp. 144–168). Hershey, PA: IGI Global. doi:10.4018/978-1-5225-0427-6.ch008

Turcu, C. E., & Turcu, C. O. (2017). Social Internet of Things in Healthcare: From Things to Social Things in Internet of Things. In C. Reis & M. Maximiano (Eds.), *Internet of Things and Advanced Application in Healthcare* (pp. 266–295). Hershey, PA: IGI Global. doi:10.4018/978-1-5225-1820-4.ch010

Unwin, D. W., Sanzogni, L., & Sandhu, K. (2017). Developing and Measuring the Business Case for Health Information Technology. In K. Moahi, K. Bwalya, & P. Sebina (Eds.), *Health Information Systems and the Advancement of Medical Practice in Developing Countries* (pp. 262–290). Hershey, PA: IGI Global. doi:10.4018/978-1-5225-2262-1.ch015

Urooj, S., & Singh, S. P. (2016). Wavelet Transform-Based Soft Computational Techniques and Applications in Medical Imaging. In P. Saxena, D. Singh, & M. Pant (Eds.), *Problem Solving and Uncertainty Modeling through Optimization and Soft Computing Applications* (pp. 339–363). Hershey, PA: IGI Global. doi:10.4018/978-1-4666-9885-7.ch016

Vasant, P. (2018). A General Medical Diagnosis System Formed by Artificial Neural Networks and Swarm Intelligence Techniques. In U. Kose, G. Guraksin, & O. Deperlioglu (Eds.), *Nature-Inspired Intelligent Techniques for Solving Biomedical Engineering Problems* (pp. 130–145). Hershey, PA: IGI Global. doi:10.4018/978-1-5225-4769-3.ch006

Waegemann, C. P. (2016). mHealth: History, Analysis, and Implementation. In A. Moumtzoglou (Ed.), M-Health Innovations for Patient-Centered Care (pp. 1-19). Hershey, PA: IGI Global. doi:10.4018/978-1-4666-9861-1.ch001

Watfa, M. K., Majeed, H., & Salahuddin, T. (2016). Computer Based E-Healthcare Clinical Systems: A Comprehensive Survey. *International Journal of Privacy and Health Information Management*, *4*(1), 50–69. doi:10.4018/IJPHIM.2016010104

Wietholter, J. P., Coetzee, R., Nardella, B., Kincaid, S. E., & Slain, D. (2016). International Healthcare Experiences: Caring While Learning and Learning While Caring. In D. Velliaris & D. Coleman-George (Eds.), *Handbook of Research on Study Abroad Programs and Outbound Mobility* (pp. 470–496). Hershey, PA: IGI Global. doi:10.4018/978-1-5225-0169-5.ch019

Witzke, K., & Specht, O. (2017). M-Health Telemedicine and Telepresence in Oral and Maxillofacial Surgery: An Innovative Prehospital Healthcare Concept in Structurally Weak Areas. *International Journal of Reliable and Quality E-Healthcare*, *6*(4), 37–48. doi:10.4018/IJRQEH.2017100105

Wójcik, A., & Chojnacki, M. (2016). Behavior and Ethical Problems in the Functioning of the Operating Theater (Case Study). In A. Rosiek & K. Leksowski (Eds.), *Organizational Culture and Ethics in Modern Medicine* (pp. 154–179). Hershey, PA: IGI Global. doi:10.4018/978-1-4666-9658-7.ch007

Wolk, K., & Marasek, K. P. (2016). Translation of Medical Texts using Neural Networks. *International Journal of Reliable and Quality E-Healthcare*, *5*(4), 51–66. doi:10.4018/IJRQEH.2016100104

Wong, A. K., & Lo, M. F. (2018). Using Pervasive Computing for Sustainable Healthcare in an Aging Population. In B. Fong, A. Ng, & P. Yuen (Eds.), *Sustainable Health and Long-Term Care Solutions for an Aging Population* (pp. 187–202). Hershey, PA: IGI Global. doi:10.4018/978-1-5225-2633-9.ch010

Wu, W., Martin, B. C., & Ni, C. (2017). A Systematic Review of Competency-Based Education Effort in the Health Professions: Seeking Order Out of Chaos. In K. Rasmussen, P. Northrup, & R. Colson (Eds.), *Handbook of Research on Competency-Based Education in University Settings* (pp. 352–378). Hershey, PA: IGI Global. doi:10.4018/978-1-5225-0932-5.ch018

Yadav, N., Aliasgari, M., & Poellabauer, C. (2016). Mobile Healthcare in an Increasingly Connected Developing World. *International Journal of Privacy and Health Information Management, 4*(2), 76–97. doi:10.4018/IJPHIM.2016070106

Yadav, S., Ekbal, A., Saha, S., Pathak, P. S., & Bhattacharyya, P. (2017). Patient Data De-Identification: A Conditional Random-Field-Based Supervised Approach. In S. Saha, A. Mandal, A. Narasimhamurthy, S. V, & S. Sangam (Eds.), Handbook of Research on Applied Cybernetics and Systems Science (pp. 234-253). Hershey, PA: IGI Global. doi:10.4018/978-1-5225-2498-4.ch011

Yu, B., Wijesekera, D., & Costa, P. C. (2017). Informed Consent in Healthcare: A Study Case of Genetic Services. In A. Moumtzoglou (Ed.), *Design, Development, and Integration of Reliable Electronic Healthcare Platforms* (pp. 211–242). Hershey, PA: IGI Global. doi:10.4018/978-1-5225-1724-5.ch013

Yu, B., Wijesekera, D., & Costa, P. C. (2017). Informed Consent in Electronic Medical Record Systems. In I. Management Association (Ed.), Healthcare Ethics and Training: Concepts, Methodologies, Tools, and Applications (pp. 1029-1049). Hershey, PA: IGI Global. doi:10.4018/978-1-5225-2237-9.ch049

Yu, M., Li, J., & Wang, W. (2017). Creative Life Experience among Students in Medical Education. In C. Zhou (Ed.), *Handbook of Research on Creative Problem-Solving Skill Development in Higher Education* (pp. 158–184). Hershey, PA: IGI Global. doi:10.4018/978-1-5225-0643-0.ch008

Zarour, K. (2017). Towards a Telehomecare in Algeria: Case of Diabetes Measurement and Remote Monitoring. *International Journal of E-Health and Medical Communications, 8*(4), 61–80. doi:10.4018/IJEHMC.2017100104

Zavyalova, Y. V., Korzun, D. G., Meigal, A. Y., & Borodin, A. V. (2017). Towards the Development of Smart Spaces-Based Socio-Cyber-Medicine Systems. *International Journal of Embedded and Real-Time Communication Systems, 8*(1), 45–63. doi:10.4018/IJERTCS.2017010104

Zeinali, A. A. (2018). Word Formation Study in Developing Naming Guidelines in the Translation of English Medical Terms Into Persian. In M. Khosrow-Pour, D.B.A. (Ed.), Encyclopedia of Information Science and Technology, Fourth Edition (pp. 5136-5147). Hershey, PA: IGI Global. doi:10.4018/978-1-5225-2255-3.ch446

Ziminski, T. B., Demurjian, S. A., Sanzi, E., & Agresta, T. (2016). Toward Integrating Healthcare Data and Systems: A Study of Architectural Alternatives. In T. Iyamu & A. Tatnall (Eds.), *Maximizing Healthcare Delivery and Management through Technology Integration* (pp. 270–304). Hershey, PA: IGI Global. doi:10.4018/978-1-4666-9446-0.ch016

Ziminski, T. B., Demurjian, S. A., Sanzi, E., Baihan, M., & Agresta, T. (2016). An Architectural Solution for Health Information Exchange. *International Journal of User-Driven Healthcare*, *6*(1), 65–103. doi:10.4018/IJUDH.2016010104

Zineldin, M., & Vasicheva, V. (2018). Reducing Medical Errors and Increasing Patient Safety: TRM and 5 Q's Approaches for Better Quality of Life. In *Technological Tools for Value-Based Sustainable Relationships in Health: Emerging Research and Opportunities* (pp. 87–115). Hershey, PA: IGI Global. doi:10.4018/978-1-5225-4091-5.ch005

About the Contributors

Simon Taukeni, Dr., is an academic, book editor and researcher. His research interest mainly is in the fields of psychology and public health.

* * *

Melisa Anderson is a recipient of the 2017 UK Global Chevening Scholarship and recently completed her Master of Science in Biomedical Sciences at the University of Glasgow, Scotland, UK. She also holds a Master of Art in Teaching from the University of the West Indies Mona and a Bachelor of Science (Honours) from the University of Technology, Jamaica. Melisa is a Chemistry Lecturer at the All American Institute of Medical Sciences Alliance Health Division and she currently serves as Manager of the Cytogenetics Laboratory in the Pathology Department at the University of the West Indies, Mona.

Lennox Anderson-Jackson holds a Caribbean Diploma in Diagnostic Radiological Science from the University of the West Indies Mona, Kingston, Jamaica; a Bachelor of Science degree with honors in Diagnostic Medical Sonography from Weber State University in Ogden, Utah, USA; and a Master of Science degree in Counselling and Consulting Psychology from the International University of the Caribbean, Kingston, Jamaica. Presently, Mr. Anderson-Jackson is pursuing the MPhil/PhD in Chemical Pathology at the University of the West Indies, Mona, Kingston, Jamaica. He has over 28 years of experience in the field of radiological science and has worked in 4 countries including Jamaica, United States of America, Cayman Islands, and Anguilla. He worked in several government hospitals and private hospitals and clinics in Jamaica including the Kingston Public Hospital (1991), the Bustamante Hospital for Children, Cornwall Regional Hospital, Montego Bay Hospital, Radiology West (2003-2013), Royale Imaging Centre (2009-2013) and Reddy's Medical Centre. He also worked as a Clinical Ultrasound Instructor at the School of Medical Radiation Technology, University of the West Indies, Mona, Jamaica in collaboration with Michner Institute in Canada (2004-2008). Mr.

Anderson-Jackson is presently the CEO and chief Medical Ultrasound Practitioner and Radiographer at the LYL Ultrasound Centre in Lucea, Hanover, Jamaica. He is a member of Who's Who amongst Students of American Universities and Colleges (Edition 1999). He was also a nominee for Crystal Crest Scholar of the year for Weber State University (1997). A Member of the Profession Supplementary to Medicine, Jamaica. He has been involved in some published articles as author and co-author. Mr. Anderson-Jackson was honoured in 2011 with the Distinguished Alumni Award by the Rusea's Old Student Association (ROSA) for achievements in the field of science and research.

Daniel Opotamutale Ashipala holds a Master of Nursing Science in Mental Health Nursing Science from the University of Namibia in Namibia. He is currently a researcher, Senior Lecturer and Head of Department for the School of Nursing in the Faculty of Health Sciences at the University of Namibia. His research interests include primary health care and health care services and nursing education, and health service management. He has published a quite number of articles on the delivery of teaching and learning in higher education studies. He has also published widely on nursing management, clinical cursing, community health nursing, mental health nursing and health policy. He is a doctoral candidate at Stellenbosch University in Cape Town, South Africa. His doctoral work focus on developing a training programme to facilitate a task shifting approach for nurses in the Namibia PHC services.

Dana C. Branson is an assistant professor for the Social Work Program, housed in the Department of Criminal Justice, Social Work, and Sociology. Dr. Branson earned her PhD in Psychology from Northcentral University in 2011, received her Master of Social Work (child and family emphasis) from the University of Kansas in 1995, and completed her undergraduate work at Southwest Baptist University, obtaining a Bachelor of Science in Psychology and Sociology, with a minor in Counseling in 1993. Dr. Branson has been a licensed practitioner (LCSW) and a member of NASW since 1997. Dr. Branson joined Southeast Missouri State after 21 years of clinical experience with substance use disorders, mental health, co-occurring disorders, and trauma-informed care. Dr. Branson's practice is focused primarily with women and adolescents and incorporates the many diverse dynamics of rural social work. Dr. Branson regularly serves as a conference presenter, providing workshops, breakout sessions, and guided discussions on vicarious trauma, adolescent substance abuse trends, and military social work. Dr. Branson has participated in international social work opportunities in Ireland and Belarus.

Jabari Brown is a Medical Technologist in the Department of Pathology, The University of the West Indies. Mona Campus, Kingston Jamaica. He graduated from the University of Technology, Jamaica with a Bachelor of Science Degree in Medical Technology. His area of research interest includes endocrine function and disorders, and effectiveness of modern treatment regimen.

D.K. Chaturvedi, Dr., is working in Dept. of Elect. Engg, Faculty of Engg, D.E.I., Dayalbagh, Agra since 1989. Presently, he is a Professor. He did his B.E. at the Govt. Engineering College Ujjain, M.P. then he did his M.Tech. and PhD from D.E.I. Dayalbagh. He is gold medalist and received young scientists fellowship from DST, Government of India in 2001-2002 for post doctorial research at Univ. of Calgary, Canada. Also, he had research collaboration with different organizations at national and international level. He is the Fellow - The Institution of Engineers (India), Fellow - Aeronautical Society of India, Fellow - IETE, Sr. Member IEEE, USA and Member of many National and International professional bodies such as IET, U.K., ISTE, Delhi, ISCE, Roorkee, IIIE, Mumbai and SSI, etc. The IEE U.K. recognized his work in the area of Power System Stabilizer and awarded honorary membership to him in 2006. He did many R&D projects of MHRD, UGC, AICTE etc. and consultancy projects of DRDO. He contributed in the national mission of ICT of Govt. of India as Virtual Power Lab Developer. He has guided 10 PhDs, 65 M.Tech. dissertations and published more than 300 international and national papers. He has chaired and co-chaired many international and national conferences. He is a referee of many international journals including IEE Proceedings and IEEE Transactions. He is Head of Dept. of Footwear Technology, Convener, Faculty Training and Placement Cell, and Advisor, IEI Students' Chapter (Elect. Engg.), D.E.I. Dayalbagh, Agra.

Tanya Heasley is originally from Essex, England, and is an award-winning coach and entrepreneur with over 18 years' experience in a successful progressive career within mental health and personal development. A trained Counsellor, Positive Psychology Coach and a specialist in Anger Management, Tanya has worked closely with teachers and support staff within education, as well as vulnerable adults in the private sector. Tanya works as a Positive Anger Coach and actively promotes the art of anger as a communicative emotion.

Eveline Kalomo, Dr., received her Bachelor of Arts degree in Social Work from the University of Namibia and obtained a Master of Arts degree in International Child Welfare from the University of East Anglia in the United Kingdom. Her doctoral studies (PhD) and master's in social work are from the University of Minnesota, School of Social Work in the United States (US). Her research interests include kinship care, population aging, gerontology, HIV/AIDS, mental health, immigrant older adults of African descent, social development and international social work. Her dissertation is a study that stemmed from her extensive work with families and children affected by AIDS in Namibia. Her study investigates the association between supports and depression of elderly caregivers raising children orphaned by AIDS in rural Namibia.

Johannes N. Mampane, PhD, is an academic and a researcher at the University of South Africa. His research interests lie in the fields of gender, health, and sexuality. He advocates for social justice, inclusivity, equality and diversity issues concerning marginalized, disenfranchised, and minority populations in society.

Donovan McGrowder, Dr., holds a Bachelor of Science (Honours) and a Doctor of Philosophy (PhD) degrees in Biochemistry and Chemistry, and Biochemistry, respectively, from the University of the West Indies, Mona, Kingston, Jamaica. Dr. McGrowder also holds a Master of Science degree from University of Westminster, London, UK, and a Master of Arts in Psychology and Counselling from St. Stephens College, Alberta, Canada. He also has post-graduate training and experience in clinical biochemistry and molecular biology. Dr. McGrowder joined the staff of The University of the West Indies, Mona, in 2001 as a research fellow in the Department of Basic Medical Sciences – Biochemistry Section and was promoted to lecturer in 2003 and senior lecturer in 2009. He is also a Consultant of Chemical Pathology at the University Hospital of the West Indies. He is a Fellow of the Institute of Biomedical Science, UK, Fellow of the Royal Society of Tropical Medicine and Hygiene, UK, and Member of the Institute of Health Promotion and Education, UK.

Joel Medusalem holds a Bachelor of Nursing Science (Cli) (Hon) from the University of Namibia, in Namibia. He is a registered nurse by profession and a researcher with an interests focused health care services and nursing education. He has a research article publication on teaching and learning in higher education studies.

Fabian Miller is a lecturer, researcher and the Head of Department of Physical Education at The Mico University College. He has participated in research in the Medical field and Sport Science field. He has worked on research in sport services in the CARIFORUM region which aim was to establish regional policies for sport services for the member states involved and to establish sport services as a viable industry in the region. His current research is aimed to establish biological passports of college/university athletes who compete in sprinting and long distance events. Mr. Miller also published peer reviewed journal articles and book chapters. He co-authored the manuscript titled "Prostate Specific Antigen Testing in a Tertiary

Teaching Hospital" and co-authored the book chapter titled "Dietary Antioxidants in the Chemoprevention of Prostate Cancer. Mr. Miller is a graduate from G.C Foster College where he completed a Diploma in Education and a Bachelor's Degree in Physical Education and Sport, he went on to pursue and complete his Masters of Science in Physical Education at The University of Technology, Jamaica and he is currently a PhD student in Biotechnology, Faculty of Science and Technology, University of the West Indies, Mona. Mr. Miller is a board member of the Social and Human Sciences Advisory Committee of Jamaica National Commission for UNESCO (Period of 2016-2019).

Omolade Okwa obtained a PhD in Parasitology (1997), M. Sc Cellular Parasitology (1992), and B. Sc (Hons) Zoology (1990) all from University of Ibadan, Nigeria. She was a recipient of a commonwealth fellowship supported by British Council tenable at Keele University, United Kingdom, Center for Entomology and Parasitology (CAEP), School of Life sciences, Keele University, Staffordshire, United Kingdom. She was a visiting Honorary Visiting Research Fellow at Keele University, United Kingdom. She is a member of Malaria Society of Nigeria (MSN), Nigerian Society of Experimental Biology (NISEB), Nigerian Society for Parasitology (NSP), Science Association of Nigeria (SAN), Zoological Society of Nigeria (ZSN) and Vice President Organisation of women in Science for the developing world, LASU chapter (OWSD). She is presently a Professor of Zoology at Lagos State University, Nigeria and Head of the department (2007-2010, 2014-2016). She has 43 scientific research publications in local and international journals, 8 scientific reviews and 4 books.

Karthikeyan Ramalingam, M.Sc. M.Phil., PhD, Associate professor, BS Abdur Rahman Crescent Institute of Science and Technology, Chennai, Tamil Nadu, India with over 19 years of laboratory knowledge, including academic, government, and industry projects handling experience with excellent supervisory skills and a strong record of scientific accomplishments and publications. He has strong scientific background in microbiology, including bacteria, fungi and Actinomyces, microbial pathogenesis, environmental microbiology, dental microbiology and cancer biology. He finished his doctoral degree from Centre of Advanced Study in Marine Biology, Annamalai University, Prangipettai, Tamil Nadu, India. He has experienced and well trained at the University of Texas Health Science Center at San Antonio, Texas, USA on different aspects of dental microbiology, characterization and application for anticariogenic agents development and he has used nanoemulsion against battlefield multi-resistant microorganism to prevent battlefield related infections. In US Naval Medical Research Unit, San Antonio, Texas, USA, he had worked in different nanoemulsion and metal nano-particles against infectious disease-causing microorganisms. Then he worked in New York University, USA, their he worked in microbial derived modified Sophorolipids (biosurfactants) against eradication of different human and plant pathogenic microorganisms. At the New York University he handled USA-NSF-SBIR project as principle investigator. He successfully completed more than 5 years of research and training in USA, and his contribution in USA, research and supervision of undergraduate and pre-doctoral students has been appreciated and acknowledged by his mentors and he got the 2012 Maria Yeung outstanding Postdoctoral Award with a cash prize at the University of Texas Health Science Center at San Antonio, Texas, USA. His major projects involve drug molecule development, including antimicrobial agents and anticancer drug development. He worked as scientific team leader in human pathogenic microbiology and environmental microbiology projects. He has strong leadership, management and communication skills including management of multi-disciplinary teams including academia, government, and industry collaborations. He has experience working with Clinical Research Organizations (CROs), Contract Research Organizations, and Academic/Industry collaborators. His technical expertise in bacteriology, biofilm-based assays, and antimicrobial assay development, including biofilm attachment substrate development. In vivo expertise in animal survival studies for infection and anticancer lead development, including mouse and rat.

Rohit Rastogi received his B.E. degree in Computer Science and Engineering from C.C.S. Univ. Meerut in 2003, the M.E. degree in Computer Science from NITTTR-Chandigarh (National Institute of Technical Teachers Training and Research-affiliated to MHRD, Govt. of India), Punjab Univ. Chandigarh in 2010. Currently he is pursuing his PhD in computer science from Dayalbagh Educational Institute, Agra under the renowned professor of Electrical Engineering Dr. D.K. Chaturvedi in area of spiritual consciousness. Dr. Santosh Satya of IIT-Delhi and Dr. Navneet Arora of IIT-Roorkee have happily consented him to co supervise. He is also working presently with Dr. Piyush Trivedi of DSVV Hardwar, India in center of Scientific spirituality. He is an Associate Professor of CSE Dept. in ABES Engineering. College, Ghaziabad (U.P. India), affiliated to Dr. A.P. J. Abdul Kalam Technical Univ. Lucknow (earlier Uttar Pradesh Tech. University). Also, he is preparing some interesting algorithms on Swarm Intelligence approaches like PSO, ACO, BCO, etc. Rohit Rastogi is involved actively with Vichaar Krnati Abhiyaan and strongly believe that transformation starts within the self.

Ndapeua Shifiona, RN, RM, D Cur (Psychiatric Nursing), is a lecturer in the Mental Health Nursing Unit, Department Community and Mental Health Nursing, Oshakati Campus, University of Namibia. She was awarded a D Cur (Psychiatric Nursing) by the University of Johannesburg, South Africa. She obtained a master's degree in Psychiatric Nursing from the University of Johannesburg, South Africa. She has a post-basic diploma in Psychiatric Nursing from the Sterkfontein College of Nursing, South Africa and a postgraduate certificate in Pharmacotherapy from the University of Namibia. She was awarded membership status by the Golden Key International Honour Society which was validated by the University of Johannesburg, South Africa. Her educational background in Psychiatric Nursing has given her a broad base from which to approach psychiatry/mental health nursing issues. She has published research articles in international journals, organized seminars and workshops; presented scientific papers in national and international conferences. Her passion is teaching and working with individuals living with mental illness.

Nestor Tomas is a lecturer at the University of Namibia, in the department of General Nursing Science, at the School of Nursing. His focus research areas include public health, behavioral changes, nursing ethics, reproductive health, public policy, health financing, online distance learning, nursing education among others. Mr. Tomas is at the earlier stage of his research career, published in international journals and seek to collaborate with other aspiring researchers around the globe. He is currently a PHD candidate at the University of South Africa.

Dwayne Ricardo Tucker is a senior medical laboratory technologist at the University of the West Indies, Mona, Jamaica since 2010. He holds a Bachelor of Science Degree in Medical Technology from the Northern Caribbean University, Manchester, Jamaica. Dwayne is a 2016 British Chevening scholar who obtained a Master of Science Degree in Oncology in 2017 from the University of Nottingham, United Kingdom. In collaboration with the Caribbean Institute for Health Research, Dwayne contributed to genetics-focused research on prostate cancer survivors of African ancestry during a fellowship at the Fox Chase Cancer Center (FCCC). He is a prospective PhD student at the University of British Columbia in Vancouver, Canada, where he will investigate molecular proteins as potential prognostic and diagnostic tools for prostate cancer. As a member of the African-Caribbean Cancer Consortium (AC3), he hopes to apply the knowledge and skills garnered from his PhD training towards improving prostate cancer prognosis and prevention within the realms of Black men worldwide.

Kurt Vaz is the Administrator in the Department of Pathology at The University of the West Indies, Mona Campus, Kingston Jamaica. He has over fifteen years of experience in clinical laboratory sciences. As a scientist he seeks to make a real difference in biomedical research and always strives to give his utmost best to patient care.

Nuuyoma Vistolina was born in the Oshana region, Namibia. She is a Senior Lecturer in the School of Nursing, University of Namibia Rundu campus. She holds a Master's Degree in Health Science Education (Stellenbosch University) obtained in 2017 and a Master's Degree in Public Health (University of the Western Cape) obtained in 2013. She is pursuing a doctoral degree in nursing education at the University of Johannesburg.

Index

F

G

H

I

K

M

N

O

P

Q

R

S

T

V

W

www.ingramcontent.com/pod-product-compliance
Lightning Source LLC
LaVergne TN
LVHW080905300926
849162LV00003B/568
* 9 7 8 1 7 9 9 8 2 1 3 9 7 *